Osteotomy About the Knee

Sam Oussedik • Sebastien Lustig
Editors

Osteotomy About the Knee

A Comprehensive Guide

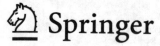

Editors
Sam Oussedik
Orthopaedic Surgery Department
University College London Hospitals
London
UK

Sebastien Lustig
Orthopaedic Surgery, Arthritis and Joint
Replacement Department
Lyon Croix-Rousse Univeristy Hospital
Lyon
France

ISBN 978-3-030-49057-7   ISBN 978-3-030-49055-3   (eBook)
https://doi.org/10.1007/978-3-030-49055-3

This Springer imprint is published by the registered company Springer Nature Switzerland AG
The registered company address is: Gewerbestrasse 11, 6330 Cham, Switzerland

Preface

We live in evermore demanding times. Our patients' functional expectations no longer taper with increasing age; the growing obesity epidemic is leading to greater rates of degenerative knee disease in ever-younger patients; access to expensive surgery in developing economies remains challenging.

Osteotomy About the Knee offers a potential solution to these clinical problems, restoring function and offering pain relief through manipulation of the limb's weight-bearing axis.

Although it has fallen into relative disuse since the advent of modern knee arthroplasty, it should form part of all knee surgeons' armamentarium, precisely to meet the challenges outlined above. Although technically demanding, the results achieved by experienced surgeons make this a reliable and reproducible option.

It is hoped that the chapters collected within this tome will provide new options for the novice and technical tips for the experienced surgeon. We have gathered together the most experienced osteotomy surgeons to share their experience, techniques, tips and results in the ultimate hope of improving the outcome for patients worldwide.

London, UK   Sam Oussedik
Lyon, France   Sebastien Lustig

Acknowledgement

The editors would like to acknowledge the contribution of Dr. Elliot Sappey-Marinier, MD, to this book and thank him for his efforts.

Contents

Part I

Basic Science

From Hippocrates to Coventry and Beyond: The History of Joint Realignment

1

M. A. Roussot, S. Huijs, and Sam Oussedik

1.1 Introduction

Joint realignment has a history dating back to thousands of years. Giant leaps have been taken through the work of some of orthopaedic's greatest pioneers. Advancements such as the introduction of anaesthesia, the development of aseptic surgical technique and surgical instrumentation, the clinical application of X-rays and its evolution into advanced imaging techniques, refinement in our understanding of limb alignment and fracture fixation and inpatient selection represent some of the cornerstones of what has now become a valuable method of improving pain and function for appropriately selected patients.

We currently have technologies such as computer guidance, robotics, advanced 3D and dynamic imaging and artificial intelligence that have brought the horizon to our fingertips and will provide a means of achieving new levels of accuracy and reproducibility.

In this chapter we will describe the history of joint realignment, focusing on the evolution of osteotomies around the knee.

1.2 Ancient Thinkers to Nineteenth Century Pioneers

The principles of deformity correction were contemplated in ancient times. The Edwin Smith Papyrus (circa 1600 BC) recorded three cases of correction of alignment for humeral fractures in ancient Egypt [1]. Hippocrates (460–370 BC) used a device later known as the Hippocratic scamnum (Fig. 1.1) to realign fractured long bones as they are healed, a technique that was further developed by Celsus and Galen [1, 2]. However, it was not until the sixteenth century that *osteoclasia*, the

M. A. Roussot · S. Huijs · S. Oussedik (✉)
University College London Hospitals NHS Trust, London, UK

© Springer Nature Switzerland AG 2020
S. Oussedik, S. Lustig (eds.), *Osteotomy About the Knee*,
https://doi.org/10.1007/978-3-030-49055-3_1

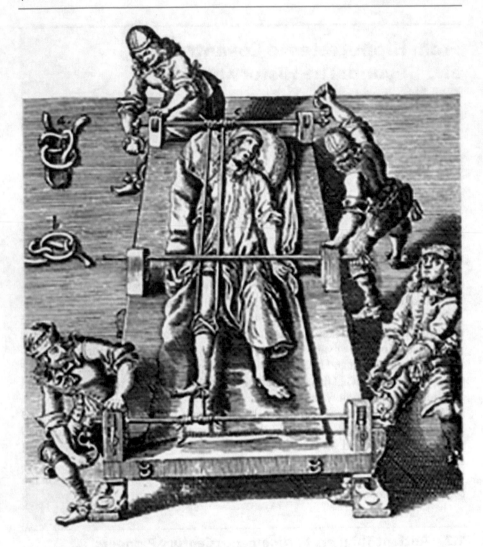

Fig. 1.1 Hippocratic scamnum. Origin unknown

deliberate fracture and stabilisation of a long bone for the purpose of deformity correction, was described [2, 3].

Despite being stifled by the lack of suitable antisepsis, anaesthesia techniques and rudimentary surgical instrumentation, in 1826, John Rhea Barton performed the first osteotomy to treat a patient with ankylosis of the hip [4]. His intention was to create an 'artificial joint' through non-union of the subtrochanteric osteotomy, thereby improving function. Almost a decade later, in 1835, he performed the first supracondylar femoral osteotomy in order to treat ankylosis of the knee [5]. During a 5-min procedure without anaesthesia, he removed a wedge of bone from the anterior

> 1835
> John Rhea Barton performs the first supracondylar femoral osteotomy

distal femur and gradually corrected the flexion deformity in a splint over several weeks (Fig. 1.2) [5]. He reported success in 12 of 14 osteotomy procedures, noting 2 deaths from 'hectic irritation and exhaustion' post-operatively [3]. His work made a profound impact on future developments with respect to osteotomy for deformity correction as well as the concepts of arthroplasty and joint range of motion.

1846
William Morton and Robert Liston perform first surgical procedures using ether anaesthesia

An important breakthrough occurred in 1846 when William Morton at Massachusetts General Hospital and Robert Liston at University College Hospital in London performed the first surgical procedures on their respective continents with the use of ether, a major milestone in the development of effective anaesthesia for surgery, permitting procedures of greater duration, complexity and accuracy [6].

In the 1850s, Langenbeck developed the less invasive technique of subcutaneous osteotomy' to treat hip and knee ankylosis and lower limb deformities. Through a small incision with minimal soft tissue disruption, he drilled a cortical window, through which he used a small saw to partially section the bone to allow manual breaking and straightening [7]. Subsequent work by surgeons including Billroth, Volkman, Pancoast and Gross further developed the instrumentation and techniques for transcutaneous osteotomy, with reportedly good results, but sepsis remained an obstacle.

Fig. 1.2 Illustration of osteotomy performed by Barton in 1837. (From Barton JR (1837) On a new treatment for certain cases of ankylosis. Am J Med Sc 21:332–340)

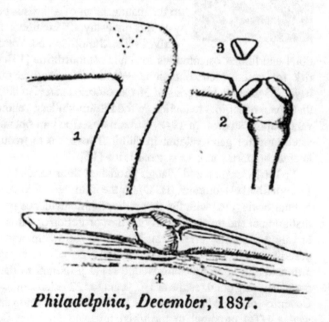

Philadelphia, December, 1837.

Lister's ground breaking work in antiseptic surgery, having applied Pasteur's principles of fermentation to the aetiology of wound sepsis [8], influenced William MacEwan of the Glasgow Royal Infirmary who described his technique of 'antiseptic osteotomy' in treating lower limb deformities such as genu valgum and genu varum in

> 1878
> William MacEwen describes "antiseptic osteotomy"

the *Lancet* in 1878 [9]. He demonstrated favourable results in a series of over 50 osteotomies [9]. In 1880, MacEwen published the first book devoted to osteotomy, which included improved antisepsis and operative technique [10], and became one of the most prolific contributors to the principles of osteotomy and deformity correction of his time. He departed from the bone- or wooden-handled chisel and developed the all metal instrument with a wedge-shaped cutting end, which he called an osteotome [11]. By 1884 he had performed over 1800 osteotomies reportedly without septicaemia or fatal wound complications [12]. The usage of and indications for osteotomies expanded over the following 75 years, although results remained mixed due to lack of internal fixation, radiographic analysis, and rudimentary immobilisation techniques [3].

1.3 Deformity Correction to the Treatment of Arthrosis

> 1940
> Osteotomies are used to treat patients with knee osteoarthritis

The next era of advancement in knee osteotomy was born from the application of principles of deformity correction to the management of arthrosis, prior to which arthrodesis was the mainstay of treatment for severe cases. In the early 1940s, Steindler and Wardle performed proximal tibial and fibular osteotomies for knee osteoarthritis [13]. Despite concerns of the risk for vascular complications, Wardle described favourable results persisting beyond 5 years in his series of 38 osteotomies and also attributed part of the immediate pain relief to a reduction in the intramedullary venous pressure suggested by venographic studies. In 1948, Brittain described an opening-wedge distal femoral osteotomy for genu valgum in children resistant to treatment and in adults with lateral compartment knee osteoarthritis [14].

In 1961, Jackson and Waugh published their series of 11 high tibial osteotomies (HTO) for the treatment of knee osteoarthritis (OA) with the first radiographic evidence of realignment and union, quantifying the correction of varus or valgus deformity after mean 31 months follow-up, and

> 1961
> Jackson and Waugh publish first radiographic evidence of realignment.

described their preferred 'ball and socket type' of osteotomy [15]. Gariépy described a transfibular lateral closing-wedge HTO proximal to the tibial tubercle in 1964, demonstrating good results at 1–7 years for 22 osteotomies [16]. This inspired Mark Coventry of the Mayo Clinic in Rochester to develop his technique of closing-wedge HTO proximal to the tibial tubercle for knee OA with varus or valgus

1965
Mark Coventry describes technique of closing wedge osteotomy staple fixation and defines principles of osteotomy.

deformity, which he secured with one or two staples and cast immobilization for 4–6 weeks (Fig. 1.3) [17]. He described several principles that remain relevant, recommending that the HTO should (1) fully correct or overcorrect the deformity, (2) be near the sight of the deformity, (3) involve bone that will heal rapidly, (4) allow early range of motion and weight-bearing, (5) permit exploration of the knee if necessary and (6) minimise risks [17]. He also highlighted that osteotomy proximal to the tibial tubercle permitted transfer of compressive forces from the quadriceps to encourage union [17]. His initial series consisted of 30 knees, with 18 of the 22 cases followed up for >1 year showing satisfactory results (relief of most pre-operative pain, >90° flexion, full active extension and no insta-

bility). Loosening was seen in two knees with smooth, rounded, stainless steel staples, no cases with Vitallium rectangular bridged staples and no vascular injuries, and one peroneal nerve palsy (compression from cast) was noted, which recovered partially. While

1970
Freeman and Swanson develop Total Condylar Prosthesis for knee arthroplasty

Coventry acknowledged that favourable results were demonstrated in selected groups of patients, especially patients with early degenerative disease with relative sparing of either the medial or lateral compartment; [18] in the 1970s, the broad variety of surgical techniques, inadequately defined indications, suboptimal fixation methods and complications such as wound infection, non-union and peroneal nerve palsy lead to mixed reports [3]. Simultaneously, knee arthroplasty was demonstrating promising results with the advent of the total condylar design [19], and many surgeons moved away from osteotomies, leaving only a small number of centres performing the procedure for several years.

1.4 Advances in Fixation Techniques

Plaster casting alone or staple fixation usually augmented with bracing or casting was used to maintain correction following osteotomy by the majority of surgeons until the 1980s [3]. During this time, loss of correction and recurrence of deformity remained a significant concern. Coventry introduced the

1971
Müller reports favourable results with use of AOT-plate

stepped staple in 1969 to improve the congruence and depth of engagement of the distal limb of the staple [20]. However, a significant advancement in fixation technique came from the application of fracture fixation principles. In 1958 the Arbeitsgemeinschaft für Osteosynthesefragen (now known as the AO foundation) was founded, and despite failures seen with early permutations of fixation devices, in 1971 Müller (one of the founding members) reported good or excellent results in 83% of patients at 1–6 years post-HTO, advocating the use of AO T-plates [21]. The potential to achieve early stable fixation

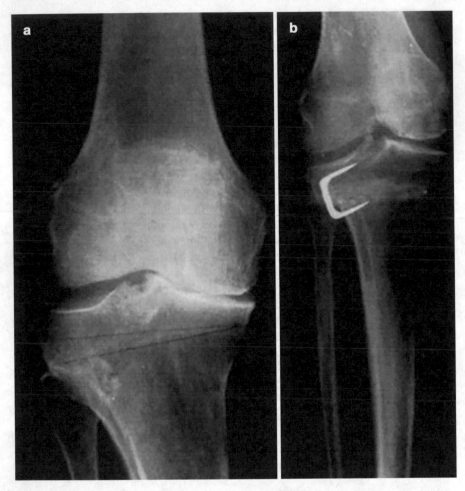

Fig. 1.3 (a) Pre- and (b) post-operative radiographs from Coventry's description of proximal tibial osteotomy technique with staple fixation in 1965. (Reproduced with permission from Wolters Kluwer Health, Inc. Coventry MB. Osteotomy of the upper portion of the tibia for degenerative arthritis of the knee. *J Bone Joint Surg Am.* 1965;47:984-90)

permitting early knee range of motion was recognised. Krackow's group showed good or excellent results in 93% of distal femoral osteotomies using the 90° AO distal femoral blade plate in 1988 [22]. Miniaci et al. used a similar device moulded from a semitubular plate for 41 HTOs with good early results, but unsatisfying mechanical axis corrections in 50% of cases, leading them to describe a new method of pre-operative planning for mechanical axis correction in 1989 [23].

During the 1990s fixation techniques developed in diversity and complexity. Following the influential work of Dror Paley in deformity correction and the use of the Illizarov technique [24], dynamic external fixation was utilised for HTOs with the advantages of early weight-bearing and potential to control the correction post-operatively [25, 26]. However, this method was technically demanding and faced challenges of patient concordance and pin tract complications [3]. A resurgence of the opening-wedge osteotomy was seen along with the development of more spe-cialised plating systems, such as spacer plates (e.g. Puddu plate, Arthrex Inc., Naples, Florida, USA) and angular stable devices such as the TomoFix plate (Mathys Inc., Bettlach, Switzerland) in the late 1990s [27, 28]. The former was a stainless plate which contained a spacer of variable size to assist in maintaining the correc-tion and the latter a titanium plate with angular stable locking screws. The TomoFix gained popularity because of improved biomechanical properties, including tor-sional strength, increased load to failure, and reduced risk of displacement in the event of propagation of the osteotomy to the opposite cortex [28–31]. Additional augmentation with bone graft or bone graft substitute was still advocated by some authors to reduce the risk of failure.

1.5   Understanding the Ideal Correction and Improvements in Pre-operative Planning

Prior to the advent of radiographic imaging, deformity analysis and correction were judged "by eye", and although the first human application of X-ray technology in 1895 by Wilhelm Conrad Röentgen gave birth to a new era of skeletal imaging, short knee films were utilised without regard to the overall axis of the limb or loca-tion of deformity. With greater use of radiographic analysis for planning and evalu-ation of correction, authors began to question the alignment targets, evolving from anatomical axis correction to mechanical axis correction measured on full leg length images, the value of which was highlighted by Harris and Kostuik in 1970 [32].

> 1979
> Fujisawa *et al* define correction target for valgus HTOs

The correction target was ill-defined until 1979, when Fujisawa et al. demonstrated arthroscopic and histological evidence of fibrocartilage regeneration in patients whose mechanical axes were corrected to a point 30–40% lateral to the midpoint of the tibial plateau in a series of 54 patients undergoing valgus HTO for osteoarthritis of the knee [33]. This became widely accepted and incorporated in the evolving methods for pre-operative planning [23, 34]. Miniaci et al. described their technique for pre-operative planning using long-leg weight-bearing films in addition to varus and val-gus stress tests in 1989 (Fig. 1.4) [23], defining the corrective angle required by projecting the target mechanical axis as defined by Fujisawa et al. Dugdale et al. described an algorithm to determine the correction taking into consideration the mechanical axis as well as the joint line separation caused by ligamentous laxity in complex cases (Fig. 1.5) [34].

The work conducted by Dror Paley (1989 onward), his description of the centre of rotation of deformity (CORA) and his methods of deter-mining the site, magnitude and direction of cor-rection required has provided greater depth to our understanding of joint realignment [24, 35]. The potential to create new deformities, such as joint line obliquity, without due consideration for these principles became apparent.

> 1989
> Miniaci *et al* describe technique for pre-operative planning of correction
> AND
> Paley describes principles of deformity correction

Fig. 1.4 Description of pre-operative planning of correction by Miniaci et al. (Reproduced with permission from Wolters Kluwer Health, Inc. Miniaci A, Ballmer FT, Ballmer PM, Jakob RP. Proximal tibial osteotomy. A new fixation device. Clin Orthop Relat Res 1989;246:250–9)

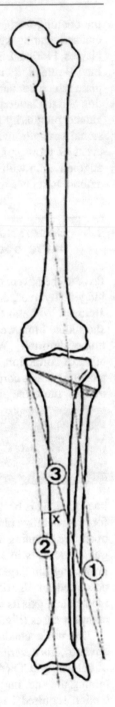

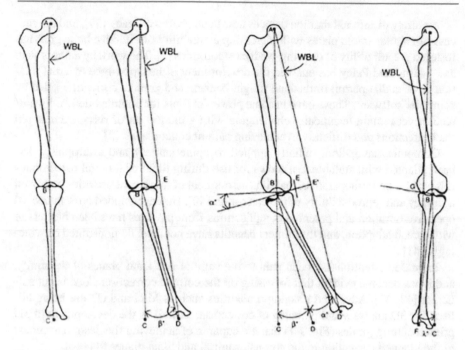

Fig. 1.5 Description of pre-operative planning of correction by Dugdale et al. (Reproduced with permission from Wolters Kluwer Health, Inc. Dugdale TW, Noyes FR, Styer DA. Preoperative planning for high tibial osteotomy. The effect of lateral tibiofemoral separation and tibiofemoral length. *Clin Orthop Relat Res.* 1992;Jan(274):248-64)

1.6   Distal Femoral or Proximal Tibial Osteotomy?

Early pioneers performed distal femoral and proximal tibial osteotomies for varus and valgus deformities with immense heterogeneity in technique and philosophy. In 1973, Shoji and Insall demonstrated the inferior outcomes of HTO for valgus deformity in comparison to HTO for varus deformity [36]. In the same year, Coventry advocated that distal femoral osteotomy was preferable to HTO for valgus deformity >12° or if the plane of the joint line was inclined >10° from the horizontal, so as to avoid resultant joint line obliquity that would cause excessive shear force and failure [18]. These findings were confirmed by case series and comparative studies in the 1980s by Maquet, McDermott et al. and Healy et al. [22, 37, 38]

1.7   Twenty-First Century Osteotomies

Since the turn of the century, the practice of osteotomy around the knee has undergone evolution in terms of fixation methods, understanding of limb alignment targets, the use of technological aids to optimise accuracy and precision of correction and the ability to monitor outcomes.

A variety of internal fixation devices now have proven efficacy [39], and the success of angular stable plates with increasing availability of effective bone graft has fostered greater utility of opening-wedge osteotomies [3]. The work by authors such as Illizarov and Paley has enabled the development of hexapod-type external fixation devices that permit immediate weight-bearing and gradual correction aided by computer software. These have become powerful tools for complex deformity correction yet remain technically challenging with a unique set of risks, such as pin tract infections and difficulty in achieving patient concordance [3].

Computer navigation, initially applied to spine surgery and arthroplasty, has been adapted with suitable workflows for use during tibial or femoral osteotomies (Fig. 1.6). The intraoperative, real time assessment of alignment provides improved accuracy and reproducibility of the correction [40]. However, added cost, increased operative duration and potential complications from pin sites have been barriers to widespread adoption, and the clinical benefits have not been demonstrated convincingly [41].

Increased attention has been paid to the sagittal and axial planes of deformity, and it has become evident that focussing on the coronal correction alone is not sufficient [42, 43]. Advanced imaging modalities such as MRI and CT are being utilised for 3D analysis and planning of correction, as well as the development of 3D printed cutting guides (Fig. 1.7) that are capable of achieving the desired accuracy of the planned correction in the coronal, sagittal and axial planes [44–46].

Defining the indications for osteotomy remains a challenge. Age and level of activity are no longer clear, defining characteristics, and some risk factors for failure such as smoking, obesity and the degree of deformity have limited supporting evidence [47–51]. While the expansion of indications and utility of partial knee arthroplasty has challenged the indications for osteotomies, analogous to that seen in the 1970s with total knee arthroplasty [52–54], there is also a growing body of evidence demonstrating the efficacy of osteotomies alone or combined with cartilage restoration procedures, and ligament reconstructions in the treatment of instability and even concomitant total knee arthroplasty [55–59].

1.7.1   What Will the Future Hold?

For decades we have been able to create large clinical datasets, which have been utilised to determine survivorship of orthopaedic procedures such as arthroplasty and to a lesser extent, osteotomies [56, 60]. However, our ability to incorporate this information into clinical decision-making is now evolving rapidly with the development of machine learning and artificial intelligence, which may offer support for patient selection and determining the optimal correction in future [61].

Robotic-assisted surgery is being used successfully for hip and knee arthroplasty. Although it has not yet been utilised clinically in the context of osteotomies, this technology has been used successfully in animal and cadaver models to assist in achieving alignment of fractured bones [62], as well as to perform osteotomies with advanced cutting modalities, such as laser and water jet cutting techniques, which may increase precision and ability to perform complex osteotomies [63–65].

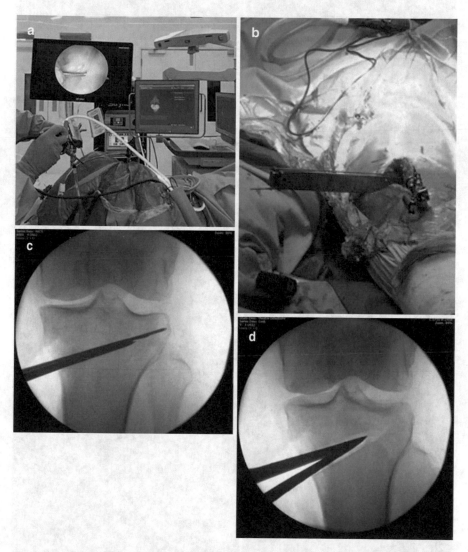

Fig. 1.6 Left knee valgus producing HTO using computer navigation. Note the use of arthroscopic assisted registration (**a**), medial opening wedge high tibial osteotomy (**b**), intra-operative fluoroscopic images (**c, d**) and navigations screen captures (**e, f**) showing correction from 7.5° varus to 1.5° valgus mechanical axis. (**g**) and (**h**) demonstrate pre-operative and post-operative X-rays

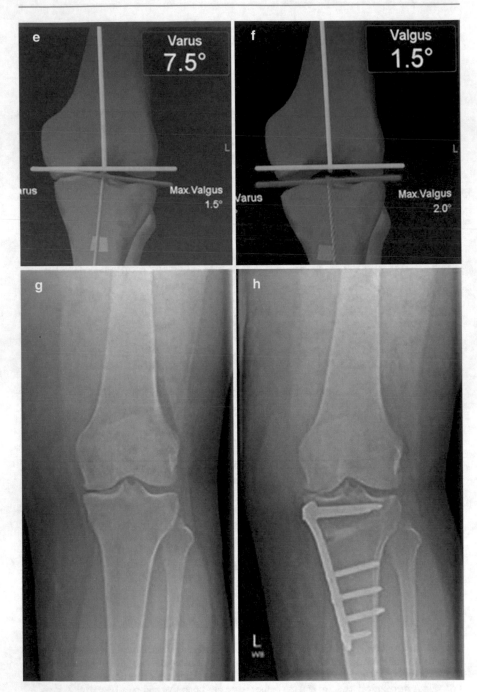

Fig. 1.6 (continued)

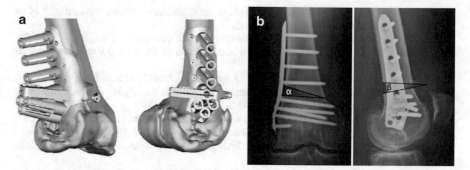

Fig. 1.7 Pre-operative planning for 3D printed cutting guide (**a**) and post-operative radiographs following osteotomy (**b**). (Reproduced with permission and copyright © of The British Editorial Society of Bone & Joint Surgery Victor J. Premanathan A. Virtual 3D planning and patient specific surgical guides for osteotomies around the knee. *Bone Joint J*. 2013;95-B(11 Supple A):153-8)

1.8   Summary and Conclusions

The evolution of joint realignment has received contributions from highly influential pioneers over thousands of years and continues to evolve rapidly. As technological aids provide increasing levels of accuracy and precision in terms of planning and surgical technique, our future challenges will be to refine the indications for osteotomies and determine the appropriate correction for each individual.

References

1. Brorson S. Management of fractures of the humerus in Ancient Egypt, Greece, and Rome: an historical review. Clin Orthop Relat Res. 2009;467(7):1907–14.
2. Dabis J, Templeton-Ward O, Lacey AE, Narayan B, Trompeter A. The history, evolution and basic science of osteotomy techniques. Strat Traum Limb Recon. 2017;12(3):169–80.
3. Smith J, Wilson A, Thomas N. Osteotomy around the knee: evolution, principles and results. Knee Surg Sports Traumatol Arthrosc. 2013;21(1):3–22.
4. Barton JR. On the treatment of anchylosis, by the formation of artificial joints. North Am Med Surg J. 1827;3:279–400.
5. Di Matteo B, Tarabella V, Filardo G, Viganò A, Tomba P, Marcacci M. John Rhea Barton: the birth of osteotomy. Knee Surg Sports Traumatol Arthrosc. 2013;21(9):1957–62.
6. Boott F. Surgical operations performed during insensibility, produced by the inhalation of sulphuric ether. Lancet. 1847;49(1218):5–8.
7. Adams W. On subcutaneous osteotomy. Br Med J. 1879;2(981):604.
8. Lister J. Illustrations of the antiseptic system of treatment in surgery. Lancet. 1867;90(2309):668–9.
9. Macewen W. Lecture on antiseptic osteotomy for genu valgum, genu varum, and other osseous deformities. Lancet. 1878;112(2887):911–4.
10. Macewen W. Osteotomy with an inquiry into the aetiology and pathology of knock-knee, bow-leg, and other osseous deformities of the lower limbs. London: Forgotten Books; 1880.
11. Macewen W. Antiseptic osteotomy in genu valgum and anterior tibial curves: with a few remarks on the pathology of knock-knee. Br Med J. 1879;2(981):607–9.
12. Jones AR. Sir William Macewen. J Bone Joint Surg Br. 1952;34(1):123–8.

13. Wardle EN. Osteotomy of the tibia and fibula in the treatment of chronic osteoarthritis of the knee. Postgrad Med J. 1964;40(467):536–42.
14. Brittain HA. Treatment of genu valgum; the discarded iron. Br Med J. 1948;2(4572):385–7.
15. Jackson J, Waugh W. Tibial osteotomy for osteoarthritis of the knee. J Bone Joint Surg Br. 1961;43(4):746–51.
16. Gariépy R. Genu varum treated by high tibial osteotomy. J Bone Joint Surg Br. 1964;46:783–4.
17. Coventry MB. Osteotomy of the upper portion of the tibia for degenerative arthritis of the knee. J Bone Joint Surg Am. 1965;47:984–90.
18. Coventry MB. Osteotomy about the knee for degenerative and rheumatoid arthritis: indications, operative technique, and results. J Bone Joint Surg Am. 1973;55(1):23–48.
19. Swanson SA, Freeman MA. A new prosthesis for the total replacement of the knee. Acta Orthop Belg. 1972;38(Suppl 1):55–62.
20. Coventry MB. Stepped staple for upper tibial osteotomy. J Bone Joint Surg Am. 1969;51(5):1011.
21. Müller W, Jani L. Experiences with 75 high tibial osteotomies. Reconstr Surg Traumatol. 1971;12(0):53–63.
22. Healy W, Anglen J, Wasilewski S, Krackow K. Distal femoral varus osteotomy. J Bone Joint Surg Am. 1988;70(1):102–9.
23. Miniaci A, Ballmer F, Ballmer P, Jakob R. Proximal tibial osteotomy. A new fixation device. Clin Orthop Relat Res. 1989;246:250–9.
24. Paley D. The principles of deformity correction by the Ilizarov technique: technical aspects. Tech Orthop. 1989;4(1):15–29.
25. Weale A, Lee A, MacEachern A. High tibial osteotomy using a dynamic axial external fixator. Clin Orthop Relat Res. 2001;382:154–67.
26. Magyar G, Toksvig-Larsen S, Lindstrand A. Open wedge tibial osteotomy by callus distraction in gonarthrosis: operative technique and early results in 36 patients. Acta Orthop Scand. 1998;69(2):147–51.
27. Stuart MJ, Beachy AM, Grabowski JJ, An K-N, Kaufman KR. Biomechanical evaluation of a proximal tibial opening-wedge osteotomy plate. Am J Knee Surg. 1999;12(3):148–53; discussion 53–4
28. Staubli AE, De Simoni C, Babst R, Lobenhoffer P. TomoFix: a new LCP-concept for open wedge osteotomy of the medial proximal tibia–early results in 92 cases. Injury. 2003;34:55–62.
29. Stoffel K, Stachowiak G, Kuster M. Open wedge high tibial osteotomy: biomechanical investigation of the modified Arthrex Osteotomy Plate (Puddu Plate) and the TomoFix Plate. Clin Biomech. 2004;19(9):944–50.
30. Agneskirchner J, Freiling D, Hurschler C, Lobenhoffer P. Primary stability of four different implants for opening wedge high tibial osteotomy. Knee Surg Sports Traumatol Arthrosc. 2006;14(3):291–300.
31. Pape D, Kohn D, Van Giffen N, Hoffmann A, Seil R, Lorbach O. Differences in fixation stability between spacer plate and plate fixator following high tibial osteotomy. Knee Surg Sports Traumatol Arthrosc. 2013;21(1):82–9.
32. Harris WR, Kostuik JP. High tibial osteotomy for osteo-arthritis of the knee. J Bone Joint Surg Am. 1970;52(2):330–6.
33. Fujisawa Y, Masuhara K, Shiomi S. The effect of high tibial osteotomy on osteoarthritis of the knee. An arthroscopic study of 54 knee joints. Orthop Clin North Am. 1979;10(3):585–608.
34. Dugdale TW, Noyes FR, Styer D. Preoperative planning for high tibial osteotomy. The effect of lateral tibiofemoral separation and tibiofemoral length. Clin Orthop Relat Res. 1992;274:248–64.
35. Paley D. Principles of deformity correction. New York: Springer; 2014.
36. Shoji H, Insall J. High tibial osteotomy for osteoarthritis of the knee with valgus deformity. J Bone Joint Surg Am. 1973;55(5):963–73.
37. Maquet P. The treatment of choice in osteoarthritis of the knee. Clin Orthop Relat Res. 1985;192:108–12.

38. McDermott A, Finklestein J, Farine I, Boynton E, MacIntosh D, Gross A. Distal femoral varus osteotomy for valgus deformity of the knee. J Bone Joint Surg Am. 1988;70(1):110–6.
39. Gao L, Madry H, Chugaev DV, Denti M, Frolov A, Burtsev M, et al. Advances in modern osteotomies around the knee. J Exp Orthop. 2019;6(1):9.
40. Neri T, Myat D, Parker D. The use of navigation in osteotomies around the knee. Clin Sports Med. 2019;38(3):451–69.
41. Wu ZP, Zhang P, Bai JZ, Liang Y, Chen PT, He JS, et al. Comparison of navigated and conventional high tibial osteotomy for the treatment of osteoarthritic knees with varus deformity: a meta-analysis. Int J Surg. 2018;55:211–9.
42. Lustig S, Scholes CJ, Costa AJ, Coolican MJ, Parker DA. Different changes in slope between the medial and lateral tibial plateau after open-wedge high tibial osteotomy. Knee Surg Sports Traumatol Arthrosc. 2013;21(1):32–8.
43. d'Entremont AG, McCormack RG, Horlick SGD, Stone TB, Manzary MM, Wilson DR. Effect of opening-wedge high tibial osteotomy on the three-dimensional kinematics of the knee. Bone Joint J. 2014;96-B(9):1214–21.
44. Victor J, Premanathan A. Virtual 3D planning and patient specific surgical guides for osteotomies around the knee. Bone Joint J. 2013;95-B(11 Supple A):153–8.
45. Jones GG, Jaere M, Clarke S, Cobb J. 3D printing and high tibial osteotomy. EFORT Open Rev. 2018;3(5):254–9.
46. Donnez M, Ollivier M, Munier M, Berton P, Podgorski JP, Chabrand P, et al. Are three-dimensional patient-specific cutting guides for open wedge high tibial osteotomy accurate? An in vitro study. J Orthop Surg Res. 2018;13(1):171.
47. W-Dahl A, Toksvig-Larsen S. Cigarette smoking delays bone healing a prospective study of 200 patients operated on by the hemicallotasis technique. Acta Orthop Scand. 2004;75(3):347–51.
48. Sherman SL, Thompson SF, Clohisy JC. Distal femoral varus osteotomy for the management of valgus deformity of the knee. JAAOS. 2018;26(9):313–24.
49. Rossi R, Bonasia DE, Amendola A. The role of high tibial osteotomy in the varus knee. JAAOS. 2011;19(10):590–9.
50. Brinkman JM, Lobenhoffer P, Agneskirchner JD, Staubli AE, Wymenga AB, van Heerwaarden RJ. Osteotomies around the knee. J Bone Joint Surg Br. 2008;90-B(12):1548–57.
51. Lobenhoffer P. Indication for unicompartmental knee replacement versus osteotomy around the knee. J Knee Surg. 2017;30(8):769–73.
52. Parratte S, Argenson J-N, Pearce O, Pauly V, Auquier P, Aubaniac J-M. Medial unicompartmental knee replacement in the under-50s. J Bone Joint Surg Br. 2009;91(3):351–6.
53. Smith WB, Steinberg J, Scholtes S, Mcnamara IR. Medial compartment knee osteoarthritis: age-stratified cost-effectiveness of total knee arthroplasty, unicompartmental knee arthroplasty, and high tibial osteotomy. Knee Surg Sports Traumatol Arthrosc. 2017;25(3):924–33.
54. Streit MR, Streit J, Walker T, Bruckner T, Kretzer JP, Ewerbeck V, et al. Minimally invasive Oxford medial unicompartmental knee arthroplasty in young patients. Knee Surg Sports Traumatol Arthrosc. 2017;25(3):660–8.
55. Cantin O, Magnussen RA, Corbi F, Servien E, Neyret P, Lustig S. The role of high tibial osteotomy in the treatment of knee laxity: a comprehensive review. Knee Surg Sports Traumatol Arthrosc. 2015;23(10):3026–37.
56. León SA, Mei XY, Safir OA, Gross AE, Kuzyk PR. Long-term results of fresh osteochondral allografts and realignment osteotomy for cartilage repair in the knee. Bone Joint J. 2019;101-B(1_Supple_A):46–52.
57. Veltman ES, van Wensen RJA, Defoort KC, van Hellemondt GG, Wymenga AB. Single-stage total knee arthroplasty and osteotomy as treatment of secondary osteoarthritis with severe coronal deviation of joint surface due to extra-articular deformity. Knee Surg Sports Traumatol Arthrosc. 2017;25(9):2835–40.
58. Dejour D, Saffarini M, Demey G, Baverel L. Tibial slope correction combined with second revision ACL produces good knee stability and prevents graft rupture. Knee Surg Sports Traumatol Arthrosc. 2015;23(10):2846–52.

59. Bonin N, Ait Si Selmi T, Donell ST, Dejour H, Neyret P. Anterior cruciate reconstruction combined with valgus upper tibial osteotomy: 12 years follow-up. Knee. 2004;11(6):431–7.
60. Niinimäki TT, Eskelinen A, Mann BS, Junnila M, Ohtonen P, Leppilahti J. Survivorship of high tibial osteotomy in the treatment of osteoarthritis of the knee. J Bone Joint Surg Br. 2012;94-B(11):1517–21.
61. Bini SA. Artificial intelligence, machine learning, deep learning, and cognitive computing: what do these terms mean and how will they impact health care? J Arthroplasty. 2018;33(8):2358–61.
62. Wang J, Han W, Lin H. Femoral fracture reduction with a parallel manipulator robot on a traction table. Int J Med Robot. 2013;9(4):464–71.
63. Sotsuka Y, Nishimoto S, Tsumano T, Kawai K, Ishise H, Kakibuchi M, et al. The dawn of computer-assisted robotic osteotomy with ytterbium-doped fiber laser. Lasers Med Sci. 2014;29(3):1125–9.
64. Baek KW, Deibel W, Marinov D, Griessen M, Bruno A, Zeilhofer HF, et al. Clinical applicability of robot-guided contact-free laser osteotomy in cranio-maxillo-facial surgery: in-vitro simulation and in-vivo surgery in minipig mandibles. Br J Oral Maxillofac Surg. 2015;53(10):976–81.
65. Suero EM, Westphal R, Zaremba D, Citak M, Hawi N, Citak M, et al. Robotic guided waterjet cutting technique for high tibial dome osteotomy: a pilot study. Int J Med Robot. 2017;13(3)

Load, Alignment, and Wear

2

Arne Kienzle, Carsten F. Perka, Georg N. Duda, and Clemens Gwinner

2.1 Basic Knee Kinematics

The human knee is the largest and one of the most biomechanically demanded joints, as it is located between the two longest lever arms of the body and its most powerful muscles. Even though flexion and extension are regarded as primary knee kinematics, a total of six independent degrees of freedom with three translations and three rotations (flexion/extension, anterior-posterior displacement, external/internal rotation, varus/valgus motions, compression/distraction, and medial/lateral shift) contribute to its overall function.

Knee flexion progresses as a combination of femoral rolling, gliding, and rotation over the underlying tibial plateau. The magnitude of each of these movements changes throughout the range of motion. Commencing with early knee flexion, the tibiofemoral contact point moves posteriorly with advancing knee flexion. Notably, this effect is much more pronounced on the lateral side, as the lateral femoral condyle rolls on a larger radius compared to the medial side [1]. This asymmetry in condylar movement causes a passive internal rotation of the tibia with flexion. Vice versa, the tibia rotates externally, the so-called screw home rotation, during terminal extension.

A. Kienzle
Center for Musculoskeletal Surgery, Charité-University Medicine, Berlin, Germany

Laboratory of Adaptive and Regenerative Biology, Brigham & Women's Hospital, Harvard Medical School, Boston, MA, USA

C. F. Perka (✉) · C. Gwinner
Center for Musculoskeletal Surgery, Charité-University Medicine, Berlin, Germany
e-mail: carsten.perka@charite.de

G. N. Duda
Centre for Sports Science and Sports Medicine, Julius Wolff Institute, Charité-University Medicine, Berlin, Germany

© Springer Nature Switzerland AG 2020
S. Oussedik, S. Lustig (eds.), *Osteotomy About the Knee*,
https://doi.org/10.1007/978-3-030-49055-3_2

Knee stability through the range of motion is ensured by both static and dynamic structures that work in concert to prevent excessive movement or instability, which may occur across multiple planes of motion.

Static stabilizers of the knee joint comprise the bony structure. In contrast, the incongruity of the skeletal architecture, as well as its articular cartilage surfaces— possessing an extremely low coefficient of friction—limits the ability to resist translation. Shape, orientation, and functional properties of the menisci improve congruence between femoral condyles and the tibial plateau and distribute compressive forces across the knee joint. Notwithstanding the importance of bony and meniscal anatomy for physiological knee kinematics, the amount of stability provided is minimal considering the large loads transferred through the knee joint. Conversely, orientation and material properties of dynamic stabilizers, including ligaments, the capsule, and musculotendinous soft tissues, are the centerpiece of knee stability. Even small changes to any of these parameters will alter the inherently complex interactions between the aforementioned structures and ultimately distort overall movement patterns of the knee, consequently impacting alignment, load distribution, and wear of the components forming the knee joint. Medical intervention is imperative in numerous cases to prevent permanent damages to the knee joint.

2.2 Load

The load distribution of the knee joint is dependent on kinematics, limb alignment, body habitus, and physical activity. These forces can be categorized into external forces (EF) and internal forces (IF). EF comprise of the body weight, ground reaction force, and acceleration/deceleration of the limb segments. IF counteract EF and are generated by active muscle contraction, ligamentous forces, and joint contact forces. Additionally, the muscular components not only provide stability, but also increase precision of movement and thus play a significant role in controlling the load distribution.

EF can be measured in a laboratory setting using motion analysis and force plates. In contrast, IF can only be estimated using analytical models of the knee joint and by assessment of isometric muscle strength [2]. For more accurate in vivo measurements of IF, prosthetic joints have been instrumented with force transducers [3]. However, knee joints have fundamentally different movement patterns after endoprosthetic replacement.

Loads of 200–400%BW (percent of body weight) have been reported for level walking [4–6], yet loads can go up to 670%BW depending on individual factors and the model used for analysis [7, 8]. Regarding daily activities, highest loads of approximately 350%BW occur during stair ascent and descent [9].

Both EF and IF can have significant impact on the wear of the components of the knee joint, with menisci and cartilage being especially at risk [10]. Additionally, long-lasting imbalances in load distribution can lead to malalignment, and preexisting malalignment can lead to load imbalances. These can result in permanent damage to vital structures for unimpaired movement. Surgical intervention is justified when permanent harm can be averted, or damaged structures offloaded, and physiological function of the knee joint can be conserved. While conservative therapy approaches such as reduction of the total load by loss of weight is generally beneficial for patients, osteotomy allows for operative adjustment of the load distribution. Both for planning surgical interventions and for satisfactory clinical outcomes, detailed knowledge on physiological load distribution is essential.

2.3   Alignment

2.3.1   Coronal Alignment

Static knee alignment is subject to a multitude of influencing factors, such as genetics, demographics, biomechanics, posture, and level of activity. Coronal alignment is advocated to play a key role in load distribution between the medial and lateral compartment as well as soft tissue tension within the knee. At the same time, unphysiological load distribution can permanently impact the biomechanical properties of the components forming the knee joint and ultimately alter its alignment. Coronal alignment can also be affected by wear, degenerative changes, and coronal laxity, mainly of the medial and lateral collateral ligament complexes.

In addition to the confusing and etymological terminology of varus (Latin for "crooked") and valgus (Latin for "twisted" or "bent"), there is paucity of uniform methodology for measuring lower extremity coronal alignment to this day [11]. Commonly, coronal alignment is defined using the hip-knee-ankle (HKA) angle, with values around 180° being regarded as physiological. Notably, no consensus has been reached whether a HKA of 180° should be referred to as neutral, as a considerable number of studies has shown that the mean HKA tends to be slightly in varus [12, 13].

Another important component of the coronal alignment is the joint line orientation [14], which is on average in 3° valgus. Thus, the angle between the mechanical axis of the femur and a tangent to the femoral condyles (femoral mechanical axis, FMA) is typically in 3° valgus and to the tibial mechanical axis (TMA) typically in 3° varus (Fig. 2.1a). This can be confounded by joint space opening, measured as the joint line convergence angle (JLCA). Consequently, the summation of FMA, TMA, and JLCA adds up to the HKA (Fig. 2.1b) [15].

In a landmark study, Hsu et al. delineated the aforementioned angles using full-length weight-bearing radiographs [13]. Foremost, they noted the HKA to be in 1.2° varus and stated that 75% of the load passed through the medial compartment during single-leg stance. This asymmetry in load distribution may explain the markedly higher prevalence of osteoarthritis (OA) with medial compartment involvement compared to the lateral compartment [16]. In spite of the outstanding importance for physiological functioning of the knee, current studies have highlighted the broad variability of coronal alignment in native as well as osteoarthritic knees [17].

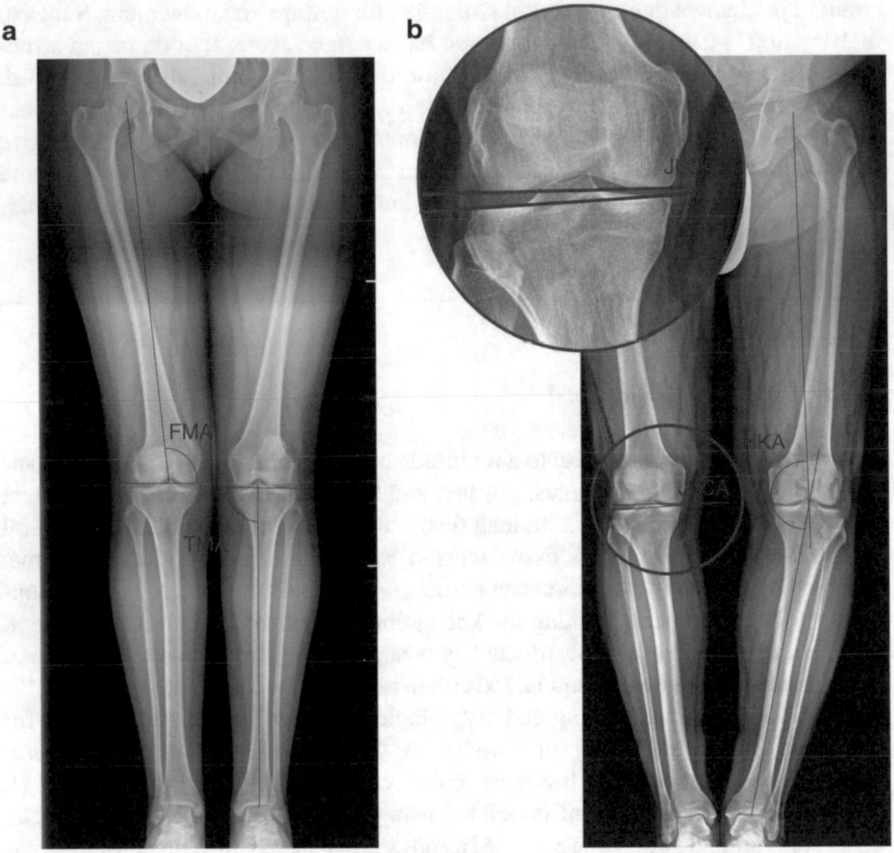

Fig. 2.1 Radiographic analysis of lower limb axial alignment. (**a**) Femoral mechanical axis (FMA; left) and tibial mechanical axis (TMA; right) in a non-arthritic valgus knee. (**b**) Joint line convergence angle (JLCA; left). The summation of FMA, TMA, and JLCA adds up to the HKA (right)

Gender-specific differences further complicate defining an exact physiological angle; in a prominent study, Bellemans et al. found 32% of men and 17% of women to have a constitutional varus with their physiological alignment at 3° or more [12]. With respect to femoral rotation, the posterior condylar axis is on average 3° internally rotated relative to the epicondylar axis in the straight knee [18]; however, again, there is considerable heterogeneity within these parameters in varus and valgus knees.

Stark malalignment can alter the load distribution, wear, and, subsequently, damage knee joint structures [19]. In such cases the alignment may be adjusted by medical intervention. While the use of externally applied knee braces has yielded mixed results [20, 21], surgical intervention such as osteotomy can significantly alter coronal alignment of the knee [22]. However, lack of a clear definition of coronal malalignment complicates the determination for medical necessity to intervene. As a significant fraction of the normal population has a natural coronal alignment of $\geq 3°$ varus, operative adjustment of the mechanical alignment to neutral may not always be desirable and would be unphysiological for these individuals [12].

2.3.2   Sagittal Alignment

Similar to coronal alignment, sagittal alignment plays an essential role in translation as well as controlling of the load distribution in the knee. Soft tissue restraints are essential to control sagittal knee laxity, with the anterior and posterior cruciate ligament being the mainstay of sagittal stability and facilitating a central pivot for internal/external rotation. However, the role of the bony geometry of the underlying tibial plateau in sagittal alignment is not as well understood.

There is an emerging consensus that the posterior inclination of the tibial plateau has a direct influence on knee kinematics [23]. This includes anteroposterior laxity, the center of rotation, and loading of the cruciate ligaments [24].

In a cornerstone study for modern osteotomy, Agneskirchner and Lobenhoffer demonstrated that a correction in sagittal tibial alignment, namely, by increasing the tibial slope (TS), can be used to counteract posterior tibial translation [25]. These results were echoed in clinical studies in which an increased tibial slope has been shown to result in greater anterior tibial translation during simple weight-bearing activities [26]. Consequently, sagittal alignment plays a significant role in the load distribution on the cruciate ligaments. Current scientific literature supports a moderate to strong association between an increased TS to an elevated risk of anterior cruciate ligament (ACL) or ACL graft injury [27–29]. Vice versa, patients with decreased TS may be prone to posterior cruciate ligament (PCL) injury [30]. Increased TS have indeed been shown to correlate with heightened posterior laxity in healthy knees [23]. Thus, elevated TS can be beneficial after PCL reconstruction as it may avoid mechanical overload of the graft [31, 32].

2.4   Wear

All structures forming the knee joint are susceptible to wear. Cartilaginous tissue is especially at risk due to its poorly vascularized nature and thus limited capacity for regeneration [10]. Once the dynamic equilibrium between the continual formation and breakdown of the cartilaginous matrix is violated and exceeds the system's ability to compensate, irreversible matrix degradation is inevitable. As the biomechanical properties of the injured cartilage are impaired, the aforementioned cascade continues to affect the surrounding cartilage, making it highly susceptible to further damage, which, over time, leads to osteoarthritic deterioration of the knee joint.

This principle of "wear and tear" is a highly simplified explanation of the multifactorial entity of OA. In fact, OA of the knee joint is a highly complex condition, with cartilage degradation, accompanying synovitis, subchondral bone remodeling,

Table 2.1 Kellgren-Lawrence classification of radiographic knee osteoarthritis [33]

Grade I	Grade II	Grade III	Grade IV
Doubtful narrowing of the joint space with possible osteophyte formation	Possible narrowing of the joint space with definite osteophyte formation	Definite narrowing of joint space, moderate osteophyte formation, some sclerosis, and possible deformity of bony ends	Large osteophyte formation, severe narrowing of the joint space with marked sclerosis, and definite deformity of bony ends

degeneration of ligaments and menisci, and hypertrophy of the joint capsule being integral parts of the pathogenesis. Thus, due to the variety of clinical presentations, it is difficult to rigorously define knee OA.

OA can be classified as either primary (idiopathic) or secondary. Although the etiology of primary OA is mostly undefined, genetic, age-related, ethnic, and bio-mechanical factors are presumed to play a key role. Common causes of secondary OA include trauma, malalignment as well as infectious, inflammatory, and bio-chemical etiologies that are relatively well understood. In cases with altered load distribution, corrective osteotomy can potentially delay or prevent development of secondary OA.

For the diagnosis of OA standardized, plain radiography remains the gold standard. Disease severity can be graded by radiographic appearance according to the Kellgren-Lawrence scale (Table 2.1), which was published in 1957 and continues to be the most commonly used classification [33]. However, despite the advantages of plain radiography, such as cost-effectiveness, availability, and inter-rater reliability, patients' clinical presentation and radiographic changes do not necessarily correlate [34].

2.5 Summary

The human knee is the largest and one of the most biomechanically demanded joints in the human body. While offering a wide range of motions, the structures forming the knee joint have to meticulously balance the compressive forces across the knee joint. Orientation, shape, and material properties of the bony structure and dynamic stabilizers, including ligaments, the capsule, and musculotendinous soft tissues, are essential for knee stability. Even small changes to any of these parameters will alter the inherently complex interactions between these structures and ultimately distort overall movement patterns of the knee, consequently impacting alignment, load distribution, and wear of the components forming the knee joint. As detailed in the following chapters, surgical intervention is imperative in numerous cases to prevent permanent damages to the knee joint.

Conflict of Interest The authors declare that they have no conflicts of interest in the authorship and publication of this contribution.

References

1. Pinskerova V, et al. Does the femur roll-back with flexion? J Bone Joint Surg Br. 2004;86(6):925–31.
2. Zheng N, et al. An analytical model of the knee for estimation of internal forces during exercise. J Biomech. 1998;31(10):963–7.
3. D'Lima DD, et al. Tibial forces measured in vivo after total knee arthroplasty. J Arthroplast. 2006;21(2):255–62.
4. Taylor WR, et al. Tibio-femoral loading during human gait and stair climbing. J Orthop Res. 2004;22(3):625–32.
5. Kuster MS, et al. Joint load considerations in total knee replacement. J Bone Joint Surg Br. 1997;79(1):109–13.
6. Morrison JB. The mechanics of the knee joint in relation to normal walking. J Biomech. 1970;3(1):51–61.
7. Mikosz RP, Andriacchi TP, Andersson GB. Model analysis of factors influencing the prediction of muscle forces at the knee. J Orthop Res. 1988;6(2):205–14.
8. Seireg A, Arvikar RJ. The prediction of muscular load sharing and joint forces in the lower extremities during walking. J Biomech. 1975;8(2):89–102.
9. Mundermann A, et al. In vivo knee loading characteristics during activities of daily living as measured by an instrumented total knee replacement. J Orthop Res. 2008;26(9):1167–72.
10. Wilson W, et al. Pathways of load-induced cartilage damage causing cartilage degeneration in the knee after meniscectomy. J Biomech. 2003;36(6):845–51.
11. Houston CS, Swischuk LE. Occasional notes. Varus and valgus—no wonder they are confused. N Engl J Med. 1980;302(8):471–2.
12. Bellemans J, et al. The Chitranjan Ranawat award: is neutral mechanical alignment normal for all patients? The concept of constitutional varus. Clin Orthop Relat Res. 2012;470(1):45–53.
13. Hsu RW, et al. Normal axial alignment of the lower extremity and load-bearing distribution at the knee. Clin Orthop Relat Res. 1990;255:215–27.
14. Hungerford DS, Krackow KA. Total joint arthroplasty of the knee. Clin Orthop Relat Res. 1985;192:23–33.
15. Cooke TD, Li J, Scudamore RA. Radiographic assessment of bony contributions to knee deformity. Orthop Clin North Am. 1994;25(3):387–93.
16. Thomas RH, et al. Compartmental evaluation of osteoarthritis of the knee. A comparative study of available diagnostic modalities. Radiology. 1975;116(3):585–94.
17. Moser LB, et al. Native non-osteoarthritic knees have a highly variable coronal alignment: a systematic review. Knee Surg Sports Traumatol Arthrosc. 2019;27(5):1359–67.
18. Koh YG, et al. Gender differences exist in rotational anatomy of the distal femur in osteoarthritic knees using MRI. Knee Surg Sports Traumatol Arthrosc. 2019; https://doi.org/10.1007/s00167-019-05730-w.
19. Gao F, et al. The influence of knee malalignment on the ankle alignment in varus and valgus gonarthrosis based on radiographic measurement. Eur J Radiol. 2016;85(1):228–32.
20. Brouwer RW, et al. Braces and orthoses for treating osteoarthritis of the knee. Cochrane Database Syst Rev. 2005;(1):CD004020.
21. Singer JC, Lamontagne M. The effect of functional knee brace design and hinge misalignment on lower limb joint mechanics. Clin Biomech (Bristol, Avon). 2008;23(1):52–9.
22. Niemeyer P, et al. Two-year results of open-wedge high tibial osteotomy with fixation by medial plate fixator for medial compartment arthritis with varus malalignment of the knee. Arthroscopy. 2008;24(7):796–804.
23. Schatka I, et al. High tibial slope correlates with increased posterior tibial translation in healthy knees. Knee Surg Sports Traumatol Arthrosc. 2018;26(9):2697–703.
24. Feucht MJ, et al. The role of the tibial slope in sustaining and treating anterior cruciate ligament injuries. Knee Surg Sports Traumatol Arthrosc. 2013;21(1):134–45.

25. Agneskirchner JD, et al. Effect of high tibial flexion osteotomy on cartilage pressure and joint kinematics: a biomechanical study in human cadaveric knees. Winner of the AGA-DonJoy Award 2004. Arch Orthop Trauma Surg. 2004;124(9):575–84.
26. Dejour H, Bonnin M. Tibial translation after anterior cruciate ligament rupture. Two radiological tests compared. J Bone Joint Surg Br. 1994;76(5):745–9.
27. Li Y, et al. Are failures of anterior cruciate ligament reconstruction associated with steep posterior tibial slopes? A case control study. Chin Med J. 2014;127(14):2649–53.
28. Webb JM, et al. Posterior tibial slope and further anterior cruciate ligament injuries in the anterior cruciate ligament-reconstructed patient. Am J Sports Med. 2013;41(12):2800–4.
29. Wordeman SC, et al. In vivo evidence for tibial plateau slope as a risk factor for anterior cruciate ligament injury: a systematic review and meta-analysis. Am J Sports Med. 2012;40(7):1673–81.
30. Bernhardson AS, et al. Posterior tibial slope and risk of posterior cruciate ligament injury. Am J Sports Med. 2019;47(2):312–7.
31. Gwinner C, et al. Tibial slope strongly influences knee stability after posterior cruciate ligament reconstruction: a prospective 5- to 15-year follow-up. Am J Sports Med. 2017;45(2):355–61.
32. Gwinner C, et al. Posterior laxity increases over time after PCL reconstruction. Knee Surg Sports Traumatol Arthrosc. 2019;27(2):389–96.
33. Kellgren JH, Lawrence JS. Radiological assessment of osteo-arthrosis. Ann Rheum Dis. 1957;16(4):494–502.
34. Bagge E, et al. Osteoarthritis in the elderly: clinical and radiological findings in 79 and 85 year olds. Ann Rheum Dis. 1991;50(8):535–9.

Principles of Alignment Correction Surgery

3

Matthieu Ehlinger, Henri Favreau, David Eichler, and François Bonnomet

3.1 Introduction

The indications for osteotomies around the knee can be grouped into three main categories:

1. The treatment of isolated single-compartmental osteoarthritis (the patellofemoral compartment will not be considered in this chapter).
2. Management of joint malalignment associated with ligament laxity and instability (more or less associated with early osteoarthritis).
3. Bone recurvatum.

Whatever the indication and the type of osteotomy performed, it is essential to know and understand the biomechanics of the lower limb.

The purpose of this chapter is to review the biomechanics of the lower limb and set the angular correction goals of these osteotomies.

M. Ehlinger (✉)
Service de Chirurgie Orthopédique et de Traumatologie, Hôpital de Hautepierre, Hôpitaux Universitaires de Strasbourg, Strasbourg Cedex, France

Laboratoire ICube, CNRS UMR 7357, Ilkirch, France
e-mail: Matthieu.ehlinger@chru-strasbourg.fr

H. Favreau · D. Eichler · F. Bonnomet
Service de Chirurgie Orthopédique et de Traumatologie, Hôpital de Hautepierre, Hôpitaux Universitaires de Strasbourg, Strasbourg Cedex, France
e-mail: henri.favreau@chru-strasbourg.fr; david.eichler@chru-strasbourg.fr; francois.bonnomet@chru-strasbourg.fr

3.2 Radiographic Assessment

Radiographic assessment has three main goals:

- To confirm the operative indication, which means that the lesion is amenable to correction by osteotomy
- To define the level of the osteotomy: DFO or HTO or both
- To determine the angular correction required

Radiographs of both limbs must be obtained and should include the following views:

- Anteroposterior (AP) and lateral views of the knee fully extended
  - AP view: assess the articular surfaces; calculate the obliquity of the joint line, particularly for the tibia, with the Levigne angle [1] which defines the epiphyseal varus and thus a local anatomy which might predispose to medial tibiofemoral osteoarthritis (Fig. 3.1).
  - Lateral view: assess the presence of a cup and measure the tibial slope provided that the first 20 cm of the proximal tibia are visible.
- Rosenberg view (45° AP view)
  - Accurately analyze the extent of cartilage wear.

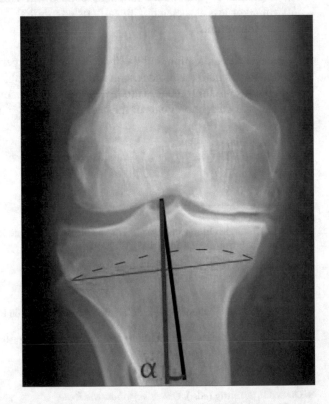

Fig. 3.1 Measurement of epiphyseal varus: the epiphyseal axis (thick red line) connects the center of the tibial spines to the middle of the line connecting the ends of the former growth cartilage plate (thin red line). Black line, mechanical axis of the tibia. α, Levigne epiphyseal angle [1]

- Merchant (sunrise) view
  - Assess patellofemoral space and the possible correlation with the frontal deformity of the lower limb.
- Stress views, in the frontal and sagittal plane
  - Assess laxity, reducibility of deformities, and the contribution of wear to the deformity.
- Full-length views
  - The AP allows specifying the frontal (coronal plane) angular deviation and the mechanical axis of the lower limb, a possible joint opening, and determines the varus deviations (intrinsic, extrinsic, global) allowing varus moment measurement.
  - It can be in a single or bipedal leg stance. To date, there is no consensus. The single leg stance reproduces walking conditions but exposes to overcorrection; the bipedal exposes to undercorrection [2]. It is possible to obtain both and average them out (Fig. 3.2).

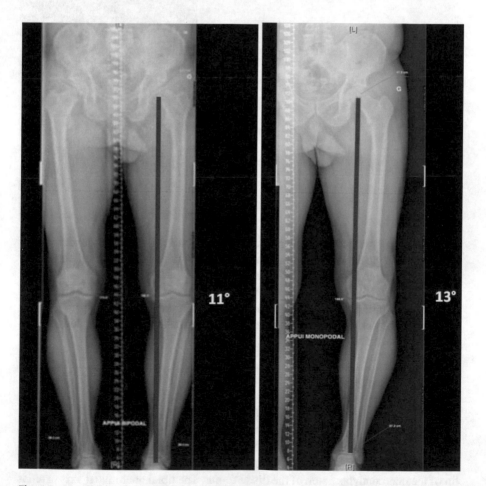

Fig. 3.2   2° difference between bipedal and left single leg stance AP full-length views

Fig. 3.3 25° recurvatum
due to an undiagnosed
postero-postero-medial
ligamentous lesion

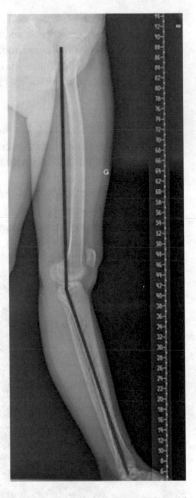

- A precise protocol must be proposed for reproducibility and comparability of pre- and postoperative measurements. Any rotation or flexion of the hip or knee can modify the angles observed.
- The lateral full-length view is especially necessary when there is a significant recurvatum, of bony or ligamentous origin (Fig. 3.3).
- Finally, an MRI can sometimes be indicated, particularly when considering associated ligamentous instability.

3.3   Femorotibial Axis

3.3.1   Static Aspect of Lower Limb Goniometry

Mechanical and anatomical axes exist for the femur and the tibia. The femoral anatomical axis runs through the intramedullary canal of the femoral diaphysis and the tip of the intercondylar notch of the distal femur. The tibial anatomical axis extends from the center of the tibial spines to the middle of the ankle mortise.

Fig. 3.4 Lower limb
mechanical axis (HKA).
Femoral head center (H),
knee center (K), ankle
center (A). Femoral
mechanical axis (HK line),
tibial mechanical axis (KA
line). HA line

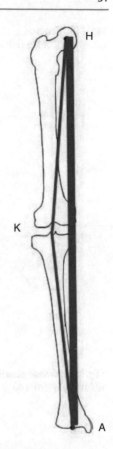

The femoral mechanical axis runs from the center of the femoral head (point H) to the tip of the intercondylar notch, with a 5–7° inclination difference than the anatomical axis.

The tibial mechanical axis overlaps with its anatomical axis.

The mechanical axis of the lower limb (Fig. 3.4), through which stresses pass, is the line connecting the center of the femoral head (point H) to the center of the ankle mortise (point A). Its position relative to the center of the knee (point K)—defined as the intersection of the tangent line to the femoral condyles in its center with the perpendicular to the tangent line to the tibial spines—determines a lower limb in varus (angle less than 180°) or valgus (angle greater than 180°). It is commonly accepted that the mechanical axis of the lower limb is 180° ± 2°, measured on the medial aspect.

Finally, it is important to measure the mechanical femoral and tibial angles.

On long-leg standing radiographs, the mechanical femoral angle (HKI) is measured between the tangent line to the femoral condyles and the femoral mechanical axis (Fig. 3.5). It is conventionally measured inwards and is approximately 92° ± 2°.

Fig. 3.5 Femoral
mechanical angle (HKI)

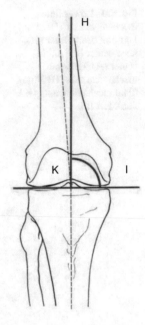

Fig. 3.6 Medial proximal
tibial angle (MPTA)

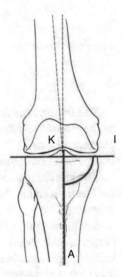

On long-leg standing AP views, the medial proximal tibial angle (MPTA) is measured between the tangent line to the tibial plates and the tibial mechanical axis (Fig. 3.6). It is conventionally measured medially and is approximately 88° ± 2°.

When an osteotomy is indicated for osteoarthritis, femoral and tibial mechanical angles are fundamental to determine the origin of the deformity and therefore the site of the correction.

3.3.2 Dynamic Aspect of Lower Limb Goniometry or Knee Biomechanics

In a single leg stance, a force (P) equal to the body weight is applied at the knee level. This weight is applied directly above the body's center of gravity—represented by S2—and is located inside the knee. To avoid dislocation of the joint, a force (L) applied by the lateral tendon-ligament complex opposes it on the lateral side (Fig. 3.7).

Equilibrium of force moments (Fig. 3.8) and the resultant force (R) (Fig. 3.9) acting on the joint surfaces of the knee are important to understand because any disturbance occurring in these two equations will have consequences for joint wear.

There is a predominance of varus stress due to the gap between the mechanical axis of the lower limb (HKA) and the gravitational axis (G) connecting S2 to the ground through the calcaneus. This deviation is called "extrinsic varizing distance" (EVE) by Thomine et al. [3] (Fig. 3.10).

Fig. 3.7 Body weight (P) and lateral complex (L)

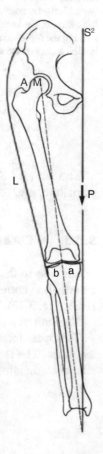

Fig. 3.8 Equation of equilibrium of forces. Body weight "*P*" multiplied by the distance "*a*" from the center of the knee is balanced with the lateral complex "*L*" multiplied by the distance "*b*" from the center of the knee

$$a \cdot |\vec{P}| = b \cdot |\vec{L}|$$

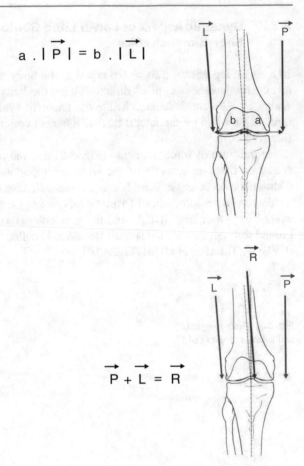

Fig. 3.9 The resultant "*R*" of the forces of the weight "*P*" and the lateral shroud "*L*" is two to three times the body weight "*P*" and is exerted slightly medial to the center of the knee, thus shifting the forces to the medial aspect of the knee

$$\vec{P} + \vec{L} = \vec{R}$$

The fact that the resultant forces act medial to the center of the knee leads to premature wear of the medial compartment (Fig. 3.11).

3.3.3 In Case of Varus Axial Deviation

In addition to the EVE, there is an intrinsic varus deviation (EVI) related to the deformation corresponding to the distance between the center of the knee and the HKA (Fig. 3.12).

The sum of the EVE and the EVI is the global varus gap (EVG).

This wear increases the varus angle, thus increasing the EVI. As a result, EVG increases. The resultant (*R*) of the forces will be applied more and more on the medial compartment, further worsening medial wear (Fig. 3.13).

Fig. 3.10 "Extrinsic varizing distance" (EVE) according to Thomine et al. [3]. The red line is the mechanical axis (HKA) of the lower limb. *P* body weight. *G* gravity line

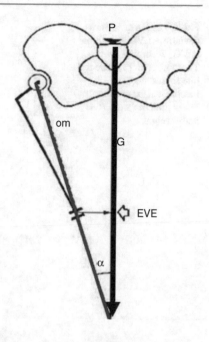

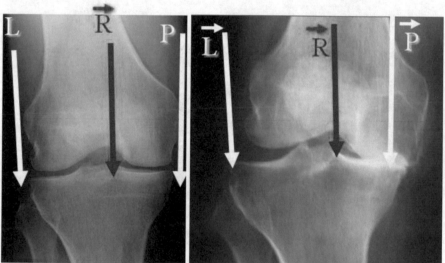

Fig. 3.11 Medial compartment wear due to the resultant "*R*" of the forces medial to the center of the knee

3.3.4 In Case of Valgus Deviation

There is no longer an EVI. The EVE automatically decreases or supersedes or even takes a negative value, letting a valgus deviation (EVL) appear, the consequences of which are reversed (Fig. 3.14).

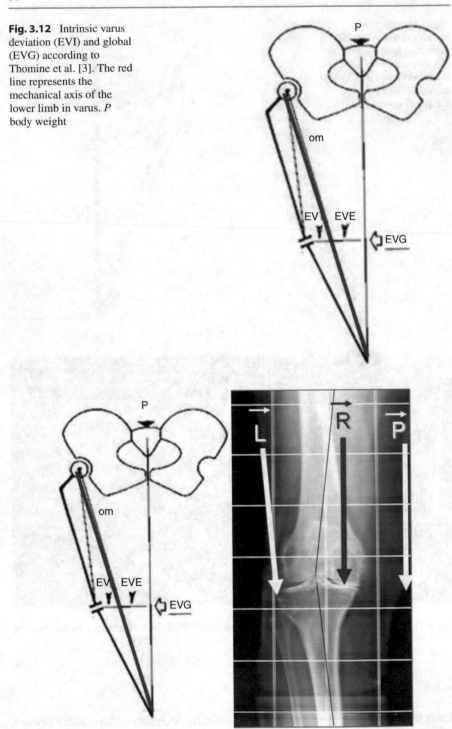

Fig. 3.12 Intrinsic varus deviation (EVI) and global (EVG) according to Thomine et al. [3]. The red line represents the mechanical axis of the lower limb in varus. *P* body weight

Fig. 3.13 Increased medial migration of the resultant (*R*) secondary to a varus deformation. *P* body weight. *L* strength of the lateral complex

Fig. 3.14 Valgus deformation (red line: mechanical axis of the lower limb passing outside the center of the knee). *P* body weight. *G* gravity line

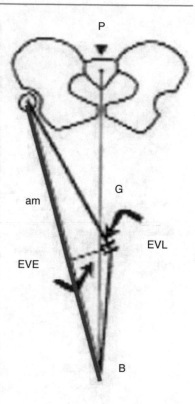

The resultant (*R*) of the forces is offset on the lateral side of the knee, causing wear on the lateral compartment (Fig. 3.15).

3.4 Practical Implication: Correction Goal

For an equivalent angular deviation, the predominance of varus stresses on a straight knee leads to a greater rise in medial wear than lateral wear. The EVI increases the effect of the varus angulation and limits that of a valgus. Thus, valgus deformity will be tolerated for a longer period of time.

The goal of a femoral or tibial osteotomy for the treatment of single-compartment osteoarthritis is to relieve the compartment affected by local mechanical stresses. This goal will be different between a varus and a valgus preoperative presentation:

- In the case of genu varum, it is necessary to compensate for the remaining EVI in case of a neutral correction. A slight valgus overcorrection of 3–6° [4] is therefore recommended. This overcorrection will also compensate for the deficit of the lateral complex (*L*), which is opposed to the force of the body weight (*P*).
- On the other hand, in the case of genu valgum, the angular targets of corrections are controversial. For some, in order to relieve the lateral compartment without overloading the medial compartment, and without disturbing the lateral complex

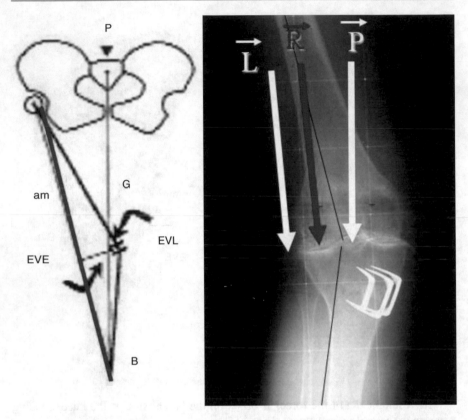

Fig. 3.15 Resultant (*R*) of the forces applied laterally on a genu valgum. *P* body weight. *L* strength of the lateral complex. *G* gravity line

(*L*) or creating an EVI, it is necessary to neutrally correct the axis to limit an EVE occurrence. An objective of 0° or 2° of varus is usually accepted [5–9]. For others, on the contrary, it is necessary to undercorrect with 2–4° of residual valgus [10, 11].

In any case, it is clearly established that valgus or varus overcorrection above 5° is harmful to long-term results [12, 13].

3.5 Practical Implication: Angular Correction Measurement

Several tools are available for measuring the angular correction to be applied to a frontal PTO when correcting a varus:

– The simplest method, but not necessarily the most accurate or precise, is to set up a corner at the osteotomy level corresponding to the desired angular correction.

Table 3.1 Correction table by Hernigou et al. [14]

Beta	4	5	6	7	8	9	10	11	12	13	14	15	16	17	18	19
M																
50	3	4	5	6	7	8	9	10	10	11	12	13	14	15	16	16
55	4	5	6	7	8	9	10	10	11	12	13	14	15	16	17	18
60	4	5	6	7	8	9	10	11	12	14	15	16	17	18	19	20
65	5	6	7	8	9	10	11	12	14	15	16	17	18	19	20	21
70	5	6	7	8	10	11	12	13	15	16	17	18	20	21	22	23
75	5	6	8	9	10	12	13	14	16	17	18	20	21	22	24	25
80	6	7	8	10	11	13	14	15	17	18	19	21	22	24	25	26

Beta **angular correction in the desired degree.** *M* **length (in millimeters) of the osteotomy. The intersection of the two gives the correction height of the osteotomy in millimeters**
For the desired beta correction of 10° with an osteotomy length $M = 60$ mm, the opening will be 10 mm

This correction will depend on the deformity measured by goniometry and the correction target.

- For a medial opening HTO, Hernigou et al. [14] defined a trigonometric table to obtain an opening height in millimeters for a given angular correction according to the length of the osteotomy (Table 3.1).
- Finally, navigation is perfectly suited, with a correction made according to the observed angulation and the desired target [15, 16].

Dugdale et al. [16] described the most common method for the angular correction measurement of a varizing DFO for a valgus deformity (Fig. 3.16).

3.6 Practical Implication: Degenerative Lesions Frontal Correction Site

In the presence of medial wear, there is usually a varus deformity. Whether the anomaly is tibial with a significant tibial epiphyseal varus; secondary to dynamic factors such as a decrease in the valgus moment due to the weakness of the lateral complex; or an increase in the varus moment due to overweight or a marked varus morphotype, the correction will be performed at the tibial level.

In the presence of lateral wear, there is usually a valgus deformity, most of the time associated with hypoplasia of the lateral condyle. This lateral osteoarthritis is often well tolerated for a long time, with a generally efficient lateral complex. Analysis of the orientation of the joint line is fundamental because it reflects the deformity. An HKA angle in valgus with a varus or neutral joint line orientation generally indicates a tibial origin, so the correction will be tibial otherwise the risk is to further increase this joint line obliquity when a femoral varus osteotomy is performed. When the joint line is valgus the correction must be femoral.

Fig. 3.16 Valgus correction calculation method for distal femoral osteotomy[16]: (**a**) Mechanical axis of the lower limb in valgus. (**b**) The correction angle corresponds to the angle between the line from the center of the femoral head to the middle of the tibial plateaux and the line from the center of the tibial plateaux to the center of the talus. (**c**) Representation of the correction of the mechanical axis by opening wedge distal femoral osteotomy

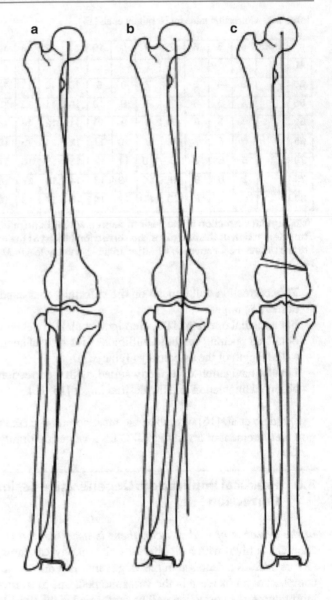

When the anomalies are both femoral and tibial, the choice of tibial correction is preferred if the correction does not induce a change in the joint line over 10°. On the other hand, a double osteotomy (femoral and tibial) is recommended, with an angular correction at each stage defined according to the angles HKI and AKI. The overall angular correction objective complies with the rules mentioned above.

3.7   Osteotomy for Frontal or Sagittal Ligament Laxity

In these indications, the ligament problem is corrected by a bony procedure, the main symptom being instability.

The coronal plane correction is most often tibial. In this frontal plane, medial or postero-medial instability will be treated with a tibial varus osteotomy. In cases of lateral and posterolateral instability, a tibial valgus osteotomy should be provided (Fig. 3.17). The angular objective of the correction will be to aim for 0–2° of valgus or varus depending on the direction of the desired correction.

In the sagittal plane, the correction site is also most often at the tibial level due to the technical difficulties of sagittal distal femoral osteotomies. The most classic case is a significant posterior laxity associated with a postero-medial or posterolateral lesion (Fig. 3.18). The angular goal will be a complete correction, considering that 1 mm corrects 1°.

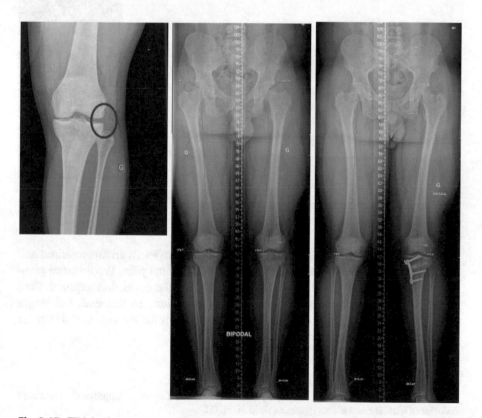

Fig. 3.17 Tibial valgus osteotomy for lateral and posterolateral laxity

Fig. 3.18 Postoperative
image of a tibial flexion
osteotomy for a 25°
recurvatum due to an
unnoticed postero-postero-
medial ligamentous lesion
shown in Fig. 3.3

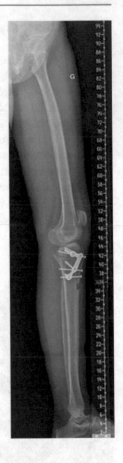

3.8　Summary

Osteotomy about the knee is a powerful tool in the surgeon's armamentarium and
can be used to deal with both instability and wear-related pain. Preoperative planning will clarify both the ideal site and magnitude of the correction required. Care
should be taken to avoid both under- or overcorrection. To this end, full-length
radiographs are mandatory, with careful measurement of the location and size of the
deformity guiding surgical correction.

Conflict of Interest　H.F., D.E.: none.

F.B.: Consultant education Amplitude®, Serf®

M.E.: Consultant education Depuy-Synthes®, Newclip®, Lepine®, Amplitude®, associated
redactor of Conférences d'Enseignement de la SOFCOT.

References

1. Levigne C, Dejour H, Brunet-Guedj E. Intérêt de l'axe épiphysiare dans l'arthrose. In: les gonarthroses. Journées Lyonnaises du genou. 1991. p. 127-41
2. Hunt MA, Birmingham TB, Jenkin TR, Giffin JR, Jones IC. Measures of frontal plane limb alignment obtained from static radiographs and dynamic gait analysis. Gait Posture. 2008;27:635–40.
3. Thomine JM, Boudjema A, Gibon Y, Biga N. Varizing axial distances in osteoarthrosis of the knee. Rev Chir Orthop Reparatice Appar Mat. 1981;67:319–27.
4. Babis GC, An KN, Chao EY, Larson DR, Rand JA, Sim FH. Upper tibia osteotomy: long term results-realignment analysis using OASIS computer soft-ware. J Orthop Sci. 2008;13:328–34.
5. Puddu G, Cipolla M, Cerullo G, Franco V, Gianni E. Which osteotomy for a valgus knee? Int Orthop. 2010;34:239–47.
6. Brouwer RW, Huizinga MR, Duivenvoorden T, van Raaij TM, Verhagen AP, Bierma-Zeinstra SM, Verhaar JA. Osteotomy for treating knee osteoarthritis. Cochrane Database Syst Rev. 2014;12:CD004019.
7. Mitchell JJ, Dean CS, Chahla J, et al. Varus-producing lateral distal femoral opening-wedge osteotomy. Arthrosc Tech. 2016;5:e799–807.
8. Quirno M, Campbell KA, Singh B, et al. Distal femoral varus osteotomy for unloading valgus knee malalignment: a biomechanical analysis. Knee Surg Sports Traumatol Arthrosc. 2017;25:863–8.
9. Forkel P, Achtnich A, Petersen W. Midterm results following medial closed wedge distal femoral osteotomy stabilized with a locking internal fixation device. Knee Surg Sports Traumatol Arthrosc. 2015;23:2061–7.
10. Zarrouk A, Bouzidi R, Karray B, Kammoun S, Mourali S, Kooli M. Distal femoral varus osteotomy outcome: is associated femoropatellar osteoarthritis consequential ? Orthop Traumatol Surg Res. 2010;96:632–6.
11. Thein R, Bronak S, Thein R, Haviv D. Distal femoral osteotomy for valgus arthritic knees. J Orthop Sci. 2012;17:745–9.
12. Marin Morales LA, Gomez Navalon LA, Zorrilla Ribot P, Salido Valle JA. Treatment of osteoarthritis of the knee with valgus deformity by means of varus osteotomy. Acta Orthop Belg. 2000;66:272–8.
13. Sharma L, Sorig J, Felson DT, Cahue S, Shamiyeh E, Dunlop DD. The role of knee alignment in disease progression and functional decline in knee osteoarthritis. JAMA. 2001;286:188–95.
14. Hernigou P, Ovadia H, Goutallier D. Mathematical modeling of open-wedge tibial osteotomy and correction table. Rev Chir Orthop Reparatrice Appar Mot. 1992;78:258–63.
15. Saragaglia D, Chedal-Bornu, Rouchy RC, Rubens-Duval B, Mader R, Pailhé R. Role of computer-assisted surgery ostéotomies around the knee. Knee Surg SportsTraumatol Arthrosc. 2016;24:3387–95.
16. Dugdale TW, Noyes FR, Styer D. Preoperative planning for high tibial osteotomy. the effect of lateral tibiofemoral separation and tibiofemoral length. Clin Orthop Relat Res. 1992;274:248–64.

Part II

Realignment Surgery (HTO/DFO)

Outcomes of Surgery for Medial Arthrosis

4

Sven Putnis, Thomas Neri, and David Parker

4.1 Introduction

The knee is comprised of three articular compartments, and of these the medial compartment is most frequently affected by isolated arthrosis. This can be attributed to 60–70% of weight-bearing load being transmitted through the medial compartment in a normally aligned knee and varus being the most common malalignment [1]. There is a greater incidence of injury to medial structures, with a higher rate of both chondral and meniscal trauma when compared to the lateral side [2]. Chondral injuries have the potential to progress, and a meniscal injury causes disruption to its intrinsic hoop stresses important for load distribution and protection of the joint [3]. Varus malalignment can be accentuated by medial compartment cartilage wear, further increasing the load distribution medially and accelerating osteoarthritis (OA).

Due to the frequency of isolated medial arthrosis, an osteotomy around the knee that can off-load the medial compartment has the potential to benefit the greatest number of patients. Determining whether coronal varus alignment is present and the forces that drive it are important steps in deciding whether an osteotomy is indicated and, if so, which is the most appropriate. To create the largest angular correction in knee alignment with the smallest osteotomy wedge, the osteotomy needs to be placed as close to the knee as possible. A high tibial osteotomy (HTO) formed either

S. Putnis (✉)
Avon Orthopaedic Centre, Bristol, UK

Sydney Orthopaedic Research Institute, Sydney, NSW, Australia

T. Neri
University hospital of Saint-Etienne, Saint-Priest-en-Jarez, France

Sydney Orthopaedic Research Institute, Sydney, NSW, Australia

D. Parker
Sydney Orthopaedic Research Institute, Sydney, NSW, Australia
e-mail: dparker@sydneyortho.com.au

© Springer Nature Switzerland AG 2020
S. Oussedik, S. Lustig (eds.), *Osteotomy About the Knee*,
https://doi.org/10.1007/978-3-030-49055-3_4

as an opening wedge on the medial side, or a closing wedge laterally are the most common osteotomies around the knee for isolated medial arthrosis.

There are examples of other osteotomies that have been described to address this pathology. Occasionally coronal varus alignment can be driven from the femur creating a case for a distal femoral osteotomy [4]. A fibula osteotomy used, either in isolation or in combination with an HTO, to off-load the medial compartment has recently gained increased interest [5].

Improvements seen in total knee arthroplasty (TKA) and medial unicompartmental knee arthroplasty (UKA) mean that results from HTOs must be closely scrutinized to review their relevance. There are several ways in which the outcomes and efficacy of osteotomy can be evaluated. In this chapter, functional outcomes are reported using patient-reported outcome measures (PROMs) and gait analyses, with subsequent development of preoperative predictors of outcome. Radiological outcome can show the coronal correction achieved and highlight the potential for unwanted changes in tibial slope or patella height. Magnetic resonance imaging (MRI) and second-look arthroscopy can evaluate interval changes in cartilage health [6]. The type and frequency of complications specific to each osteotomy is analyzed to further guide choice. Long-term follow-up aims to determine the progression of OA and tackles the question that all knee surgeons and their patients want to know: how long will this procedure be effective and can it therefore be used to avoid the need for knee arthroplasty?

This chapter summarizes the best available evidence to guide surgeon choice with regard to the two main types of HTO, medial opening wedge (Fig. 4.1) and lateral closing wedge (Figs. 4.2 and 4.3).

4.2 High Tibial Osteotomy (HTO)

4.2.1 Functional Outcome

4.2.1.1 Patient-Reported Outcome Measures (PROMs)

It has become mandatory for clinical research papers to report on how patients evaluate their own recovery and outcome. Several different evaluation scores have been validated and are in current use. In general, HTO patients' expectations are relief of medial knee pain, improved function, and an improved longer-term prognosis. There is an expectation of a return to a high level of function, and there is consensus across the literature of this occurring, with the majority of patients reporting significant improvements in their clinical outcome [7–12].

Prospective studies have seen significant improvements after opening wedge HTO. In a study of 52 knees [11] in an age group of 31–64 years (mean 47), with a mean angular correction of 8° stabilized with an internal locking plate (Puddu Instruments, Arthrex, Naples, Florida) and iliac crest bone autograft, all five subscores of the Knee Injury and Osteoarthritis Outcome Score (KOOS) increased significantly during the first year by 40–131% from preoperative values. The improvement was maintained throughout the 10-year follow-up for those with a surviving osteotomy. Seven patients required TKA conversions, with a survival rate

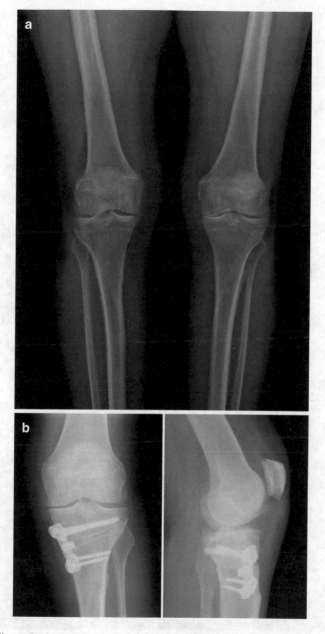

Fig. 4.1 Radiographs demonstrating (**a**) left knee medial arthrosis and (**b**) postoperative opening wedge correction

at 5 years of 94% and at 10 years 83% [11]. A Larger retrospective series has reinforced this data, with Kaplan-Meier analysis demonstrating 97.7% survival at 5 years and 80% at 10 years in a cohort of 210 patients over an 11-year period [13].

Similar study designs with closing wedge osteotomies also demonstrate improvements in PROMs. The Western Ontario and McMaster Universities Arthritis

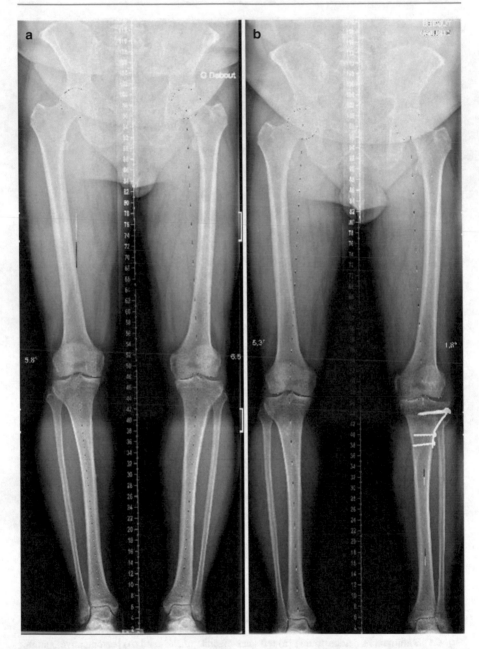

Fig. 4.2 Full-length radiographs demonstrated alignment correction using a closing wedge HTO from (**a**) preoperatively to (**b**) 1-year postoperatively

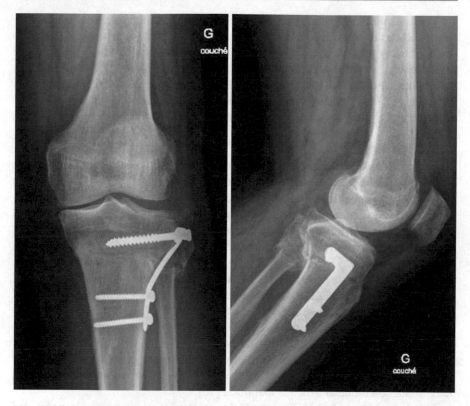

Fig. 4.3 Postoperative radiographs after closing wedge HTO combined with proximal fibula osteotomy

(WOMAC) score covers pain, stiffness, and physical function. In a cohort of 298 patients, a decrease from 48.0 ± 17.2 to 23.6 ± 19.7 ($p < 0.001$) was observed over a mean follow-up period of 5.2 ± 1.8 years, with a 5-year survival of 93% [14]. Ten-year outcomes from 95 patients demonstrated WOMAC and Knee Society Score (KSS) improving significantly between preoperative (mean 61; 32–99) and 5 (mean 88; 35–100, $p = 0.001$) and 10 years (mean 84; 38–100, $p = 0.001$). Older patients were found to have better functional outcomes overall, despite their higher revision rate [10].

PROMs improvements have been seen in studies comparing opening and closing wedge techniques. A randomized controlled trial over 2 years saw an improvement in each KOOS subscore in the range of 30–80%, with scores starting to plateau at 12 months postoperatively. A range of other PROMs scores were also used in this comprehensive study with combined improvements in mean Oxford Knee Score (OKS: from 26–37), Lysholm (from 48–72), Tegner Activity Scale (from 2.3–3.0), and University of California, Los Angeles (UCLA) activity scale (from 5.5 to 6.2) over the 2-year study period [9].

These results have been consolidated in a 2014 Cochrane Review which analyzed PROMs to conclude that a valgus-producing HTO reduces pain and improves knee function in patients with medial compartmental gonarthrosis [12]. These improvements in outcome were also noted in a comprehensive 2017 meta-analysis, which saw significant improvements in Hospital for Special Surgery (HSS) knee score (across four studies), visual analogue scale (VAS) for knee pain (across five studies), and Lysholm score (across four studies) [8].

4.2.1.2 Gait Analysis

An increased knee adduction moment is seen during gait in patients with knee OA and varus malalignment when compared to a normal population, and this has been shown to correlate with pain and can also lead to progression of OA [15]. It is therefore desirable to demonstrate that a HTO can reduce this. This can be evaluated with gait analysis to provide objective evidence of the positive biomechanical effect of the procedure. This can also provide guidelines for the degree of correction required to achieve the desired effects.

A 2017 systematic review and meta-analysis found 4 Level 2 studies and 8 Level 3 studies, with a total of 237 opening wedge and 143 closing wedge HTOs. Overall findings were of an increase in walking speed and stride length, with a decrease in adductor moment and lateral thrust when compared to the preoperative value in basic gait variables. Changes in co-contraction of the medial-sided muscles after surgery differed depending on the frontal plane alignment. However, no clear relationship between the magnitude of mechanical axis correction and the change in knee adduction moment axis was identified [16].

Leitch et al. looked at HTO patients during level walking and stair ascent and concluded that an opening wedge HTO is associated with sustained changes in knee moments in all three planes, suggesting substantial alterations to the loads on the knee during ambulation. Mean changes at 12 months postoperatively suggested decreases in the peak knee adduction, flexion, and internal rotation moments. These decreases were observed despite increases in walking speed. Both pre- and postoperatively, the peak knee adduction moment was significantly lower during stair ascent than during level walking ($p = 0.001$), while the flexion and internal rotation moments were significantly higher ($p < 0.01$). This study found a direct correlation between magnitude of change in the mechanical axis angle and gait, with a Pearson correlation between a decrease in varus and adduction moment ($p = 0.027$) and internal rotation moment ($p = 0.011$). As a control, there were no changes in the knee moments on the non-surgical limb [17].

A further study by Morin et al. demonstrated an improved perception of walking. It was carried out in 21 prospective and consecutive patients (14 men and 7 women, with a median age of 52). Gait was analyzed preoperatively and at 1 year postoperatively and compared to a healthy control group. They first demonstrated that patients with medial compartment OA had altered gait relative to the control population. Their walking speed was slower, step length was shorter, and single-leg stance time was shorter, while the double-leg stance time was longer (all $p < 0.001$). Step width was comparable between the two groups preoperatively, but it was wider in the patient group postoperatively ($p = 0.003$). After a correction from preoperative median of 7° varus [range 1–11] to 3° valgus [range 0–6], time–distance parameters of gait did not significantly change. However, using a subjective grading system (poor, fair, good, or excellent) according to the patients' overall perception of walking both before and after the procedure, there was an improvement so that it was no longer different from controls [18].

Gradual coronal and sagittal realignment can be achieved with the use of an external fixator to stabilize the HTO. McClelland et al. describe potential advantages of this approach in a study of 36 patients who after osteotomy underwent dynamic opening wedge correction using a Garches external fixator. They allowed patients to fully weight-bear with correction over approximately 5 weeks until the patients feel that the medial compartment of their knee was off-loaded and that the alignment "felt normal" for them. Gait analysis subsequently revealed a statistically significant change in adductor moment ($p < 0.001$) which was maintained at mean 6 years follow-up [19].

4.2.2 Radiological and Macroscopic Outcomes

4.2.2.1 Radiological Mechanical Axis

After the work of Fujisawa et al. [20], the concept that the weight-bearing line should pass through a point 62% of the way along the entire tibial plateau width as measured from the most medial point was developed (named the Fujisawa point). Located just lateral to the lateral tibial spine, this corresponds to an overall mechanical axis of 3–5° of valgus. More valgus may be introduced with the aim to increase survivorship [21], or less if there is lateral compartment pathology. Whatever the indication and aim of the procedure, the desired amount of correction needs to be achieved accurately and maintained. Stabilization of an osteotomy is reliant on adequate fixation. A randomized controlled study demonstrated that there was no effect on correction even after immediate weight-bearing through an opening wedge osteotomy gap fixed with a procedure-specific locking plate (Tomofix, Synthes, Switzerland). The mean mechanical femorotibial angle was corrected from 6° of varus to 4° of valgus in the group allowed to immediately weight-bear and from 5° of varus to 3° of valgus in the group who commenced full weight-bearing at 2 months. They reported no loss of the desired correction in any patient [22].

With the wide variety of different fixation and grafting techniques, comparison between studies can be difficult. Nerhus et al. published a detailed study assessing radiological outcomes after opening and closing wedge HTO, with opening wedges fixed with an internal locking plate (Puddu Instruments, Arthrex, Naples, Florida) with iliac crest autograft and closing wedges fixed with two staples. They saw alteration of preoperative hip-knee-ankle (HKA) axis of -6.2 ± 3.5 and -6.0 ± 2.6 to 0.6 ± 2.6 and 0.4 ± 2.3 for closing and opening wedge HTO, respectively. There was similar loss of alignment seen in both groups with a planned correction of 9.7 ± 3.3 and 9.7 ± 3.0 resulting in an achieved correction of 6.8 ± 2.9 and 6.4 ± 2.4 at 6 months postoperatively [9]. In a study where both opening and closing wedge osteotomies were supported with the same internal locking plate (Numélock II system, Stryker, Switzerland), and the desired HKA correction was 4° of valgus, preoperative HKA varus angles of 4.3° and 4.1° were measured at 3.8° and 4.4° of valgus, respectively, for opening and closing HTO at 1-year follow-up [23].

4.2.2.2 MRI Evaluation

HTO provides coronal realignment and subjective improvements in pain and quality of life, but there is also the potential benefit of allowing articular cartilage preservation and possible regeneration. Accurate T2-mapping is possible in all areas after implantation of a titanium fixation device and in most areas after implantation of a cobalt chrome fixation device [24]. The effect on cartilage over time has been studied in ten patients who underwent opening wedge HTO with preoperative and postoperative (6-month, 1-year, and 2-year) MRI using delayed gadolinium-enhanced (dGEMRIC) methods with hand segmentation and T1-Gd relaxation times reflective of glycosaminoglycan content. A decrease in T1-Gd values on the medial side were observed for all patients at 6 months and remained reduced for all but two participants at 1 and 2 years after HTO. The positive changes in the T1-Gd of the medial tibial plateau were responsible for the positive overall change in the appearance of the medial compartment [6]. Changes in the subchondral bone structure have also been seen on MRI evaluation of 22 HTO cases, with a significant decrease in trabecular number ($p < 0.05$), significantly more pronounced medially than laterally ($p < 0.001$) at a mean of 1.5 years [25].

4.2.2.3 Arthroscopic Evaluation

By utilizing a second-look arthroscopy at the time of plate removal, studies have provided information regarding the condition of the articular cartilage after HTO [20, 26, 27]. Kim et al. evaluated 104 patients at 2 years post-surgery. They found improvements in previous cartilage lesions in the medial femoral condyle and the medial tibial plateau in 54 knees (51.9%) and 36 knees (34.6%), respectively. Overall partial or total regeneration was also seen in the medial femoral condyle in 75 knees (72%) and medial tibial plateau in 57 knees (55%). While overall clinical improvements were seen, this study could not correlate these with rates of cartilage regeneration [27]. Kumagai et al. performed a similar study with a 2-year second-look arthroscopy on 131 knees and found newly formed femoral cartilaginous tissue in 71% of patients and tibial in 51% of patients but again without correlation with clinical outcome [26]. Both studies did, however, correlate cartilage regeneration with a low patient body mass index (BMI).

4.2.3   Survivorship

4.2.3.1 Timeline for Conversion to TKA

Long-term studies are required to give an accurate estimate of conversion rate to TKA. An article published 20 years ago by Naudie et al. provided an early insight, with a 10- to 22-year follow-up of 106 HTO patients with a mean survival rate of

73% of patients at 5 years, 51% of patients at 10 years, 49% at 15 years, and 30% at 20 years [28]. Four years later a further study demonstrated a better overall 10-year survival rate of 74%, which improved to 90% in patients who had large valgus corrections (radiographic valgus angle at 1 year between 8° and 16°) [21]. More recent studies have looked at opening and closing wedge HTO separately, with 10-year survival similar at 75% but improving to 90% with an opening wedge technique [29]. A detailed comparison is found in the "Opening Versus Closing Wedge HTO" section of this chapter below.

Using a probabilistic state-transition computer model with health states defined by pain, postoperative complications, and subsequent surgical procedures, with health outcome as quality of life years (QALYs), it has been demonstrated that in 50 to 60-year-old patients, HTO is a cost-effective option when compared with UKA and TKA. This is based on HTO survivorship, with a calculation that if the HTO annual conversion rate increased to 2.6% from a baseline value of 2.3% annually, then TKA becomes a more cost-effective strategy [30].

Reassuringly, there is evidence of the subsequent TKA functioning similarly to a primary TKA, including those with a valgus mechanical axis [31]. A 2015 systematic review looked at the outcome after conversion to TKA, finding two studies with Level 3 evidence and eight studies with Level 4 evidence. Comparative studies did not demonstrate statistically significant clinical or radiologic differences with similar revision rates [32]. New Zealand registry data has also demonstrated no significant difference in mean OKS between primary TKA and TKA for a failed osteotomy, even among patients younger than 65 years [33].

4.2.3.2 Revision Surgery

There is evidence to suggest that technical issues are seen during TKA surgery after a closing wedge HTO. A previous systematic review found that procedures such as a quadriceps snip, tibial tubercle osteotomy, and lateral soft tissue release were more frequently needed, and because of loss of proximal tibial bone geometry in the closing wedge HTO group, concerns such as decreased bone stock and tibial stem impingement in the lateral tibial cortex were noted [32].

There may therefore be a concern regarding a difference in difficulty and subsequent outcome of a TKA upon progression of OA when choosing the type of HTO. The difference in the postoperative angular deformities of the proximal tibia between opening and closing wedge HTO is, however, small and has been shown to be clinically irrelevant with little influence on the subsequent TKA difficulty. The amount of bony deformity, and subsequent technical challenge, will depend on the degree of previous correction. Preoperative planning is important, as there is a risk of interference between TKA tibial implant and endosteal bone, especially after a closing wedge [34]. Additionally, a closing wedge has been shown to more often require a two-stage approach with initial hardware removal and a new surgical incision for the TKA. Despite these issues, the reported 5-year clinical outcomes of TKA following closing wedge were comparable with those previously undergoing an opening wedge [35].

4.2.3.3 Prognostic Factors

With the increase in uptake of Surgical Registries such as The UK Knee Osteotomy Registry (UKKOR), increasingly accurate information on the conversion rate to TKA will become available. The cost-effectiveness of joint preservation HTO has already been discussed, emphasizing the need to establish which patients have the best HTO longevity [30]. In 2004, The International Society of Arthroscopy, Knee Surgery and Orthopaedic Sports Medicine (ISAKOS) was the first to formulate a list of patient factors which were "ideal," "possible," and "not-suited" to HTO (Table 4.1) [36].

Studies have demonstrated that patients with less advanced medial OA have better clinical results, and it is no surprise that the conversion rate is lower in this group [11, 37]. Deciding at an early stage who will benefit from an HTO is therefore important. Furthermore, in a series of 210 patients, those with cartilage loss amenable to concurrent cartilage treatment (microfracture, chondroplasty, matrix-induced autologous chondrocyte implantation) at the time of surgery had reduced conversion to TKA by a factor of 5.3 ($p = 0.025$) [13].

Further variables have been identified that are significantly related to a poor outcome: an age greater than 56 years ($p = 0.008$) and a limitation <120° in postoperative knee flexion ($p < 0.001$). Alongside lower grades of OA, patients with only mild

Table 4.1 Ideal, possible, and patients not suited for HTO according to the International Society of Arthroscopy, Knee Surgery and Orthopaedic Sports Medicine (ISAKOS) [36]

Ideal	Possible	Not suited
Isolated medial joint line pain	Moderate patellofemoral arthritis	Bicompartmental (medial and lateral) OA
Normal lateral and patellofemoral components		Meniscectomy in the compartment to be loaded by the osteotomy
Age (years) 40–60	Age 60–70 or <40	
Malalignment <15°	Flexion contracture <15°	Fixed flexion contracture >25°
Metaphyseal varus, i.e., TBVA >5°		
High-demand activity but no running or jumping	Wish to continue all sports	Obese patients
BMI < 30		
	Previous infection	
Full range of movement		
Normal ligament balance	ACL, PCL, or PLC insufficiency	
IKDC (A) B, C, D/Ahlback I–IV		
No cupula		
Non-smoker		
Some level of pain tolerance		

BMI body mass index, *TBVA* tibial bone varus angle, *IKDC* International Knee Documentation Committee osteoarthritis classification, *ACL* anterior cruciate ligament, *PCL* posterior cruciate ligament, *PLC* posterolateral corner, *OA* osteoarthritis preoperative symptoms and excellent preoperative KSS ($p < 0.001$) have also been shown to function better and for longer [37]. Similar guidance was given in a 10-year follow-up of 95 patients undergoing closing wedge osteotomy with improved survival associated with age <55 years, preoperative WOMAC scores >45, and a BMI <30 [10].

One predictor of early conversion to TKA has been seen in patients returning for postoperative follow-up. If the KOOS quality of life (QoL) subscore recorded at 2 years was under 44, patients had a 11.7 times higher risk for later TKA than those with QoL ≥44 ($p = 0.017$) [11].

4.2.4 Complications

HTO may be a technically challenging procedure, particularly for lower volume surgeons, and there have been reports of a significant rate of complications after HTO, despite the majority of these being minor.

A multicenter trial of 209 opening wedge HTO found an overall complication rate of 29.7%. Most complications were minor, with the most common being an undisplaced lateral hinge fracture. Major complications (need for hardware removal 4.8%, deep wound infection 1.9%, loss of correction 1%, nonunion 0.5%, and early conversion to arthroplasty 0.5%) occurred in 8.6%, and those patients showed significantly worse clinical outcomes (WOMAC, $p = 0.001$) [38].

A retrospective study of 115 patients found that while serious complications appeared rare, a similarly high overall complication rate of 31% was seen. This included minor wound infections (9.6%), major wound infections (3.5%), metalwork irritation necessitating plate removal (7%), nonunion requiring revision (4.3%), vascular injury (1.7%), and compartment syndrome (0.9%). No thromboembolic complications were observed. There was no correlation with complication rate and BMI, implant type, type of bone graft used, or patient age at surgery [39].

4.2.5 Opening Versus Closing Wedge HTO

The most recent Cochrane Review was published in 2014. This was an update from the 2009 publication and covered a total of 21 studies, including randomized and controlled clinical trials involving 1065 people. It concluded that valgus high tibial osteotomy reduces pain and improves knee function in patients with medial compartmental osteoarthritis of the knee and clearly goes on to state that there was no evidence to suggest a significant difference between opening and closing wedge HTO technique.

Since this publication, there have been several new studies which have aimed to determine the difference between the two approaches. Duivenvoorden et al. randomized 92 patients, with a 6-year follow-up. Complications of nonunion, loss of correction, and iliac crest morbidity were only seen in the opening wedge HTO group, but conversion to TKA was 8% versus 22% found in closing wedge HTO

($p = 0.05$). In the surviving osteotomies, no difference in clinical outcomes or radiographic alignment was seen [13]. The same group published a long-term retrospective study with a larger cohort of 412 patients revealing a 75% probability of survival of closing wedge HTO after 10 years versus 90% in the opening wedge HTO group ($p < 0.05$). They did however emphasize that according to the Osteoarthritis Research Society International (OARSI) criteria, equal numbers in both groups were "in need for prosthesis." [29]

Nerhus et al. performed a prospective randomized controlled trial with a 2-year follow-up. Their outcome measures were a selection of PROMs and a knee examination for range of motion. There were no differences in the time course of the clinical improvement between the closing and opening wedge techniques for HTO with continued improvement in physical function for between 6 months and 1 year after HTO regardless of the technique used [40].

Not all studies have revealed similar clinical results. Van Egmond et al. randomized 50 patients, and while they found very similar results in their outcomes, with the same number requiring conversion to arthroplasty (5 in each group at mean 7.9 years), and similar overall PROMs, further analysis of specific categories within the PROMs demonstrated significantly superior outcomes for a closing wedge HTO in VAS for satisfaction and WOMAC pain and stiffness subscales. They felt this was evidence enough to justify their statement of better clinical results after a closing HTO. One suggested explanation was the development of patella baja after an opening wedge HTO, leading to patellofemoral complaints and worse results [41]. Overall these studies have not managed to find a clear difference in clinical outcomes.

Further research has also looked at the anatomical changes that occur after each type of osteotomy and the potential for a change in subsequent knee function. Two effects have emerged: the effect of an osteotomy on posterior tibial slope and the effect on patella height. By using more updated evidence than the Cochrane Review, and including these parameters, Wu et al. performed a new comprehensive meta-analysis of 22 studies. Alongside clinical results demonstrating no difference between groups ($p > 0.05$), 11 of these studies had results regarding posterior slope, and 7 looked at patella height. This summary of the change in these radiological parameters was interesting, demonstrating that despite no difference in the mean angle of correction, the opening wedge HTO group showed a wider range of motion than the closing wedge HTO group ($p = 0.003$). There was a greater posterior tibial slope angle ($p < 0.001$) and a decrease in patellar height than the closing wedge HTO group ($p < 0.001$) [8]. It is worth noting that the changes in tibial slope were often small, with 1–2° decrease in a closing wedge and a similar increase after an opening wedge. These types of small changes may only become clinically relevant in patients with ACL deficiency or exert their effect over a long time period and therefore may only be seen in longer-term clinical studies.

The findings of a potential unwanted change in sagittal alignment with an increased posterior slope have led to some concerns in performing an opening wedge HTO in an ACL deficient knee, with advice to carefully plan the osteotomy orientation to avoid inadvertently increasing the posterior tibial slope in this patient group [42]. Increasing tibial slope may also produce or exacerbate a flexion contracture which is undesirable. A cadaveric study designed to answer the concern in ACL deficient patients demonstrated that a closing wedge shows more reproducible neutralization of posterior tibial slope and decreased anterior tibial translation in ACL deficiency compared with an opening wedge. However, additional findings were that a closing wedge is associated with increased external tibial axial rotation and lateral patellar tilt, which may adversely affect the patellofemoral joint [43]. An alteration in patella height may lead to a change in contact pressures, with further recent evidence of a progression in patellofemoral OA in those patients with a large opening wedge correction ($\geq$13 mm, $p = 0.019$) [44].

In summary, both opening and closing wedge osteotomies are likely to be effective realignment options in the majority of patients, with surgical precision in achieving the appropriate correction the most important variable, and surgeon preference guided by assessment of a number of different anatomical factors.

4.3   Alternative Osteotomies for Medial Arthrosis

4.3.1   Distal Femoral Osteotomy

Understanding the changes that occur in the skeleton to drive medial arthrosis is important when planning surgery. Cooke et al. in 1997 compared radiographs of healthy adult participants and those with medial compartment knee OA and concluded that varus malalignment and progression of OA were driven by a reduced valgus angle at the distal femur and an increased condylar plateau angle [45]. More recently a larger study of 797 normal and 454 OA-affected knees, with subdivision of the normal subjects by age and the OA-affected subjects by limb alignment, provided further speculation of knee OA progression. They concluded that, based on the alignment changes with age in normal knees, initiation and early progression of OA may be mediated mainly by the switch from lateral to medial bowing deformity of the femoral shaft accompanied by a decrease in the femoral neck angle [46]. Given these femoral driving forces, despite the normal physiological valgus of the distal femur, it is important to ensure that medial compartment arthrosis with overall varus coronal alignment does not have a correctable femoral component. While unusual, if a varus deformity is localized within the femur, it is preferable to correct it with a lateral closing wedge distal femoral osteotomy [4], which can also be performed in combination with a HTO [47].

4.3.2   Fibula Osteotomy

Fibula osteotomies have been used in combination with closing wedge osteotomies to allow hinge reduction (Fig. 4.4), and there have now been publications reporting the positive results of an isolated fibula osteotomy to off-load medial compartment OA, with the hypothesis that it removes the splinting effect of the fibula on the

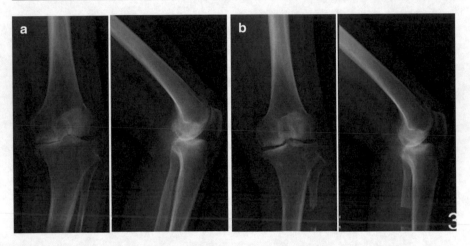

Fig. 4.4 (a) Preoperative AP and lateral radiographs of a 64-year-old woman showing a severe degree of medial compartment osteoarthritis and knee varus deformity. (b) Postoperative AP and lateral radiographs following proximal fibula osteotomy showing the recovered medial joint space, improved alignment, and a fibular defect [48]

lateral side of the knee, allowing load to be more evenly distributed across the weight-bearing surface. The largest clinical series' have come from China, with Yang et al. presenting the results from 110 patients in severe pain from medial compartment OA, with radiographic evidence of significant varus, and in whom conservative management has failed. An osteotomy of the fibula is performed 6–10 cm below the fibula head, with removal of a 2 cm length of bone. With a minimum of 2-year follow-up (range 24–189), significant improvements in both the radiographic appearance (mean correction of 3° valgus, with a 5 mm decrease in lateral joint space) and clinical function (mean VAS $p < 0.001$, mean KSS $p < 0.005$) were reported alongside long-term pain relief. Four patients required early conversion to TKA (at mean 12.4 months, range, 7–17 months) [48]. A more recent study has added further evidence with 47 patients undergoing fibula osteotomy over a 4-month period demonstrating significant pain relief and improved joint function at a mean of 13.4 months postoperatively, with no observed postoperative complications including wound infection, delayed healing, or nerve damage [5].

A recent cadaveric study has nicely demonstrated a possible explanation for these clinical findings. Researchers found significantly lower pressure readings in the medial compartment of the knee after a proximal fibular osteotomy, leading the authors to surmise that this approach may reduce knee pain and improve function in patients with medial compartment knee osteoarthritis [49].

Liu et al. analyzed their series of 111 high fibula osteotomies and found the best clinical results were seen in those patients with the best preoperative KSS clinical score, those with less medial space narrowing, and when a smaller angle is seen between the distal femoral condyles and the tibial plateau [50].

These results give potential for fibula osteotomy to have a place in the treatment of medial arthrosis and provide a basis for further long-term clinical studies.

4.4 Conclusions

HTO is the most common osteotomy around the knee, and there is a good evidence base that it provides significant improvement in clinical outcome and function, in appropriately selected patients, with evidence that off-loading the medial compartment may also facilitate cartilage regeneration. Recent improvements in patient selection and surgical technique have demonstrated reduced complications, improved outcomes, and excellent survivorship, without significant effect on subsequent arthroplasty.

References

1. Arden N, Nevitt MC. Osteoarthritis: epidemiology. Best Pract Res Clin Rheumatol. 2006;20:3–25.
2. Majewski M, Susanne H, Klaus S. Epidemiology of athletic knee injuries: a 10-year study. Knee. 2006;13:184–8.
3. Badlani JT, Borrero C, Golla S, Harner CD, Irrgang JJ. The effects of meniscus injury on the development of knee osteoarthritis: data from the osteoarthritis initiative. Am J Sports Med. 2013;41:1238–44.
4. van der Woude JAD, Spruijt S, van Ginneken BTJ, van Heerwaarden RJ. Distal femoral valgus osteotomy: bone healing time in single plane and biplanar technique. Strategies Trauma Limb Reconstr. 2016;11:177–86.
5. Wang X, et al. Proximal fibular osteotomy: a new surgery for pain relief and improvement of joint function in patients with knee osteoarthritis. J Int Med Res. 2017;45:282–9.
6. Parker DA, Beatty KT, Giuffre B, Scholes CJ, Coolican MRJ. Articular cartilage changes in patients with osteoarthritis after osteotomy. Am J Sports Med. 2011;39:1039–45.
7. Duivenvoorden T, et al. Comparison of closing-wedge and opening-wedge high tibial osteotomy for medial compartment osteoarthritis of the knee: a randomized controlled trial with a six-year follow-up. J Bone Joint Surg Am. 2014;96:1425–32.
8. Wu L, Lin J, Jin Z, Cai X, Gao W. Comparison of clinical and radiological outcomes between opening-wedge and closing-wedge high tibial osteotomy: a comprehensive meta-analysis. PLoS One. 2017;12:e0171700.
9. Nerhus TK, et al. Radiological outcomes in a randomized trial comparing opening wedge and closing wedge techniques of high tibial osteotomy. Knee Surg Sports Traumatol Arthrosc. 2017;25:910–7.
10. Howells NR, Salmon L, Waller A, Scanelli J, Pinczewski LA. The outcome at ten years of lateral closing-wedge high tibial osteotomy: determinants of survival and functional outcome. Bone Joint J. 2014;96-B:1491–7.
11. Ekeland A, Nerhus TK, Dimmen S, Thornes E, Heir S. Good functional results following high tibial opening-wedge osteotomy of knees with medial osteoarthritis: a prospective study with a mean of 8.3years of follow-up. Knee. 2017;24:380–9.
12. Brouwer RW, et al. Osteotomy for treating knee osteoarthritis. Cochrane Database Syst Rev. 2014:CD004019. https://doi.org/10.1002/14651858.CD004019.pub4.
13. Figueroa F, et al. Symptomatic relief in medial opening wedge high tibial osteotomies for the treatment of knee osteoarthritis is influenced by concurrent procedures and preoperative pain level. J ISAKOS Jt Disord Amp Orthop Sports Med. 2018;3:8.
14. Huizinga MR, Gorter J, Demmer A, Bierma-Zeinstra SMA, Brouwer RW. Progression of medial compartmental osteoarthritis 2-8 years after lateral closing-wedge high tibial osteotomy. Knee Surg Sports Traumatol Arthrosc. 2017;25:3679–86.
15. Baliunas AJ, et al. Increased knee joint loads during walking are present in subjects with knee osteoarthritis. Osteoarthr Cartil. 2002;10:573–9.

16. Lee SH, Lee O-S, Teo SH, Lee YS. Change in gait after high tibial osteotomy: a systematic review and meta-analysis. Gait Posture. 2017;57:57–68.
17. Leitch KM, Birmingham TB, Dunning CE, Giffin JR. Medial opening wedge high tibial osteotomy alters knee moments in multiple planes during walking and stair ascent. Gait Posture. 2015;42:165–71.
18. Morin V, et al. Gait analysis following medial opening-wedge high tibial osteotomy. Knee Surg Sports Traumatol Arthrosc. 2018;26:1838–44.
19. McClelland D, et al. Medium- and long-term results of high tibial osteotomy using Garches external fixator and gait analysis for dynamic correction in varus osteoarthritis of the knee. Bone Joint J. 2016;98-B:601–7.
20. Fujisawa Y, Masuhara K, Shiomi S. The effect of high tibial osteotomy on osteoarthritis of the knee. An arthroscopic study of 54 knee joints. Orthop Clin North Am. 1979;10:585–608.
21. Sprenger TR, Doerzbacher JF. Tibial osteotomy for the treatment of varus gonarthrosis. Survival and failure analysis to twenty-two years. J Bone Joint Surg Am. 2003;85-A:469–74.
22. Lansdaal JR, et al. Early weight bearing versus delayed weight bearing in medial opening wedge high tibial osteotomy: a randomized controlled trial. Knee Surg Sports Traumatol Arthrosc. 2017;25:3670–8.
23. Gaasbeek RDA, Nicolaas L, Rijnberg WJ, van Loon CJM, van Kampen A. Correction accuracy and collateral laxity in open versus closed wedge high tibial osteotomy. A one-year randomised controlled study. Int Orthop. 2010;34:201–7.
24. Verschueren J, et al. Possibility of quantitative T2-mapping MRI of cartilage near metal in high tibial osteotomy: a human cadaver study. J Orthop Res. 2018;36:1206–12.
25. Gersing AS, et al. Longitudinal changes in subchondral bone structure as assessed with MRI are associated with functional outcome after high tibial osteotomy. J ISAKOS. 2018;3:205–12.
26. Kumagai K, et al. Factors affecting cartilage repair after medial opening-wedge high tibial osteotomy. Knee Surg Sports Traumatol Arthrosc. 2017;25:779–84.
27. Kim K-I, et al. Change of chondral lesions and predictive factors after medial open-wedge high tibial osteotomy with a locked plate system. Am J Sports Med. 2017;45:1615–21.
28. Naudie D, Bourne RB, Rorabeck CH, Bourne TJ. The Install Award. Survivorship of the high tibial valgus osteotomy. A 10- to 22-year followup study. Clin Orthop Relat Res. 1999;(367):18–27.
29. Duivenvoorden T, et al. Adverse events and survival after closing- and opening-wedge high tibial osteotomy: a comparative study of 412 patients. Knee Surg Sports Traumatol Arthrosc. 2017;25:895–901.
30. Konopka JF, Gomoll AH, Thornhill TS, Katz JN, Losina E. The cost-effectiveness of surgical treatment of medial unicompartmental knee osteoarthritis in younger patients: a computer model-based evaluation. J Bone Joint Surg Am. 2015;97:807–17.
31. Saragaglia D, et al. Computer-assisted total knee replacement after medial opening wedge high tibial osteotomy: medium-term results in a series of ninety cases. Int Orthop. 2016;40:35–40.
32. Han JH, et al. Total knee arthroplasty after failed high tibial osteotomy: a systematic review of open versus closed wedge osteotomy. Knee Surg Sports Traumatol Arthrosc. 2016;24:2567–77.
33. Pearse AJ, Hooper GJ, Rothwell AG, Frampton C. Osteotomy and unicompartmental knee arthroplasty converted to total knee arthroplasty: data from the New Zealand Joint Registry. J Arthroplast. 2012;27:1827–31.
34. Kuwashima U, et al. Comparison of the impact of closing wedge versus opening wedge high tibial osteotomy on proximal tibial deformity and subsequent revision to total knee arthroplasty. Knee Surg Sports Traumatol Arthrosc. 2017;25:869–75.
35. Ehlinger M, et al. Total knee arthroplasty after opening- versus closing-wedge high tibial osteotomy. A 135-case series with minimum 5-year follow-up. Orthop Traumatol Surg Res. 2017;103:1035–9.
36. Rand J, Neyret P. ISAKOS meeting on the management of osteoarthritis of the knee prior to total knee arthroplasty. 2005.
37. Bonasia DE, et al. Medial opening wedge high tibial osteotomy for medial compartment overload/arthritis in the varus knee: prognostic factors. Am J Sports Med. 2014;42:690–8.

38. Han S-B, et al. Complications associated with medial opening-wedge high tibial osteotomy using a locking plate: a multicenter study. J Arthroplast. 2018; https://doi.org/10.1016/j.arth.2018.11.009.
39. Woodacre T, et al. Complications associated with opening wedge high tibial osteotomy—a review of the literature and of 15 years of experience. Knee. 2016;23:276–82.
40. Nerhus TK, et al. No difference in time-dependent improvement in functional outcome following closing wedge versus opening wedge high tibial osteotomy: a randomised controlled trial with two-year follow-up. Bone Joint J. 2017;99-B:1157–66.
41. van Egmond N, van Grinsven S, van Loon CJM, Gaasbeek RD, van Kampen A. Better clinical results after closed- compared to open-wedge high tibial osteotomy in patients with medial knee osteoarthritis and varus leg alignment. Knee Surg Sports Traumatol Arthrosc. 2016;24:34–41.
42. Herman BV, Giffin JR. High tibial osteotomy in the ACL-deficient knee with medial compartment osteoarthritis. J Orthop Traumatol. 2016;17:277–85.
43. Ranawat AS, et al. Comparison of lateral closing-wedge versus medial opening-wedge high tibial osteotomy on knee joint alignment and kinematics in the ACL-deficient knee. Am J Sports Med. 2016;44:3103–10.
44. Tanaka T, et al. Deterioration of patellofemoral cartilage status after medial open-wedge high tibial osteotomy. Knee Surg Sports Traumatol Arthrosc. 2018; https://doi.org/10.1007/s00167-018-5128-7.
45. Cooke D, et al. Axial lower-limb alignment: comparison of knee geometry in normal volunteers and osteoarthritis patients. Osteoarthr Cartil. 1997;5:39–47.
46. Matsumoto T, et al. A radiographic analysis of alignment of the lower extremities—initiation and progression of varus-type knee osteoarthritis. Osteoarthr Cartil. 2015;23:217–23.
47. Nakamura R, Kuroda K, Takahashi M, Katsuki Y. Additional distal femoral osteotomy for insufficient correction after high tibial osteotomy. BMJ Case Rep. 2018;2018:bcr2018224514.
48. Yang ZY, et al. Medial compartment decompression by fibular osteotomy to treat medial compartment knee osteoarthritis: a pilot study. Orthopedics. 2015;38:e1110–4.
49. Baldini T, et al. Medial compartment decompression by proximal fibular osteotomy: a biomechanical cadaver study. Orthopedics. 2018;41:e496–501.
50. Liu B, et al. Proximal fibular osteotomy to treat medial compartment knee osteoarthritis: preoperational factors for short-term prognosis. PLoS One. 2018;13:e0197980.

Outcomes of Surgery for Lateral Arthrosis

5

Vikram Kandhari and Myles R. J. Coolican

5.1 Introduction

The normal alignment of knee joint varies but is approximately 5–7° of tibio-femoral valgus which results in approximately 30–40% of body weight being borne by the lateral compartment [1]. Increased knee valgus leads to overloading of lateral compartment and the development of lateral compartment arthrosis [2]. Increased valgus at the knee joint is most commonly within the distal femur leading to knee joint line obliquity [3, 4].

Periarticular knee osteotomy is an attractive treatment option for management of isolated lateral compartment knee arthrosis especially in young patients and those whose work or recreation demands a high activity level. Realigning the valgus deformed knee decreases the rate of progression of lateral compartment knee arthrosis, relieves symptoms, and facilitates patients' return to higher level of activity [5].

The aim of periarticular osteotomy for the painful valgus aligned knee is to relieve knee pain by producing a more neutral alignment and at the same time correcting joint line obliquity. This reduces progression of lateral compartment knee arthrosis. In addition, osteotomy allows patients to engage in heavy work and to continue higher levels of recreational activities after surgery, a significant advantage of osteotomy over total knee arthroplasty (TKA) especially in the young active patients [5, 6].

Periarticular osteotomies used for correction valgus knee alignment for lateral compartment knee arthrosis can either be femoral (lateral opening wedge or medial closing wedge) or tibial (lateral opening wedge or medial closing wedge). It is of paramount importance for the clinician to be aware of the functional and

V. Kandhari · M. R. J. Coolican (✉)
Sydney Orthopaedic Research Institute, Sydney, NSW, Australia
e-mail: myles@mylescoolican.com.au

© Springer Nature Switzerland AG 2020
S. Oussedik, S. Lustig (eds.), *Osteotomy About the Knee*,
https://doi.org/10.1007/978-3-030-49055-3_5

radiological outcomes and potential complications of each before choosing. Compared to varus osteoarthritis, valgus deformed knees are much less common, and accordingly there is a paucity of published literature on outcomes of osteotomy for valgus knees. In this chapter we'll comprehensively summarize the clinical and radiological features of valgus arthritis, present our technique for surgery, and discuss outcomes and complications of osteotomy for the valgus knees with lateral compartment arthrosis.

5.2 Distal Femur Varus Osteotomy

The literature agrees that deformity within the distal femur is the cause of valgus deformity in majority of the cases with lateral overload contributing to the subsequent development of lateral arthritis. In these patients, distal femur varus osteotomy is the considered procedure of choice to correct the valgus deformity by distally advancing the lateral femoral condyle and reducing progression of lateral compartment arthrosis. It is advocated in patients with >12° of tibio-femoral valgus deformity and >10° of joint line obliquity [4]. There are two techniques of distal femur varus osteotomy—medial closing wedge distal femur osteotomy and lateral opening wedge distal femur osteotomy. The clinical and radiological outcomes and survivorship (Fig. 5.1) of the individual techniques are discussed below.

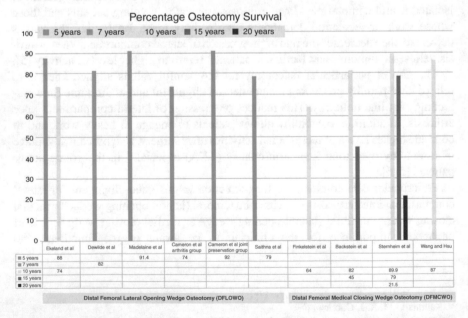

Percentage Osteotomy Survival

	Ekeland et al	Dewilde et al	Madelaine et al	Cameron et al arthritis group	Cameron et al joint preservation group	Saithna et al	Finkelstein et al	Backstein et al	Sternheim et al	Wang and Hsu
■ 5 years	88		91.4	74	92	79				
■ 7 years		82								
10 years	74						64	82	89.9	87
■ 15 years								45	79	
■ 20 years									21.5	

Distal Femoral Lateral Opening Wedge Osteotomy (DFLOWO)	Distal Femoral Medial Closing Wedge Osteotomy (DFMCWO)

Fig. 5.1 Survivorship—distal femoral osteotomy: image depicts comparative survivorship reported by the included studies of distal femoral lateral opening and medial closing wedge osteotomy for isolated lateral compartment arthrosis in valgus knees

5.3 Distal Femur Lateral Opening Wedge Osteotomy (DFLOWO)

DFLOWO has recently gained popularity over the conventional distal femoral medial closing wedge osteotomy due to technical advantages: controlled incremental correction available with navigation and the benefit of a single bone cut. A review of English language literature identified ten published case series on DFLOWO. We did not find any published randomized control trials or case-control studies. A lack of consistency in reporting of the surgical technique, method of fixation, rehabilitation protocols, patient outcome measures, and the duration of reported follow-up has made direct comparison between studies impossible.

An important consideration in treating younger patients with arthritic knees with osteotomy is survivorship—with conversion to total knee arthroplasty (TKA) as the end point. We have divided the literature on outcomes of DFLOWO with respect to the mean duration of follow-up: For mid- to long-term follow-up (mean duration of follow-up >60 months), there are seven studies [7–13], and for short- to mid-term follow-up (mean duration of follow-up 36–59 months), there are three studies [14–16].

5.4 Outcomes of Mid- to Long-Term Follow-up Studies

We found seven published studies on DFLOWO reporting on outcomes at mid- to long-term follow-up in the English literature. Ekeland et al. [7] reported on outcomes of DFLOWO in a case series of 24 patients with mean follow-up of 94 months [48–122.4]. Mean age was 48 years [31.4–62.1]. At latest follow-up, all sub-scores of KOOS were significantly improved on the pre-op values ($p < 0.001$) with more improvement noticed in the first 6 months for routine activities and over a year for sports and recreational activities. At 10 years, six knees (25%) had been converted to total knee replacement at mean 6.4 years (4–11.8 years) after osteotomy. Fourteen of the 18 patients sustained the improved KOOS scores (74%) at 10 years. The knees converted to TKA had a preoperative lower range of KOOS scores and higher radiographic grades of osteoarthritis. Range of motion decreased from mean of 126° pre-op to 114° at 3 months follow-up and was regained at 6 months follow-up. Post-traumatic malunion and reduced knee flexion occurred in one patient after fall resulting in a fracture. One patient had stiffness at 3 months and underwent arthroscopic arthrolysis to regain preoperative range of motion. Three patients had delayed union, two of whom were taking of NSAIDs which may have adversely effected bone healing. Two patients suffered a compression fracture of the medial hinge of osteotomy in the initial postoperative period resulting in overcorrection of 4°. In both cases the osteotomy healed, and both had good outcome at 10 years. The 5- and 10-year survival of the osteotomy was 88% and 74%, respectively. The postoperative angular correction in patients who were converted to TKA and those who were not was similar. Plate removal was required in 8 patients (44%). BMI did not affect conversion to TKA with the average BMI being comparable in both groups.

There was no correlation between the Kellgren-Lawrence grading on pre-op radiograph and BMI. The authors concluded that DFLOWO is an effective treatment option for lateral compartment arthrosis in young patients with a genu valgum deformity.

de Andrade et al. [8] reported on the outcomes of a novel V-shaped DFLOWO in their series of 15 patients with mean age of 49.8 years at a mean follow-up of 81.4 months (43–132 months). At final follow-up, the Knee Society rating system had five excellent, six good, one fair, and three poor scores. Excellent and good results were evident in 73% of the patients like the study by Ekeland et al. [7]. Seven (46%) of their 15 patients were in the desired range of correction (2° varus to 3° valgus) at final follow-up. The patients' age at the time of surgery, follow-up period, and postoperative anatomical angle did not have any correlation with outcomes.

Das et al. in 2008 [9] reported on 12 patients of DFLOWO with mean age of 55 (46–71) years at 74 (51–89) months follow-up with outcome measures including the Lysholm and Hospital for Special Surgery (HSS) scores. At 74 months, the Lysholm scores improved from 64 to 77, the HSS knee score from 42 to 64, and the HSS function score from 58 to 72. Implant removal was necessary in 7 of 12 patients at 25 months post-surgery predominantly due to iliotibial band irritation. Three patients deteriorated after osteotomy, and two of them underwent TKA at 37 and 42 months for persistent pain. These patients had more advanced lateral compartment osteoarthritis among the group on pre-op radiographs and higher grade of medial compartment osteoarthritis compared to the other patients in the cohort. One patient had pre-op valgus of 21° secondary to malunited condylar fracture in childhood. Inferior functional results were evident in the patients having higher medial compartment arthrosis on pre-op imaging and those patients who underwent a larger correction.

In the series by Thein et al. [10], for patients with mean age 46.7 ± 10.7 years at surgery, mean Oxford Knee Score doubled from 13.1 pre-op to 26 at mean follow-up of 6.5 years. Their series had a surprisingly high subjective satisfaction rate of 6.6/10 despite the low Oxford scores. They did not find any progression of radiographic arthritis on the final follow-up. No significant correlation was reported between age, BMI, and radiographic findings pre-surgery on outcome measures at follow-up. Poorer results in their study were attributed to older age at the time of surgery, patients undergoing bilateral osteotomies, and those with possible secondary gain.

Dewilde et al. [11] reported on the outcome of opening wedge distal femoral osteotomy for lateral arthritis of the knee in 16 patients with mean age of 47 (30–51) years using the Puddu plate and calcium phosphate bone substitute. They reported outcomes at a mean duration of 5.6 (2.5–10.5) years. Knee Society knee scores improved from 43 to 78, and 18 of 19 patients were satisfied. At latest follow-up, Hospital for Special Surgery knee scores improved from 65 to 84. They did not find any radiographic progression of osteoarthritis and reported a survivorship of 82% at 7 years. Though not statistically significant, more conversion to TKA was observed in patients with under-correction to a neutral mechanical axis [TKA group: 3.1° valgus Vs Non TKA group: 1.9° valgus]. Although bone formation was observed in all the osteotomies with the use of calcium phosphate bone substitute without any implant failures during the follow-up period, it took 47 ± 26 months for complete resorption and conversion to bone. The authors recommended slight overcorrection past a neutral mechanical axis and inferred that the mid-term results of DFLOWOs were comparable to distal femoral medial closing wedge osteotomy.

Two of the included mid-term studies by Madelaine et al. [12] and Cameron et al. [13] reported survivorship at 60 months. Madelaine et al. [12] reported 29 patients with mean age of 44.4 years. Functional knee scores improved from 50.4 pre-op to 68.5 at follow-up with a reported a survivorship of 91.4% at 60 months. There were four complications (14%). One patient each had nonunion, delayed union, stiffness, and failure of fixation within 1 year of surgery, and all the patients required surgery. Removal of hardware was performed in 23 (79%) of the patients for discomfort at a mean time of 25.3 months post-surgery. Five patients were revised to TKA at 166.6 months post-surgery. Overall 25 patients (86%) were satisfied or very satisfied at the time of last follow-up. The authors recommended on use of angled blade plates over locking plates for internal fixation of the osteotomy site.

Cameron et al. [13] reported the outcomes of DLFOWO in series of 38 patients with mean follow-up of 5 (2–12) years. In their series DLFOWO was performed for two separate indications—advanced lateral compartment arthritis and for joint preservation (isolated osteochondral lesions of lateral compartment with valgus alignment). Though the postoperative IKDC score was comparable in both the groups at the final follow-up after osteotomy [62—joint preservation and 67—arthritis group], 5-year survivorship for osteotomy was 92% in joint preservation group and 74% in arthritis group. The survivorship in the arthritis group in this study was much inferior to the 5-year survivorship of osteotomy reported in the other studies at similar mean follow-up after DLFOWO. One patient had nonunion of the osteotomy site.

5.5   Outcomes of Short- to Mid-Term Follow-up Studies

We found three studies [14–16] reporting on outcomes of DFLOWO at short- to mid-term follow-up.

Zarrouk et al. [14] and Saithna et al. [15] report the outcomes at maximum mean follow-up of 54 months. Zarrock et al. [14] reported on 22 osteotomies in 20 patients with mean age of 53 (27–66) years. There was significant improvement in KSS and functional score from 49.8 to 74.23 and 50.68 to 72.85, respectively ($p \leq 0.001$), at mean follow-up of 54 (36–132) months. At the last follow-up, 80% of the patients were satisfied. The mean pain score at last follow-up significantly improved by mean of 26 (12.72–38.4) points over their pre-op value ($p < 0.001$). The mean mobility scores marginally decreased from 23.22 before surgery to 21.95 at last follow-up. There was a trend of better clinical results in the group with constitutional valgus deformity compared p with other etiologies for valgus knee deformity including poliomyelitis, post-trauma, and multiple epiphyseal dysplasia; however the number was not sufficient for statistical comparison. The clinical results of the patients who had correction between 0° and 6° of valgus were better than the patients who had under-correction or overcorrection of the valgus deformity, but the difference was not statistically significant ($p = 0.616$). In their cohort 9 (45%) of the total patients had patellofemoral arthrosis before intervention, but at their last follow-up, results were comparable with or without patellofemoral arthrosis. In seven of the nine patients, patella re-centering was observed during follow-up after osteotomy, and the Insall-Salvati ratio increased from 1.07 to 1.15. Patella re-centering was evident in patients with normal axis as shown by their HKA (hip-knee-ankle) angle. The authors reported 8-year survival rate of 91% (CI 69–100%).

Saithna et al. [15] published outcome series of 21 DFLOWO osteotomies with mean age of 41 (28–58) years at mean follow-up of 4.5 (1.6–9.2) years. Four patients were converted to TKA at 20, 25, 40, and 70 months of follow-up (mean 3.3 years). The cumulative survivorship was 79% (95% CI 0.49–1.09) at 5 years. For the remaining 17 patients, all the reported outcome measures showed a trend toward improvement, with IKDC score (p—0.0312) and pain subdomain of KOOS score (p—0.0076) showing statistical difference at last follow-up comparted to their pre-op values. Sixteen of the 17 knees underwent reoperation during the follow-up period. Ten reoperations were for the removal of implants due to localized discomfort. Two patients had persistent symptoms for which they underwent arthroscopy, while two patients had loss of correction, one had metal malposition with infection, and one had nonunion. All four of these patients required further surgery.

Jacobi et al. [16] in their follow-up series published results of 14 patients who underwent DFLOWO at mean age of 46 ± 3.1 years (28–63) with a mean follow-up of 45 ± 3.4 months (26–64). The authors also presented their experience with use of Tomofix plate for DFLOWO. Two patients had delayed union, one eventually united and other required intervention with bone graft and additional stabilization with medial plate. The authors did not find the use of iliac crest bone graft or the size of correction influenced healing time. All the KOOS sub-scores including the final score improved at the last follow-up. Significant improvement was noted in the total score from pre-op value of 31 ± 17 (8–60) to a follow-up score of 69 ± 22 (38–100) (p—0.002). Although the Tomofix plate provided excellent stability at the osteotomy site, 12 patients (86%) required plate removal for local irritation. Despite the need for implant removal, the study reported a high satisfaction index of $73 \pm 18\%$ at last follow-up.

5.6 Distal Femur Lateral Closing Wedge Osteotomy (DFLCWO)

DFLCWO is an alternative method of correction of valgus deformity of knee. DLCWO is more technically demanding in that it requires precise removal of a bony wedge to achieve an exact correction of alignment and it requires two converging bony cuts. Published literature for DFLCWO includes results for a relatively longer follow-up compared to DFLOWO. Again, like for DFLOWO, all the published literature comprises of case series (Level IV evidence) with no randomized control trials or case-control studies (Level I and III evidence, respectively). We describe the published results for DFLCWO divided into mean reported follow-up periods—long-term follow-up (>10 years), mid-term follow-up (5–10 years), and short-term follow-up. In our literature search, there were four published studies reporting outcomes at long-term follow-up (17–20) and three (21–23) at mid-term follow-up and seven studies reporting outcomes at short-term follow-up. One of the case series by Mathew et al. does not report the mean duration of follow-up but describes a range of 1–8 years. We have included this study in the mid-term follow-up group.

5.7   Outcomes of Long-Term Follow-up Studies

Finkelstein et al. [17] published results for 21 DFLCWO at long-term follow-up. At 10 years, they reported a survival rate of 64%. Seven of the 21 DFLCWO were converted to TKA in the follow-up period, and 1 patient died of natural causes unrelated to the knee. The clinical scores improved significantly at the last follow-up compared to their pre-op value ($p < 0.0001$) with the greatest improvement evident in pain relief.

Backstein et al. [18] published results of 38 DFLCWO performed in patients with mean age of 44.1 (20–67) years. Twenty-four (60%) of the total had good or excellent results. Three (7.5%) had fair and 3 (7.5%) poor results. Twelve (30%) of the total 38 knees required TKA during the follow-up period and were considered as failure of osteotomy. The mean Knee Society objective scores improved from 18 (range, 0–74) to 87.2 (range, 50–100) for the 30 knees available for assessment at last follow-up. The mean Knee Society function score improved from 54 (range, 0–100) to 85.6 (range, 40–100). They describe one patient with preoperative Knee Society score of zero suffered from a neurologic condition and had associated valgus knee deformity, severe pain, and almost no ability to ambulate. The 10-year survival rate in this series was 82% (95% confidence interval, 75–89%), and the 15-year survival rate was 45% (95% confidence interval, 33–57%).

Kosashvili et al. [19] published results of 33 DFLCWO at mean follow-up of 15.1 (10–25) years. The osteotomy was performed at a mean age of 45.5 (24–63) years. Modified Knee Society scores improved significantly from a mean of 36.8 pre-op to 77.5 at 1-year post-surgery ($p < 0.01$). Twenty-eight (84.8%) patients had good or excellent knee function scores. At a follow-up of 10 years, the modified Knee Society scores significantly deteriorated to 66 (25–91) from the 1-year score ($p < 0.01$). The scores were still significantly more than the recorded pre-op score ($p < 0.01$). Eighteen (54%) had good or excellent outcomes at 10 years of follow-up. Two DFLCWO were converted to TKA at 6 and 8 years of follow-up. Both were morbidly obese and had undergone bilateral DFLCWO. One side of each patient required conversion to TKA. At the last mean follow-up of 15.1 years, the modified Knee Society score significantly declined to 59 (15–91) ($p < 0.008$), and only 10 knees (30.3%) had good or excellent results. Sixteen (48.5%) of all knees failed at 15.6 years mean follow-up.

Sternheim et al. [20] in their series of 45 DFLCWO had survival rate of 89.9%, 78.9%, and 21.5% at 10, 15, and 21 years, respectively. Mean modified Knee Society scores improved from 36.1 pre-op to 74.4 at 1-year follow-up and decreased to 60.5 at latest follow-up.

5.8 Outcomes of Mid-Term Follow-up Studies

Mathews et al. [21] reported on the outcomes of 21 DFLCWO at follow-up of 1–8 years. In their series they used the same technique of DFLCWO but used either plaster cast immobilization or internal fixation with staples or a blade plate. In their series 57% of the patients had significant complications including knee stiffness (48%), non-/delayed union (19%), infection (10%), and fixation failure (5%). Five (19%) were converted to TKA with 5 years. They inferred that better clinical outcomes are evident in the patients with isolated lateral compartment involvement and have rigid internal fixation.

Edgerton et al. [22] published results of 24 DFLCWO at mean follow-up of 8.3 (5–11) years. The average age at the time of osteotomy was 55 years. The mean pre-op HSS knee score was 58 (27–82), and 6 knees were having good 5 fair and 13 poor scores. At last follow-up, mean HSS knee score improved to 78 (40–94), with excellent result in 8 (33%) knees, good in 9 (38%), fair in 3 (13%), and poor in 1. Overall 75% of the patients were satisfied at last follow-up, and analysis of HSS knee score showed that the probability of having a satisfactory outcome after surgery is significantly better in patients having higher pre-op HSS knee scores ($p < 0.04$). Also, patients having valgus under-correction had poorer outcomes and tended to be less satisfied than the ones achieving neutral or varus alignment at follow-up. They noted that higher degrees of pre-op valgus and valgus under-correction were an important cause of failure and conversion. Better clinical results were evident in the patients with isolated lateral compartment involvement compared to those with bi- or tricompartmental involvement. Overall 15 (63%) of the patients had complications including pin tract infection, loss of correction and failure of fixation, and delayed/nonunion. The major reason for loss of correction was use of Hoffman fixator or staples for stabilization rather than rigid internal fixation. The majority (86%) of DFLCWO having delayed or nonunion had satisfactory outcomes.

Wang and Hsu [23] reported the clinical results in 30 patients at mean follow-up of 99 (61–169) months. The mean age of patients at the time of surgery was 53 (31–64) years. At the last follow-up, 25 (83%) of the included patients had satisfactory results, 2 had fair results, and 3 patients were converted to total knee arthroplasty. The mean knee scores significantly improved from 46 (20–63) pre-op to 88 (65–99) post-op ($p < 0.001$). Although the overall mean range of motion improved from 121° pre-op to 124° post-op, 5 patients with satisfactory results had a decrease in knee range post-op. The mean post-op tibio-femoral angle was 1.2° valgus, and it did not change over the follow-up period. The osteotomy united in 29/30 knees over the follow-up period at a mean duration of 4.7 months. Thirteen patients from the cohort underwent hardware removal after union at the osteotomy site. The cumulative 10-year survival rate for the patients was 87%. Eight of the 30 patients with associated severe patellofemoral arthritis had significant reduction in knee pain and improvement in function after the osteotomy. Their mean knee scores increased from 48 pre-op to 90 after the procedure (mean improvement, 42 points; $p < 0.001$). Postoperatively authors also found an improvement in patellofemoral maltracking in 7/8 patients.

5.9 Outcomes of Short-Term Follow-up Studies

Seven studies [24–30] evaluated reported the outcomes of DFLCWO at short-term follow-up. Out of these seven studies, five were published before 2000 and used older surgical techniques. Most of the studies reported favorable outcomes and excellent results in patients at the short-term follow-up. The case series by Forkel et al. [29] is the most recent published series reporting on the short-term outcome of the patients. All the included patients underwent removal of hardware. Sixteen of the 22 followed patients had symptomatic irritation from hardware. There were no other reported complications at the last follow-up. Overall and all subgroup scores of KOOS significantly improved at the last follow-up compared to their pre-op values. Also, the visual analog scores for pain significantly improved compared to their pre-op value ($p < 0.001$). Tegner activity score showed a non-significant improvement compared to the pre-op value. Six patients did not participate in sports after surgery, 15 participated in recreational sports, and 1 participated in basketball at competitive level.

Kazemi et al. [30] in their published series of 40 patients compared the results of use of angled blade plate and locking compression plate for stabilization of medial closing wedge distal femoral osteotomy. The authors found a higher rate of non-union in the group with use of locking compression plates; they recommended use of angled blade plates for stabilization of medial distal femoral closing wedge osteotomies.

5.10 Other Described Osteotomies

5.10.1 Proximal Tibial Medial Closing Wedge/Lateral Opening Wedge Osteotomy

One of the expected outcomes following osteotomy about the knee is to create a joint line which is approximately parallel to the floor. Femoral osteotomy will alter the joint obliquity, while tibial will not, and, accordingly, the decision as to whether to perform the osteotomy above or below the knee will depend to a large extent on the patient's preoperative joint obliquity which should be assessed on weight-bearing films. Other factors which play a role in choosing the level of osteotomy include the extent of deformity and the center of rotation of angulation [CORA]. In cases with valgus deformity <12° and the CORA is within the proximal tibia, a tibial osteotomy is preferred over the distal femoral osteotomy [31]. This clinical picture may be seen in patients with valgus deformity secondary to prior trauma or in cases with deformity secondary to previous lateral meniscectomy. Another difference and potential added advantage of high tibial osteotomy over distal femoral osteotomy is that tibial osteotomy will correct deformity through the entire range of motion, while distal femoral osteotomy unloads the knee joint only in extension [32]. Assessment of the patient's alignment through range can be performed prior to osteotomy with computer navigation and is an added advantage of choosing navigation to plan and execute osteotomy.

5.10.2 Proximal Tibial Medial Closing Wedge Osteotomy (PTMCLWO)

Few published studies evaluate the clinical outcomes of valgus deformity correction with proximal tibial medial closing wedge osteotomy. The only case series which reports the mid- to long-term clinical outcomes of PTMCWO was published by Coventry [4] who described 31 consecutive PTMCWOs at a mean follow-up of 9.4 (2–17) years. They reported no or mild pain in 24 (77%) knees, moderate pain in 6 knees, and severe pain in 1 knee at the last follow-up. Six patients were converted to TKA at average follow-up of 9.8 years.

5.10.3 Proximal Tibial Lateral Opening Wedge Osteotomy (PTLOWO)

Three published case series report clinical outcomes of PTLOWO. Marti et al. [33] presented outcomes of 34 PTLOWO with mean age of 43 (17–76) years at the time of surgery at long-term mean follow-up of 11 (5–21) years. Mean Insall Knee Score for the included patients was 84 (54–99) at last follow-up. Outcomes were graded as excellent in 9 patients (26%), good in 21 patients (62%), fair in 3 patients (9%), and poor in 1 patient (3%). There was no significant difference in the pre-op and post-op range of motion. Five knees showed evidence of moderate instability at follow-up, but none of the patients showed progression of osteoarthritis or loss of correction in the follow-up period. One patient had superficial wound infection, and three had neurapraxia of the common peroneal nerve, all of which recovered within 1 year of follow-up. There were no cases of deep infection or nonunion.

Collins et al. [32] reported the clinical and radiological outcomes of 24 PTLOWOs and result of gait analyses of 12 PTLOWOs at mean follow-up of 52 months. Statistically significant clinical improvements were identified in the lower extremity functional scale [mean change (95%CI) = 10 (2.4, 17.6)] and in the KOOS score [mean change (95%CI) = 10.9 (0.5, 21.4)]. Mechanical axis was corrected from 2.4 ± 2.4 valgus to 0 ± 2.6 varus ($p < 0.001$). The pcak knee adduction moment in gait analyses significantly improved redistributing the dynamic knee joint load to the medial compartment. Two patients required conversion to total knee arthroplasty during the study period. Their results supported the idea that proximal tibial lateral opening wedge osteotomy is a viable treatment option for valgus knee deformity with lateral compartment arthrosis requiring smaller degrees of correction.

A recent study by Mirouse et al. [34] reported outcomes of PTLOWO for 19 patients who underwent surgery at mean age of 54.5 years and mean follow-up of 4.3 (2–9) years. Their results differed with the finding of Collins et al. In their series PTLOWO produced unsatisfactory medium-term outcomes, with failure rate of 52%. At a mean follow-up of 4.3 (2–9) years, significant improvements were seen in the Knee Society knee and function scores from baseline ($p < 0.05$), 10/19 patients having global Knee Society score <140 were considered as failures. Seven of the 10 failures underwent TKA after a mean follow-up of 5.0 ± 2.7 years. The authors inferred that global IKS score of <140 at final follow-up predicted conversion to TKA. In their series, patients with HKA angle outside the 180–183° range and joint line obliquity >10° during follow-up were associated with poor outcomes of PTLOWO.

5.10.4 Novel Osteotomies

Wagner [35] and Abdi et al. [36] have published on novel techniques of performing distal femoral osteotomy and correction of valgus deformity in patients of isolated lateral compartment arthrosis. Though both noted clinical and radiological improvement in series of patients operated in each study, these techniques are not widely practiced. There is, at this time, insufficient evidence for a recommendation of either of these techniques, but interested readers can refer to the articles for further details.

5.11 Results of Navigated Osteotomies for Valgus Knee Deformities

One of the recent studies by Saragaglia and Chedal-Bornu [37] reports on the combined outcomes of DFLOWO, DFMCWO, and of double osteotomies (proximal tibial and distal femoral) performed at mean age of 42.4 ± 14.3 (15–63) years. They utilized computer navigation to assess the intra-operative correction obtained. Results of osteotomies performed in 25 knees in 23 patients were reviewed at mean follow-up of 50.9 ± 38.8 months (6–144). The mean Lysholm score was 92.9 ± 4 (86–100), the mean KOOS score was 89.7 ± 9.3 (68–100), the mean Knee Society knee score was 88.7 ± 11.4 (60–100), and function score was 90.6 ± 13.3 (55–100). Twenty-two patients were satisfied or very satisfied with the outcome; one patient was dissatisfied. None of the patients required conversion to TKA. The preoperative goal of mechanical axis correction was achieved in 86.2% of the patients and was maintained at last follow-up. They concluded that excellent mid-term clinical and radiological outcomes of periarticular knee osteotomy could be achieved with computer assistance and navigation. Only one patient had a transient paralysis of common fibular nerve which recovered without sequelae.

5.12 Choosing Between Medial Closing or Lateral Opening Wedge Distal Femoral Osteotomies

Among the commonly performed DFLCWO and DFLOWO, there is a paucity of literature directly comparing the clinical and radiological results of one over another. The most recent published literature which aids in the decision-making is a systematic review by Kim et al. [38]. They concluded that the clinical and radiological outcomes and survivorship are similar. While the opening wedge procedure is technically less demanding with a single bone cut, it does require bone grafting. Closing wedge osteotomy is technically more complex in that it requires precise pre-op planning and accurate execution of osteotomy to achieve desired correction and is difficult to titrate during surgery. The choice of one technique over another is largely dependent on surgeon's experience during training and availability of resources, particularly bone graft or substitute and navigation.

5.13 Return to Sport

Voleti et al. [39] studied the return to sport in athletic population after distal femoral osteotomy for valgus knees with lateral compartment arthrosis. The series included 13 patients (8 males and 5 females) with a mean age at surgery of 24 years (range 17–35 years). The average body mass index was 27.4 kg/m^2 (range 23–31 kg/m^2). Six patients underwent medial closing wedge osteotomy, and 7 underwent lateral opening wedge osteotomy. The mean preoperative valgus (tibio-femoral angle) significantly decreased from 7° (range 5°–13°) to 0° (range 0°–2° varus) ($p < 0.0001$). The mean alignment correction was 8° (range 5°–13°). The outcomes were reported at mean follow-up of 43 months (range 24–74 months). Four patients returned to soccer, 2 to softball, 2 to jogging, 1 to rugby, 1 to basketball, 1 to ice hockey, 1 to volleyball, and 1 to rowing. All 13 patients successfully returned to their sport of choice performing athletic activity at least 4 days a week at a mean of 11 months (range 9–13 months). All 13 patients demonstrated an significant improvements in both Marx Activity Scale and IKDC scores after surgery [mean improvement in Marx Activity Scale was 7 ± 2 points ($p < 0.0001$) with a mean final score of 11 (range 8–14); mean improvement in IKDC score was 36 ± 8 points ($p < 0.0001$) with a mean final IKDC score of 89 (range 78–96)]. Major complications, including thrombosis, arthrofibrosis, nonunion, and infection, were not seen in any of the patients. One patient required hardware removal for symptomatic plate irritation of the iliotibial band at 2 years after surgery.

5.14 Gait Analysis

van Egmond et al. [40] recently published a study analyzing the clinical and radiological outcomes and improvements in the gait analyses of 12 patients who underwent varus producing osteotomies for valgus knees with lateral compartment arthrosis. While all the osteotomies were closing wedge, five were distal femoral and three proximal tibial, and there were four patients who required double osteotomies (distal femoral and proximal tibial). For gait analyses they compared the findings to ten normal knees. The knee adduction moment in patients undergoing osteotomy increased significantly postoperatively ($p < 0.05$) and was comparable to the control group signifying effective distribution of transmitted load to the medial compartment. They noted significant improvements in patient reported outcome measures irrespective of the type of closed wedge osteotomy performed. Varus producing closing wedge osteotomy of the distal femur and proximal tibia can achieve significant improvements in the clinical outcomes and kinematics of the knee after correction of valgus deformity for lateral compartment arthrosis.

5.15 Outcomes of Conversion to Total Knee Arthroplasty

Three published studies [41–43] report on the outcomes of TKA performed in patients who had previously undergone osteotomy for correction of valgus deformity. These studies conclude the clinical outcomes after TKA in patients with prior osteotomy of distal femur are like those after primary TKA at midterm follow-up. However, there are increased technical difficulties during surgery including exposure of knee, the presence of retained hardware, and alteration to local bony anatomy adding to the difficulty with implantation of the prosthesis. There may be an increased need for use of more constrained implants to counter the residual laxity of knees. Either staged or simultaneous removal of previous hardware should be considered by the operating surgeon. In patients undergoing simultaneous removal of hardware, the use of a stemmed femoral prosthesis to bypass the empty screw holes is recommended. Gaillard et al. [42] suggest implanting the femoral component in residual tolerable varus to counter the lateral soft tissue laxity which may decrease the need for constrained implants. An extramedullary guide or computer navigation may be needed if retained hardware blocks access to the intramedullary canal. It is important to take care to prevent injury to patellar tendon which is reported to have a significantly higher chance of injury in patients undergoing TKA after varus osteotomy of distal femur. As with any knee surgery where there are prior incisions and hardware, wound problems and deep sepsis are seen more commonly.

Fig. 5.2 Pre-op and post-op alignment views: (**a**) pre-op weight-bearing alignment view depicting the valgus alignment of right lower limb. (**b**) Post-op weight-bearing alignment view depicting corrected neutral mechanical alignment of the right lower limb

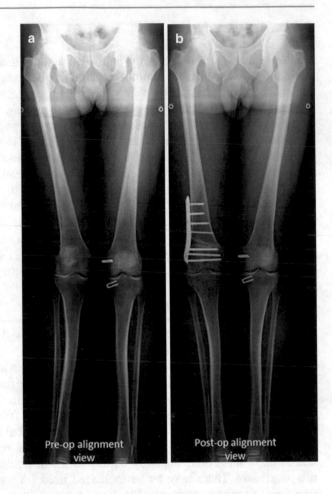

5.16 Senior Author's Preferred Surgical Technique

The senior author's preferred osteotomy for correction of the painful valgus knee with lateral arthritis in young patients is a distal femoral lateral opening wedge osteotomy. Prior to surgery, weight-bearing long and standard films are used to assess alignment, wear patterns, and joint obliquity (Figs. 5.2 and 5.3). These investigations may dictate that alternatives are required, for example, an old lateral plateau malunion may be managed with either a medial closing or lateral opening wedge tibial osteotomy. Preoperative MRI confirms the medial compartment is satisfactory and allows assessment of wear patterns—typically distally on the lateral femoral condyle. Surgery is performed under fluoroscopic guidance with navigation utilized to guide the correction achieved. We routinely use diagnostic arthroscopy prior to osteotomy to register data points for alignment and to manage any other treatable intra-articular lesions that may contribute to the patient's symptoms.

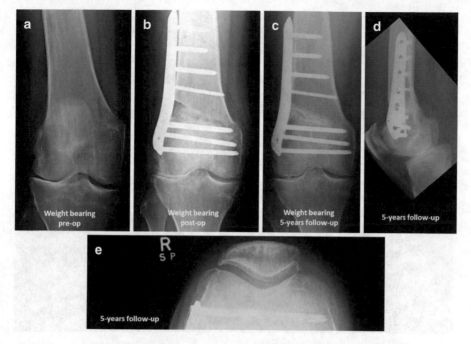

Fig. 5.3 X-rays knee: (**a**) preoperative weight-bearing anteroposterior view of the right knee in valgus showing lateral compartment arthritis. (**b**) Postoperative anteroposterior view of right knee depicting correction of valgus deformity with lateral opening wedge distal femoral osteotomy and bone grafting. (**c**) 5 years follow-up weight-bearing anteroposterior view of right knee showing maintained correction of the right knee and bony union of the osteotomy site. (**d**) 5 years follow-up lateral view of the right knee depicting well healed distal femoral osteotomy. (**e**) 5 years follow-up merchant's view of patella showing central position of the patella in the trochlear groove and mild patellofemoral arthritis

The surgery is performed in supine position with the feet the distal end of operating table and a knee side support is used for intra-operative stabilization of lower limb. A tourniquet is used only during the arthroscopy and is deflated prior to the lateral skin incision. After preparation and free sterile draping of the lower limb, femoral and tibial trackers are inserted, and the center of the femoral head is registered. A diagnostic arthroscopy is performed, and any arthroscopically treatable intra-articular causes of knee pain are addressed. Registrations of landmarks are then completed including the center of distal femur and proximal tibia as well as the femoral condyle and tibial plateau and the malleoli. The alignment is recorded both at maximal extension and at 90°. These are recorded on a whiteboard. Significantly, maximum extension is a surrogate for the sagittal plane—if this remains unaltered at the end of the procedure, there has been no change in the sagittal plane. After completion of arthroscopy, the tourniquet is deflated, and open surgical procedure for osteotomy is begun.

A lateral skin incision of 12–15 cm is made from the level of the lateral knee joint line proximally. The fascia lata is incised immediately posterior to the iliotibial

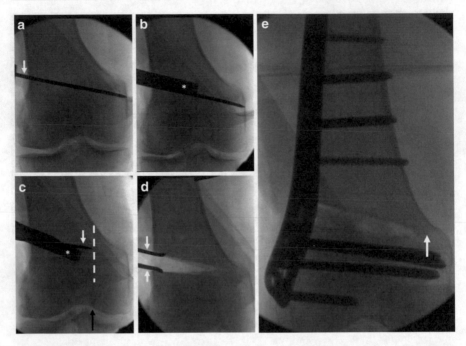

Fig. 5.4 Surgical technique: (**a**) intra-operative fluoroscopic image of right knee showing oblique lateral to medial placement of the guide wire (with arrow) at the planned level of osteotomy. (**b**) Intra-operative fluoroscopic image of right knee depicting the posterior placement of Hohmann's retractor (white*) for protection of posterior neurovascular structures. (**c**) Intra-operative fluoroscopic image of right knee depicting the medial extent of the osteotomy (dashed vertical white line) performed using osteotome (white arrow) corresponding to the lateral cortical margin of the medial femoral condyle (black arrow). (**d**) Intra-operative fluoroscopic image of right knee showing the opening of the osteotomy site using laminar spreader (white arrows). (**e**) Intra-operative fluoroscopic image of right knee showing lateral plate fixation of distal femoral osteotomy and bone grafting of osteotomy site

band, and vastus lateralis is exposed and elevated anteriorly off the lateral intermuscular septum. Utilizing fluoroscopic guidance, a guide wire is passed from the middle of the lateral femoral surface just proximal to the superior pole of the patella and slightly oblique to the axial plane, aiming slightly distally toward the adductor tubercle (Fig. 5.4). Before the osteotomy is carried out, subperiosteal dissection is performed behind the femur in line with the intended osteotomy to separate the posterior neurovascular structures from the posterior femoral surface. A blunt-tipped Hohmann's retractor is placed between the posterior soft tissues and the posterior surface of femur to protect the neurovascular structures (Fig. 5.4), and an anterior Hohmann protects the anterior extensor mechanism.

Utilizing fluoroscopy and a sagittal saw, the osteotomy is commenced through metaphyseal bone from lateral to medial immediately proximal to the guide wire. While the saw is utilized for osteotomy of the lateral and anterior femur, a sharp osteotome is used to perform osteotomy of the posterior cortex with the blunt nosed Hohmann retractor protecting at all times the posterior neurovascular structures. It is important to leave a medial hinge of intact bone with the saw and osteotome passing up to but not beyond the lateral margin of the medial femoral condyle on the medial side of the intercondylar notch (Fig. 5.4). This landmark is easily seen on fluoroscopy. While this may have the appearance on the AP projection of the osteotomy passing only two-thirds of the distance across the femur, the cross-sectional area of the distal femur means that there is only a small amount of bone keeping the hinge together. Extending the osteotomy further than the medial wall of the intercondylar notch will result in an unstable medial hinge.

After osteotomy is performed, the alignment is corrected to neutral mechanical axis under the guidance of navigation using a laminar spreader at the site of osteotomy with care to not alter the femur in the sagittal plane (Fig. 5.4). Once correction is achieved, the wedge-shaped bone void is measured and filled with allograft, and the osteotomy is stabilized with a Tomofix plate (Fig. 5.4). The neutral mechanical limb alignment is confirmed, and the wound is closed in layers. We aim for a correction of 0° mechanical axis—possibly 1–1.5° of varus in patients older than 55 and with more marked wear—and we avoid altering the slope in the sagittal plane (Fig. 5.2).

Postoperatively the limb is held in full extension in a limited range of motion brace which is opened to allow a range of 0–30° on the first postoperative day. Part of weight-bearing mobilization is allowed with support—initially one-quarter of body weight as tolerated by the patient and increasing by one-quarter body weight every 2 weeks. At 2 weeks, the brace is opened to allow a range of 0–90°, and gradual flexion is allowed with supervision by a physiotherapist till the 6-week mark when the brace is discontinued. Crutches continue as needed, and further supervised physiotherapy continues upgrading range of motion and a strengthening program.

5.17   Conclusions

Periarticular knee osteotomy is an attractive treatment option for young and active patients with isolated lateral compartment knee arthrosis. Distal femoral osteotomy is advocated in young active patients with >12° of tibio-femoral valgus deformity, >10° of joint line obliquity, and isolated lateral compartment osteoarthritis.

While good results are frequently observed, predictors of reduced symptom relief and shorter survivorship before conversion to TKA include older age at osteotomy, performance of bilateral osteotomies, and the presence of medial compartment osteoarthritis at the time of osteotomy.

It is recommended to overcorrect the preoperative valgus knee alignment to 1–2 varus which results in better clinical and radiological outcomes and facilitates easier conversion to TKA. This angular correction also decreases the rate of use of constrained implants.

Implant prominence causing soft tissue irritation is seen more commonly than with tibial osteotomy, and the need for removal of hardware should be discussed with the patient preoperatively.

For young active patients with <12° of tibio-femoral valgus, <10° of joint line obliquity, and deformity arising from proximal tibia, deformity correction and osteotomy can be performed at the level of proximal tibia.

Distal femoral lateral opening wedge osteotomy is less technically demanding and facilitates controlled intra-operative correction of the mechanical alignment of knee.

Significant improvements in the gait patterns and mechanical loading of the knee can be effectively achieved with periarticular knee osteotomy.

Young active patients with valgus knees and isolated lateral compartment arthrosis can return to the same level of sports participation as pre-op after correction of the valgus knee deformity with periarticular knee osteotomy.

The clinical results and survivorship of distal femoral varus osteotomy for isolated lateral compartment osteoarthritis of valgus knee deteriorate significantly between 10 and 15 years of follow-up.

Use of computer-assisted navigation for correction of mechanical alignment of valgus knee with isolated lateral compartment osteoarthritis facilitates accurate correction of mechanical alignment of knee. The clinical and radiological results and survivorship of navigated periarticular knee osteotomies are excellent in the short-mid-term follow-up. Further studies are required to evaluate their outcomes and survivorship at long-term follow-up.

References

1. Haddad FS, Bentley G. Total knee arthroplasty after high tibial osteotomy: a medium-term review. J Arthroplast. 2000;15(5):597–603.
2. Felson DT, Niu J, Gross KD, et al. Valgus malalignment is a risk factor for lateral knee osteoarthritis incidence and progression: findings from the Multicenter Osteoarthritis Study and the Osteoarthritis Initiative. Arthritis Rheum. 2013;65:355–62.
3. Rosso F, Margheritini F. Distal femoral osteotomy. Curr Rev Musculoskelet Med. 2014;7:302–11.
4. Coventry MB. Proximal tibial varus osteotomy for osteoarthritis of the lateral compartment of the knee. J Bone Joint Surg Am. 1987;69:32–8.
5. Hanssen AD, Stuart MJ, Scott RD, Scuderi GR. Surgical options for the middle-aged patient with osteoarthritis of the knee joint. JBJS. 2000;82-A(12):1768–81.
6. Chahla J, Mitchell JJ, Liechti DJ, et al. Opening-and closing-wedge distal femoral osteotomy: a systematic review of outcomes for isolated lateral compartment osteoarthritis. Orthop J Sports Med. 2016;4:2325967116649901.
7. Ekeland A, Nerhus TK, Dimmen S, Heir S. Good functional results of distal femoral opening-wedge osteotomy of knees with lateral osteoarthritis. Knee Surg Sports Traumatol Arthrosc. 2016;24(5):1702–9.
8. de Andrade MAP, DCFF G, Portugal AL, de Abreu e Silva GM. Distal femoral varusing for osteoarthritis of valgus knee: a long-term follow-up. Rev Bras Ortop. 2009;44(4):346–50.
9. Das D, et al. Distal femoral opening-wedge osteotomy for lateral compartment osteoarthritis of the knee. Open Access Surg. 2008;1:25–9.

10. Thein R, Haviv B, Bronak S, Thein R. Distal femoral osteotomy for valgus arthritic knees. J Orthop Sci. 2012;17(6):745–9.
11. Dewilde TR, Dauw J, Vandenneucker H, Bellemans J. Opening wedge distal femoral varus osteotomy using the Puddu plate and calcium phosphate bone cement. Knee Surg Sports Traumatol Arthrosc. 2013;21(1):249–54.
12. Madelaine A, Lording T, Villa V, Lustig S, Servien E, Neyret P. The effect of lateral opening wedge distal femoral osteotomy on leg length. Knee Surg Sports Traumatol Arthrosc. 2016;24(3):847–54.
13. Cameron JI, McCauley JC, Kermanshahi AY, Bugbee WD. Lateral opening-wedge distal femoral osteotomy: pain relief, functional improvement, and survivorship at 5 years. Clin Orthop Relat Res. 2015;473(6):2009–15.
14. Zarrouk A, Bouzidi R, Karray B, Kammoun S, Mourali S, Kooli M. Distal femoral varus osteotomy outcome: is associated femoropatellar osteoarthritis consequential? Orthop Traumatol Surg Res. 2010;96(6):632–6.
15. Saithna A, Kundra R, Getgood A, Spalding T. Opening wedge distal femoral varus osteotomy for lateral compartment osteoarthritis in the valgus knee. Knee. 2014;21(1):172–5.
16. Jacobi M, Wahl P, Bouaicha S, Jakob RP, Gautier E. Distal femoral varus osteotomy: problems associated with the lateral open-wedge technique. Arch Orthop Trauma Surg. 2011;131(6):725–8.
17. Finkelstein JA, Gross AE, Davis A. Varus osteotomy of the distal part of the femur. A survivorship analysis. J Bone Jt Surg. 1996;78(9):1348–52.
18. Backstein D, Morag G, Hanna S, Safir O, Gross A. Long-term follow-up of distal femoral varus osteotomy of the knee. J Arthroplast. 2007;22(4):2–6.
19. Kosashvili Y, Safir O, Gross A, Morag G, Lakstein D, Backstein D. Distal femoral varus osteotomy for lateral osteoarthritis of the knee: a minimum ten-year follow-up. Int Orthop. 2010;34(2):249–54.
20. Sternheim A, Garbedian S, Backstein D. Distal femoral varus osteotomy: unloading the lateral compartment: long-term follow-up of 45 medial closing wedge osteotomies. Orthopedics. 2011;34(9):e488–90.
21. Mathews J, Cobb AG, Richardson S, Bentley G. Distal femoral osteotomy for lateral compartment osteoarthritis of the knee. Orthopedics. 1998;21(4):437–40.
22. Edgerton BC, Mariani EM, Morrey BF. Distal femoral varus osteotomy for painful genu valgum. A five-to-11-year follow-up study. Clin Orthop Relat Res. 1993;(288):263–9.
23. Wang J-W, Hsu C-C. Distal femoral varus osteotomy for osteoarthritis of the knee. J Bone Joint Surg Am. 2005;87(1):127–3.
24. McDermott AG, Finklestein JA, Farine I, Boynton EL, MacIntosh DL, Gross A. Distal femoral varus osteotomy for valgus deformity of the knee. J Bone Joint Surg Am. 1988;70(1):110–6.
25. Healy WL, Anglen JO, Wasilewski SA, Krackow KA. Distal femoral varus osteotomy. J Bone Joint Surg Am. 1988;70(1):102–9.
26. Learmonth ID. A simple technique for varus supracondylar osteotomy in genu valgum. J Bone Joint Surg Br. 1990;72(2):235–7.
27. Stähelin T, Hardegger F, Ward JC. Supracondylar osteotomy of the femur with use of compression. Osteosynthesis with a malleable implant. J Bone Joint Surg Am. 2000;82(5):712–22.
28. Johnson EW Jr, Bodell LS. Corrective supracondylar osteotomy for painful genu valgum. Mayo Clin Proc. 1981;56(2):87–92.
29. Forkel P, Achtnich A, Metzlaff S, Zantop T, Petersen W. Midterm results following medial closed wedge distal femoral osteotomy stabilized with a locking internal fixation device. Knee Surg Sports Traumatol Arthrosc. 2015;23(7):2061–7.
30. Kazemi SM, Minaei R, Safdari F, Keipourfard A, Forghani R, Mirzapourshafiei A. Supracondylar osteotomy in valgus knee: angle blade plate versus locking compression plate. Arch Bone Jt Surg. 2016;4(1):29–34.
31. Phillips MJ, Krackow KA. High tibial osteotomy and distal femoral osteotomy for valgus or varus deformity around the knee. Instr Course Lect. 1998;47:429–36.

32. Collins B, Getgood A, Alomar AZ, Giffin JR, Willits K, Fowler PJ, et al. A case series of lateral opening wedge high tibial osteotomy for valgus malalignment. Knee Surg Sports Traumatol Arthrosc. 2013;21(1):152–60.
33. Marti RK, Verhagen RAW, Kerkhoffs GMMJ, Moojen TM. Proximal tibial varus osteotomy: indications, technique, and five to twenty-one-year results. J Bone Joint Surg Am. 2001;83(2):164–70.
34. Mirouse G, Dubory A, Roubineau F, Poignard A, Hernigou P, Allain J, et al. Failure of high tibial varus osteotomy for lateral tibio-femoral osteoarthritis with <10° of valgus: outcomes in 19 patients. Orthop Traumatol Surg Res. 2017;103(6):953–8.
35. Wagner M. Die suprakondyl re Femurosteotomie zur Korrektur des Genu valgum. Oper Orthopädie Traumatol. 2003;15(4):387–401.
36. Abdi R, Hajzargarbashi R, Ebrahimzadeh MH. Single cut distal femoral varus osteotomy (SCFO): a preliminary study. Arch Bone Jt Surg. 2017;5(5):322–7.
37. Saragaglia D, Chedal-Bornu B. Computer-assisted osteotomy for valgus knees: medium-term results of 29 cases. Orthop Traumatol Surg Res. 2014;100(5):527–30.
38. Kim YC, Yang J-H, Kim HJ, Tawonsawatruk T, Chang YS, Lee JS, et al. Distal femoral varus osteotomy for valgus arthritis of the knees: systematic review of open versus closed wedge osteotomy. Knee Surg Relat Res. 2018;30(1):3–16.
39. Voleti PB, Wu IT, Degen RM, Tetreault DM, Krych AJ, Williams RJ. Successful return to sport following distal femoral varus osteotomy. Cartilage. 2019;10(1):19–25.
40. van Egmond N, Stolwijk N, van Heerwaarden R, van Kampen A, Keijsers NLW. Gait analysis before and after corrective osteotomy in patients with knee osteoarthritis and a valgus deformity. Knee Surg Sports Traumatol Arthrosc. 2017;25(9):2904–13.
41. Nelson CL, Saleh KJ, Kassim RA, Windsor R, Haas S, Laskin R, et al. Total Knee Arthroplasty After Varus Osteotomy Of The Distal Part Of The Femur. J Bone Joint Surg Am. 2003;85(6):1062–5.
42. Gaillard R, Lording T, Lustig S, Servien E, Neyret P. Total knee arthroplasty after varus distal femoral osteotomy vs native knee: similar results in a case control study. Knee Surg Sports Traumatol Arthrosc. 2017;25(11):3522–9.
43. Kosashvili Y, Gross AE, Zywiel MG, Safir O, Lakstein D, Backstein D. Total knee arthroplasty after failed distal femoral varus osteotomy using selectively stemmed posterior stabilized components. J Arthroplast. 2011;26(5):738–43.

Outcomes of Surgery for Sagittal Instability

6

Stefano Pasqualotto, Marco Valoroso,
Giuseppe La Barbera, and David Dejour

6.1 Introduction

Stability of the knee is controlled by both soft tissue and bony elements, which are responsible for the overall balance of the joint in both coronal and sagittal planes.

While deformities in the coronal plane are a well-known knee pathology with established therapeutic options, bony anatomical impairments influencing sagittal balance of the knee joint are less common and are responsible for flexion/extension deformities or an altered position of the tibia with regard to the femur. Notably, an excessive anterior tibial translation is more commonly observed in early flexion, whereas excessive posterior tibial translation, also called tibial sag, is better recognized in late flexion [1–3].

The main actors in the control of sagittal stability of the knee are anterior cruciate ligament (ACL), posterior cruciate ligament (PCL), posteromedial and posterolateral structures, the menisci, and the posterior tibial slope (PTS).

Focusing on PTS, several studies have underlined how a high PTS represents a risk factor for an ACL injury since, in presence of a compressive load, a high PTS is responsible for a higher tibiofemoral anterior shear force and an increased load in the ACL [4–11].

S. Pasqualotto
IRCCS Ospedale Sacro Cuore Don Calabria, Negrar, Italy

M. Valoroso · G. La Barbera
S.C. Ortopedia e Traumatologia, Ospedale di Circolo di Varese, Varese, Italy

D. Dejour (✉)
Lyon-Ortho-Clinic, Clinique de la Sauvegarde, Lyon, France

© Springer Nature Switzerland AG 2020
S. Oussedik, S. Lustig (eds.), *Osteotomy About the Knee*,
https://doi.org/10.1007/978-3-030-49055-3_6

6.2   Posterior Tibial Slope

PTS is genetically determined; nonetheless extrinsic factors such as direct physical trauma [12], fractures, osteomyelitis, patellar tendon graft harvesting, tibial tubercle transplantation before epiphyseal fusion [13], Osgood-Schlatter's disease [14], prolonged immobilization, tibial wire traction [15], radiotherapy, poliomyelitis [16], and growth disturbance of the bony components could alter its development, increasing or decreasing it [17, 18].

6.2.1   How to Measure Posterior Tibial Slope

Several techniques have been described to calculate PTS. In the author's preferred method, PTS is defined as the angle between the line perpendicular to the tibial diaphyseal axis and the line tangent to the most superior points at the anterior and posterior edges of the medial tibial plateau (angle β in Fig. 6.1), calculated on X-rays with a true lateral view of the knee [19]. According to this method, the physiological PTS measures approximately 7°. Other methods, however, report the use of different longitudinal axes [20, 21] (Fig. 6.1) such as:

- The anterior tibial cortex (angle α).
- The posterior tibial cortex (angle γ).
- The anatomic fibular axis (angle δ).

As these axes are not parallel, PTS values differ depending on the reference axis. Methods to calculate PTS were also described using CT scan or MRI such as:

- The midpoint method proposed by Hashemi et al. [22], which connects the midpoints of two anteroposterior tibial lines within the proximal end of the tibia.
- The circle method described by Hudek et al. [23], which connects the center of two circles within the proximal tibia.

However, with true lateral views, conventional radiography did not differ from CT scan and MRI images in determining the exact PTS [24].

In addition to bony structure, sagittal stability of the knee is granted also by soft tissues. In particular, since the posterior meniscal horn is thicker than the anterior one, meniscal slope (MS), defined as the angle formed by a tangent line from the most superior border of anterior and posterior horn of the meniscus and the longitudinal axis of the tibia, may play a role in the sagittal balance [25–27]. Shifting the PTS to a more horizontal plane, the posterior meniscal horn acts like a wedge between the posterior femoral condyle and the posterior tibial plateau, restraining anteroposterior tibial translation and reducing the stress on the ACL [28, 29].

Fig. 6.1 The four methods to measure PTS. Reference axis for PTS measurement and related complementary angles: White: medial tibial plateau; Green: anterior tibial cortex (α); Orange: tibial diaphyseal axis (β); Blue: posterior tibial cortex (γ); Yellow: fibular diaphyseal axis (δ)

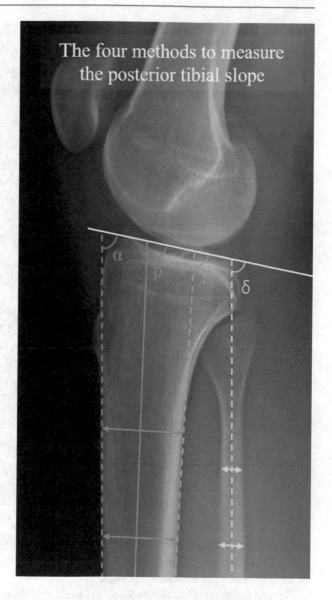

6.3 How to Assess Sagittal Instability of the Knee

A true lateral view of the knee, obtained with the patient in monopodal weight-bearing with the knee flexed by 20° and with the superimposition of the posterior femoral condyles, allows not only the measurement of the PTS but also of the "static" anterior tibial translation (ATT) [19]. This could be defined as the distance between two lines tangent respectively to the posterior femoral condyles and the

Fig. 6.2 Measurement of anterior tibial translation (ATT) in monopodal weight-bearing X-rays. The posterior tibial cortex is the reference (line A). Two lines are traced parallel to line A and tangent to posterior part the medial tibial plateau (line B) and medial femoral condyle (line C)

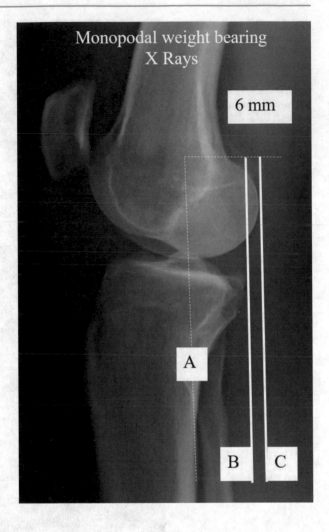

tibial plateau and parallel to the reference line, represented by the tangent to the posterior tibial cortex. This measure represents the anterior displacement of the tibia in weight-bearing conditions (Fig. 6.2).

Several techniques have been described to assess "dynamic" ATT, including both a radiographic-based device and manual or automatic devices such as KT-1000™ and KT-2000™ knee ligament arthrometer (MEDmetric Corp, San Diego, CA), the Rolimeter® (Aircast Europa, Neubeuern, Germany), and the GNRB® (Genourob, Laval, France).

In the authors' preferred method, dynamic ATT is quantified with the knee flexed by 20°, using the Telos™ stress radiography device (Metax, Hungen-Obbornhofen, Germany) with an anterior-directed force of 150 N and calculating the side-to-side difference (SSD) between the injured and the healthy knee [30] (Fig. 6.3).

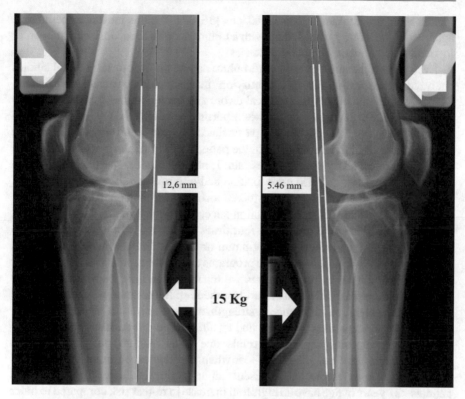

Fig. 6.3 Evaluation of "dynamic" ATT, calculating the side-to-side difference, using stress X-rays with the Telos™ (Telos GmbH, Marburg, Germany)

Moreover, stress radiography techniques represent a valid tool not only for the assessment of the ATT but also for the quantification of posterior tibial translation (PTT) on the femur in case of posterior cruciate ligament (PCL) tear and nowadays represent an essential and objective element within the PCL treatment algorithm [31, 32].

6.4   Deflexion Osteotomy

Anterior sagittal balance of the knee is mainly governed by ACL, menisci, and PTS, with the ACL representing the primary restraint to ATT. ACL tears represent the most common cause of sagittal imbalance with an incidence ranging approximately from 30 to 78 per 100,000 person-years [33]. Nowadays, ACL reconstruction is an effective surgery with 75–97% of patients reporting good to excellent outcomes [34]; nonetheless the re-rupture rate ranges from 1% to 11% [33], even though some series reported a 34% of re-tear rate [35].

Failure of an ACL reconstruction is of great concern for the orthopedic surgeon and could have significant implication for the health of the knee with a greater incidence of chondral and meniscal lesions [36, 37]. For this reason, a methodical approach is mandatory when facing with a failure of an ACL reconstruction in order to identify and correct the potential causes.

Even though the etiology of a graft failure can be multifactorial, several studies analyzed predisposing factors, identifying intrinsic and extrinsic risk factors. Considering extrinsic factors, technical errors are among the most common causes of failure [36, 38], with several studies reporting rates of 24–64% [39]. Technical errors include tunnel malposition, in particular the femoral one, advocated to be the primary cause of failure in 45–79% of the patients [39]; diagnostic errors, in which an injury to a secondary or tertiary restraint is not diagnosed, reported in more than 15% of failures [34]; and also graft fixation and/or graft tension.

Graft choice and size are not considered technical errors; nonetheless, they play an important role in ACL reconstruction success. The use of irradiated allograft, indeed, is associated with more than four times greater risk of failure compared to autograft [40, 41]; a graft diameter of 8 mm or less is correlated with an increased risk of re-tear [42–45]. Rehabilitation programs could also represent a risk factor for ACL graft failure. An early and aggressive rehabilitation may load excessively the graft, inducing a plastic deformity and lengthening. In the same way, the presence of a dynamic valgus, an imbalance in strength, and pre-activation between the hamstring and quadriceps muscle groups and an altered core proprioception and stability with poor repositioning of the trunk, due to an inappropriate rehabilitation program, increase the risk of ACL re-tear when the athletes return on the field [46].

Among intrinsic factors, age represents an important risk factor for re-tear since patients <21 years of age have an eightfold increase in re-tear risk compared to older patients [47]. In the same way, the presence of generalized joint laxity and joint-specific laxity with knee hyperextension are considered important risk factors for ACL re-tear [48]. Taking into account bony structures, the presence of a narrower intercondylar notch, a smaller notch-width index, and the presence of an A-shape notch are well-known risk factors for ACL graft tear.

In the last 20 years, particular attention has been paid to PTS as a possible risk factor for ACL tear and re-tear. Several studies and meta-analysis reported higher values of PTS to be linked with a higher risk for ACL tear and re-tear [10, 11, 49–52]. Both medial and lateral posterior inclinations of the tibial plateau are associated with an increased risk of graft failure. Particularly, a steeper medial PTS seems to be responsible for an increased static and dynamic ATT [9, 19], whereas a higher lateral tibia plateau slope is related to an increased rotatory instability [53, 54].

6.4.1 Biomechanical Effects

A correlation between PTS and ACL injury was reported in veterinarian literature where anterior closing-wedge osteotomies have been used to treat anterior knee laxity in dogs since the 1980s [55, 56].

Shifting these concepts to human knees, several biomechanical studies were conducted analyzing the effects of PTS on sagittal instability. PTS is indeed responsible for ATT, when a compressive load or quadriceps muscle force is applied to the tibiofemoral joint [21]. Therefore, an increased PTS exacerbates ATT, altering knee kinematics and modifying the distribution of contact pressures [57].

In the early 1990s, Dejour and Bonnin [19] observed that a 10° increase in PTS resulted in a 6-mm increase in ATT in both normal and ACL-deficient knees, during monopodal stance. Subsequently, in 2003 Liu and Maitland recorded an increase in ATT during walking after increasing the PTS from 4° to 12°, using a two-dimensional mathematical knee model [58]. Similarly, Shelburne et al. [59] in a computer model showed that increasing PTS, a nearly linear increase in anteriorly directed shear forces and ATT in activities of daily living (standing, squatting, and walking), is registered. In a cadaveric study, Giffin et al. [60] observed an anterior shift of the tibial resting position after a 5-mm anterior-opening-wedge tibia osteotomy. Likewise, Agneskirchner et al. evaluated knee joint kinematics after an anterior-opening-wedge osteotomy of the proximal tibia. The authors reported that as the PTS becomes steeper, the ATT becomes larger concluding that a higher PTS led to an increase in the anterior translation [57].

A more anterior position of the tibia relative to the femur should also increase strain on the ACL [4]. However, studies analyzing the effects of PTS-modifying osteotomies on ACL produce inconsistent and conflicting results. Several authors [60–63] were not able to identify higher values of ACL in situ forces when the PTS was increased via a tibia osteotomy. On the other hand, Shelburne et al. [59] reported a correlation between ACL strain and PTS during standing and walking, predicting a 26% increase in ACL force when the PTS was increased by 5° relative to the nominal value. Similarly, McLean et al. in a dynamic cadaver simulation of single-leg landing recorded a peak anteromedial ACL bundle strain to correlate with peak anterior tibial acceleration and with PTS. Specifically, for every 1° increase in PTS, the peak anterior tibial acceleration increased by 1.11 m/s^2, and the anteromedial bundle strain increased by 0.6% [64]. Recently, Bernhardson et al. [65] conducted a study on ten fresh-frozen cadaveric knees analyzing the effects of altering PTS on ACL forces, concluding that increased PTS had a linear correlation with ACL graft force when the knee was axially loaded. Analogous results were obtained also by Yamaguchi et al., who observed a significant reduction in ACL forces and ATT after a PTS-reducing osteotomy of the proximal tibia [66].

6.4.2   Indications and Contraindications for Tibial Deflexion Osteotomy

The ideal indications for an anterior closing-wedge high tibial deflexion osteotomy are knees with anterior instability, requiring second or third ACL revision surgery, presenting a PTS angle more than 12° [67, 68].

This procedure is contraindicated in case of hyperextension of the knee (>10°), multiligamentous knee injury, varus deformity greater than 5°, and grade IV bicompartmental osteoarthritis according to Kellgren and Lawrence [69, 70].

6.4.3   Clinical Results

In literature, the outcomes of deflexion osteotomy associated with ACL revision surgery are reported by few studies. These papers present several limitations such as small samples and short-term follow-up. However, reports of different techniques achieving good results in terms of knee stability and return to normal activities are encouraging [67, 70, 71].

Dejour et al. observed a series of 22 knees with chronic anterior instability correlated with an excessive PTS (average 16.5°). In this sample, there were 4 isolated tibial deflexion osteotomies and 18 osteotomies associated with ACL revision. The authors reported better clinical results in the latter group. Moreover, PTS was corrected to an average of 7° postoperatively, and the ATT in monopodal stance decreased from 12.5 mm preoperatively to 3 mm at last follow-up [71].

Sonnery-Cottet et al. reported the results of tibial deflexion osteotomy combined with tibial tubercle osteotomy and second revision ACL in five patients presenting increased PTS. The authors observed a PTS reduction from an average 13.6° preoperatively to 9.2° postoperatively, and the average differential anterior laxity decreased from 10.4 to 2.8 mm. At a mean follow-up of 31.6 months, all patients presented stable knee with good clinical outcomes at Lysholm and IKDC. Moreover, patients returned to their previous sport activity level and no re-ruptures were recorded [70]. Finally, Dejour et al. reported nine patients in which a second revision ACL reconstruction was performed with tibial deflexion osteotomy (Fig. 6.4). At a mean follow-up of 2 years, all the cases had stable knees with full range of motion, good clinical outcomes at Lysholm score, and healed osteotomies at X-ray. Moreover, the subjective patient satisfaction was excellent in four patients, good in

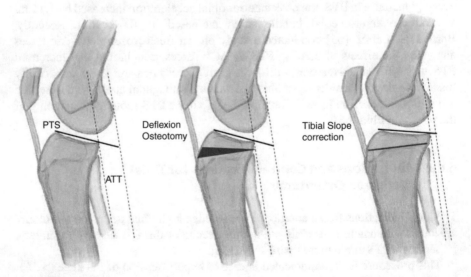

Fig. 6.4 Schematic draw of the deflexion osteotomy which corrects the posterior tibial slope (PTS) and therefore diminishes the shear forces experienced by the ACL

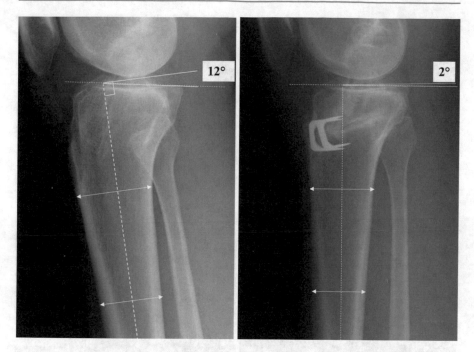

Fig. 6.5 Correction of the PTS after deflexion osteotomy: from 12° preoperatively (left) to 2° after the osteotomy (right)

three patients, and fair in two. From a radiological point of view, PTS decreased from 13.2° preoperatively to 4.4° postoperatively (Fig. 6.5) with a mean side-to-side anterior tibial translation decreased from 11.7 ± 5.2 mm preoperatively to 4.3 ± 2.5 mm postoperatively [67] (Fig. 6.6).

6.5   Flexion (Antirecurvatum) Osteotomy

Sagittal knee imbalance could also be found in hyperextended knees. Constitutional genu recurvatum is considered physiological when hyperextension of the tibia on the femur affects both knees and it is less than 15°. However, genu recurvatum is considered pathological when it is asymmetrical and acquired.

Three possible patterns are described in the literature, based on bony deformity and/or soft tissue involvement [18]:

- *Genu recurvatum with alterations of the bony elements*: in this condition, the deformity is purely osseous, and it is most commonly located in the tibial metaphysis with an inversion of the normal PTS. More rarely the lateral femoral condyle may be hypoplastic.
- *Genu recurvatum with stretching of the soft tissue elements*: this condition can be post-traumatic or a consequence of gradual stretching of the posterior structure;

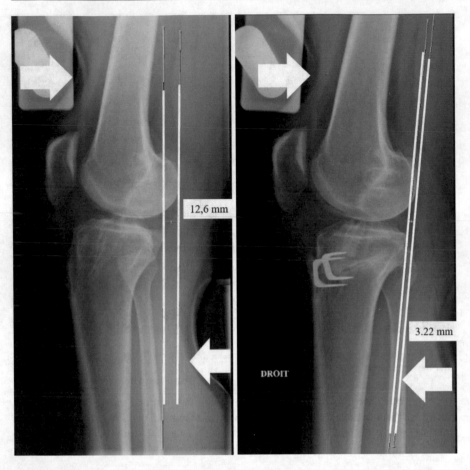

Fig. 6.6 Correction of the "dynamic" ATT with the ACL revision combined with the deflexion osteotomy: from 12,6 mm preoperatively (left) to 3,22 mm postoperatively (right)

moreover, this condition could be global, involving all the posterior soft tissues, or asymmetrical, causing posterolateral instability.

- *Genu recurvatum with bony and soft tissue alterations (mixed type)*: in this case, the original problem is a structural problem in the bony elements followed by gradual soft tissue stretching (poliomyelitis).

Genu recurvatum is a debilitating condition since the joint is very unstable. Active locking of the knee is impaired, limiting sports and also activities of daily living such as walking on uneven ground. This condition weakens not only the tibiofemoral compartment but also the patellofemoral joint; the patellofemoral lever arm is therefore abolished, compromising quadriceps function, whose contraction tends to exacerbate the recurvatum deformity. As a consequence, quadriceps muscle tends to atrophy and patients develop anterior knee pain. Moreover, recurvatum produces a pseudopatella alta and poor engagement with the trochlea, though this phenomenon is counterintuitive because gait requires knee flexion, and the patella engages beyond 20° of flexion [18, 72].

6.5.1   Biomechanical Effects

Variations of the PTS influence not only the ATT and ACL strain but also the posterior tibial translation and the forces acting on the PCL during both static and dynamic conditions.

In PCL-deficient knees, the tibia sags posteriorly at high flexion angles, where the PCL is most functional [73]. Agneskirchner et al. [57] showed that with a 5° increase in the anatomical slope, posterior tibial translation (PTT) after PCL section was completely neutralized and even turned into slight anterior translation. This was confirmed by Giffin et al. [60] who found that increases of 4–5° in PTS in a normal knee result in a ATT during resting position of 2–3 mm, which increases under axial compressive loads. Similarly, Petrigliano et al. [74] found that in PCL- and PLC-deficient knee, an increase of PTS by 5° via osteotomy determines a significant reduction in medial compartment PTT during posterior drawer test, whereas decreasing it by 5° significantly increases medial compartment PTT during both posterior drawer test and reverse pivot shift.

Only few studies analyzed PCL behavior in relation to variation of PTS. Shelburne et al. [59] with a computer model of the lower limb predicted an 11% decrease in PCL force and a 38% decrease in PLC force during squatting activity, when PTS was increased by 5°. In a biomechanical study conducted on seven fresh-frozen cadaver knees, Singerman et al. [75] showed a significant increase in PCL strain while decreasing PTS from 10° to 5°. Similarly, Bernhardson et al. [76] in ten fresh-frozen knee specimens found that PCL in situ forces decrease as the PTS becomes flat both in unloaded and loaded states. These results confirmed those obtained in a clinical study where the authors concluded that a decreased PTS represents a risk factor for PCL tear, since a leveled PTS of approximately <6° may increase PCL strain and lead to a higher rate of PCL injury [77].

6.5.2   Indications for Flexion Osteotomies

The two main indications for a PTS-increasing osteotomy are represented by pathological knee recurvatum and posterior or posterolateral instability of the knee.

In the former indication, the surgical correction is based on the clinical evidence of an asymmetric recurvatum deformity exceeding 15° associated with knee instability in single-leg stance and corroborated by a careful radiographic analysis (PTS, ATT).

In the latter one, since PCL anatomical reconstructions have been unable to restore resting position or PTT to the intact position [78], flexion osteotomy could be a good solution in the treatment of isolated PCL or combined PCL/PLC injuries in patients with a PTS < 6°.

6.5.3   Clinical Studies of Antirecurvatum Osteotomies

The literature includes few studies reporting outcomes of antirecurvatum osteotomies.

The first publication concerning the correction of genu recurvatum is attributed to Lecuire et al. [72] who reported the results of anterior-opening-wedge tibial osteotomy associated with a tibial tubercle detachment reporting very satisfactory results in patients with purely osseous deformity and suggesting to associate a capsular repair in case of mixed type.

On the other hand, Bowen et al. [12] reported very good result with a closing-wedge osteotomy in the treatment of genu recurvatum from premature physeal closure. The authors suggested to use a closing-wedge tibial osteotomy because of its stability, rapid healing, and ability to alleviate retropatellar compression by displacing the TT anteriorly.

Contrary to the results published by Bowen et al., in 1986, Vicenzi et al. [79] concluded that anterior-opening wedge with detachment of tibial tuberosity was the surgical procedure with the best results in the treatment of purely osseous genu recurvatum, whereas the poor results obtained in mixed type suggested the addition of a reconstruction of the posterior capsule.

Consistent with the results published in their previous study, Moroni et al. observed excellent or good clinical outcomes in 86% of patients with osseous deformities, whereas patients without purely osseous deformity had a relative risk of fair or poor results 13 times higher. The risk of less satisfactory results was 36 times higher when an antirecurvatum osteotomy was performed distal to the tibial tuberosity because of an abnormal anterior prominence at the tibial diaphysis and a less satisfactory correction [80].

Similarly, Balestro et al. [81] reported a 92% of satisfaction rate of an anterior-opening-wedge tibial osteotomy associated with a tibial tubercle osteotomy in the treatment of genu recurvatum. Consistent with the previous studies, best results were obtained when a purely osseous deformity was present. Furthermore, Jung et al. reported in three cases of mixed-type genu recurvatum the inability to completely address the posterior sagittal instability only with a PTS-increasing osteotomy and the need to add a PCL and/or PLC reconstruction to restore the sagittal balance of the knee [82].

Van Raaij et al. [83] proposed an anterior-opening-wedge osteotomy of the proximal tibia to treat anterior knee pain in knees with idiopathic hyperextension. The authors supposed that the osteotomy could end the repetitive impingement by readdressing knee extension. Excellent overall functional results were reported in 83% of patients, with a 9.4° increase in PTS and a corresponding decrease in patellar height according to Blackburne-Peel method. In 2017, Kim et al. [84] reported good and excellent results in five patients treated with an oblique anterior-opening-wedge osteotomy at the level of the anterior tibial tuberosity, obtaining an accurate correction of the PTS, maintenance of patellar height, and an improvement of posterior instability.

6.6   Conclusions

Sagittal imbalance is an important consideration in knee pathology. Abnormal values of PTS have been recognized, among bony alterations, as one of the most important causes of sagittal instability. Therefore, these anatomical impairments have to be identified and addressed since different techniques of sagittal osteotomies offer effective treatments for certain indications and should be considered as adjuvant or principal procedures for unstable knees with ligament lesions.

References

1. Grood ES, Stowers SF, Noyes FR. Limits of movement in the human knee. Effect of sectioning the posterior cruciate ligament and posterolateral structures. J Bone Joint Surg Am. 1988;70(1):88–97.
2. Castle TH Jr, Noyes FR, Grood ES. Posterior tibial subluxation of the posterior cruciate-deficient knee. Clin Orthop Relat Res. 1992;284:193–202.
3. Logan M, Williams A, Lavelle J, Gedroyc W, Freeman M. The effect of posterior cruciate ligament deficiency on knee kinematics. Am J Sports Med. 2004;32(8):1915–22.
4. Butler DL, Noyes FR, Grood ES. Ligamentous restraints to anterior-posterior drawer in the human knee: a biomechanical study. J Bone Joint Surg Am. 1980;62(2):259–70.
5. Brandon ML, Haynes PT, Bonamo JR, Flynn MI, Barrett GR, Sherman MF. The association between posterior-inferior tibial slope and anterior cruciate ligament insufficiency. Arthroscopy. 2006;22(8):894–9.
6. Hashemi J, Chandrashekar N, Mansouri H, Gill B, Slauterbeck JR, Schutt RC Jr, Dabezies E, Beynnon BD. Shallow medial tibial plateau and steep medial and lateral tibial slopes: new risk factors for anterior cruciate ligament injuries. Am J Sports Med. 2010;38(1):54–62.
7. Alentorn-Geli E, Mendiguchia J, Samuelsson K, Musahl V, Karlsson J, Cugat R, Myer GD. Prevention of non-contact anterior cruciate ligament injuries in sports. Part I: Systematic review of the systematic review of risk factors in male athletes. Knee Surg Sports Traumatol Arthrosc. 2014;22(1):3–15.
8. Zeng C, Yang T, Wu S, Gao SG, Li H, Deng ZH, Zhang Y, Lei GH. Is posterior tibial slope associated with noncontact anterior cruciate ligament injury? Knee Surg Sports Traumatol Arthrosc. 2016;24(3):830–7.
9. Dejour D, Pungitore M, Valluy J, Nover L, Saffarini M, Demey G. Preoperative laxity in ACL-deficient knees increases with posterior tibial slope and medial meniscal tears. Knee Surg Sports Traumatol Arthrosc. 2019;27(2):564–72.
10. Lee CC, Youm YS, Cho SD, Jung SH, Bae MH, Park SJ, Kim HW. Does posterior tibial slope affect graft rupture following anterior cruciate ligament reconstruction? Arthroscopy. 2018;34(7):2152–5.
11. Song GY, Zhang H, Zhang J, Liu X, Xue Z, Qian Y, Feng H. Greater static anterior tibial subluxation of the lateral compartment after an acute anterior cruciate ligament injury is associated with an increased posterior tibial slope. Am J Sports Med. 2018;46(7):1617–23.
12. Bowen JR, Morley DC, McInerny V, MacEwen GD. Treatment of genu recurvatum by proximal tibial closing-wedge/anterior displacement osteotomy. Clin Orthop Relat Res. 1983;(179):194–9.
13. Fielding JW, Liebler WA, Krishne Urs ND, Wilson SA, Puglisi AS. Tibial tubercle transfer: a long-range follow-up study. Clin Orthop Relat Res. 1979;(144):43–4.
14. Jeffreys TE. Genu recurvatum after Osgood-Schlatter's disease; report of a case. J Bone Joint Surg Br. 1965;47:298–9.

15. Bjerkreim I, Benum P. Genu recurvatum: a late complication of tibial wire traction in fractures of the femur in children. Acta Orthop Scand. 1975;46:1012–9.
16. Rainault JJ. Le recurvatum grave du genou poliomyélitique. Rev Chir Orthop. 1962:561–77.
17. Bonin N, Ait Si Selmi T, Dejour D, Neyret P. Knee para-articular flexion and extension osteotomies in adults. Orthopade. 2004;33:193–200.
18. Dejour D, Bonin N, Locatelli E. Tibial antirecurvatum osteotomies. Oper Techn in Sport Med. 2000;8:67–70.
19. Dejour H, Bonnin M. Tibial translation after anterior cruciate ligament rupture. Two radiological tests compared. J Bone Joint Surg Br. 1994;76:745–9.
20. Brazier J, Migaud H, Gougeon F, Cotten A, Fontaine C, Duquennoy A. Evaluation of methods for radiographic measurement of the tibial slope. A study of 83 healthy knees. Rev Chir Orthop Reparatrice Appar Mot. 1996;82:195–200.
21. Feucht MJ, Mauro CS, Brucker PU, Imhoff AB, Hinterwimmer S. The role of the tibial slope in sustaining and treating anterior cruciate ligament injuries. Knee Surg Sports Traumatol Arthrosc. 2013;21:134–45.
22. Hashemi J, Chandrashekar N, Gill B, et al. A critical look at the geometry of the tibial plateau and its influence on the biomechanics of the tibiofemoral joint. J Bone Joint Surg Am. 2008;90(12):2724–34.
23. Hudek R, Schmutz S, Regenfelder F, Fuchs B, Koch PP. Novel measurement technique of the tibial slope on conventional MRI. Clin Orthop Relat Res. 2009;467(8):2066–72.
24. Utzschneider S, Goettinger M, Weber P, Horng A, Glaser C, Jansson V, Müller PE. Development and validation of a new method for the radiologic measurement of the tibial slope. Knee Surg Sports Traumatol Arthrosc. 2011;19(10):1643–8.
25. Hudek R, Fuchs B, Regenfelder F, Koch PP. Is noncontact ACL injury associated with the posterior tibial and meniscal slope? Clin Orthop Relat Res. 2011;469:2377–84.
26. Cinotti G, Sessa P, Ragusa G, Ripani FR, Postacchini R, Masciangelo R, Giannicola G. Influence of cartilage and menisci on the sagittal slope of the tibial plateaus. Clin Anat. 2013;26(7):883–92.
27. Lustig S, Scholes CJ, Leo SP, Coolican M, Parker DA. Influence of soft tissues on the proximal bony tibial slope measured with two-dimensional MRI. Knee Surg Sports Traumatol Arthrosc. 2013;21:372–9.
28. Jenny JY, Rapp E, Kehr P. Proximal tibial meniscal slope: a comparison with the bone slope. Rev Chir Orthop Reparatrice Appar Mot. 1997;83(5):435–8.
29. Muhr G. Meniscus and instability. Langenbecks Arch Chir. 1987;372:259–61.
30. Panisset JC, Ntagiopoulos PG, Saggin PR, Dejour D. A comparison of Telos™ stress radiography versus Rolimeter™ in the diagnosis of different patterns of anterior cruciate ligament tears. Orthop Traumatol Surg Res. 2012;98(7):751–8.
31. James EW, Williams BT, LaPrade RF. Stress radiography for the diagnosis of knee ligament injuries: a systematic review. Clin Orthop Relat Res. 2014;472(9):2644–57.
32. Pache S, Aman ZS, Kennedy M, Nakama GY, Moatshe G, Ziegler C, LaPrade RF. Posterior cruciate ligament: current concepts review. Arch Bone Jt Surg. 2018;6(1):8–18.
33. Gans I, Retzky JS, Jones LC, Tanaka MJ. Epidemiology of recurrent anterior cruciate ligament injuries in National Collegiate Athletic Association Sports: the injury surveillance program, 2004–2014. Orthop J Sports Med. 2018;6(6):2325967118777823.
34. Samitier G, Marcano AI, Alentorn-Geli E, Cugat R, Farmer KW, Moser MW. Failure of anterior cruciate ligament reconstruction. Arch Bone Jt Surg. 2015;3(4):220–40. Review.
35. Allen MM, Pareek A, Krych AJ, Hewett TE, Levy BA, Stuart MJ, Dahm DL. Are female soccer players at an increased risk of second anterior cruciate ligament injury compared with their athletic peers? Am J Sports Med. 2016;44(10):2492–8.
36. MARS Group, Wright RW, Huston LJ, Spindler KP, Dunn WR, Haas AK, Allen CR, Cooper DE, DeBerardino TM, Lantz BB, Mann BJ, Stuart MJ. Descriptive epidemiology of the multicenter ACL revision study (MARS) cohort. Am J Sports Med. 2010;38(10):1979–86.
37. Borchers JR, Kaeding CC, Pedroza AD, Huston LJ, Spindler KP, Wright RW, MOON Consortium and the MARS Group. Intra-articular findings in primary and revision anterior

cruciate ligament reconstruction surgery: a comparison of the MOON and MARS study groups. Am J Sports Med. 2011;39(9):1889–93.

38. Trojani C, Sbihi A, Djian P, Potel JF, Hulet C, Jouve F, Bussière C, Ehkirch FP, Burdin G, Dubrana F, Beaufils P, Franceschi JP, Chassaing V, Colombet P, Neyret P. Causes for failure of ACL reconstruction and influence of meniscectomies after revision. Knee Surg Sports Traumatol Arthrosc. 2011;19(2):196–201.

39. Morgan JA, Dahm D, Levy B, Stuart MJ, MARS Study Group. Femoral tunnel malposition in ACL revision reconstruction. J Knee Surg. 2012;25(5):361–8.

40. Kaeding CC, Pedroza AD, Reinke EK, Huston LJ, MOON Consortium, Spindler KP. Risk factors and predictors of subsequent ACL injury in either knee after ACL reconstruction: prospective analysis of 2488 primary ACL reconstructions from the MOON cohort. Am J Sports Med. 2015;43(7):1583–90.

41. Engelman GH, Carry PM, Hitt KG, Polousky JD, Vidal AF. Comparison of allograft versus autograft anterior cruciate ligament reconstruction graft survival in an active adolescent cohort. Am J Sports Med. 2014;42(10):2311–8.

42. Magnussen RA, Lawrence JT, West RL, Toth AP, Taylor DC, Garrett WE. Graft size and patient age are predictors of early revision after anterior cruciate ligament reconstruction with hamstring autograft. Arthroscopy. 2012;28(4):526–31.

43. Mariscalco MW, Flanigan DC, Mitchell J, Pedroza AD, Jones MH, Andrish JT, Parker RD, Kaeding CC, Magnussen RA. The influence of hamstring autograft size on patient-reported outcomes and risk of revision after anterior cruciate ligament reconstruction: a Multicenter Orthopaedic Outcomes Network (MOON) Cohort Study. Arthroscopy. 2013;29(12):1948–53.

44. Conte EJ, Hyatt AE, Gatt CJ Jr, Dhawan A. Hamstring autograft size can be predicted and is a potential risk factor for anterior cruciate ligament reconstruction failure. Arthroscopy. 2014;30(7):882–90.

45. Snaebjörnsson T, Hamrin Senorski E, Ayeni OR, Alentorn-Geli E, Krupic F, Norberg F, Karlsson J, Samuelsson K. Graft diameter as a predictor for revision anterior cruciate ligament reconstruction and KOOS and EQ-5D values: a cohort study from the Swedish National Knee Ligament Register based on 2240 patients. Am J Sports Med. 2017;45(9):2092–7.

46. Acevedo RJ, Rivera-Vega A, Miranda G, Micheo W. Anterior cruciate ligament injury: identification of risk factors and prevention strategies. Curr Sports Med Rep. 2014;13(3):186–91.

47. Maletis GB, Chen J, Inacio MC, Funahashi TT. Age-related risk factors for revision anterior cruciate ligament reconstruction: a cohort study of 21,304 patients from the Kaiser Permanente Anterior Cruciate Ligament Registry. Am J Sports Med. 2016;44(2):331–6.

48. Kim SJ, Kumar P, Kim SH. Anterior cruciate ligament reconstruction in patients with generalized joint laxity. Clin Orthop Surg. 2010;2(3):130–9.

49. Andrade R, Vasta S, Sevivas N, Pereira R, Leal A, Papalia R, Pereira H, Espregueira-Mendes J. Notch morphology is a risk factor for ACL injury: a systematic review and meta-analysis. J ISAKOS. 2016;1:70–81.

50. Salmon LJ, Heath E, Akrawi H, Roe JP, Linklater J, Pinczewski LA. 20-Year outcomes of anterior cruciate ligament reconstruction with hamstring tendon autograft: the catastrophic effect of age and posterior tibial slope. Am J Sports Med. 2018 Mar;46(3):531–43.

51. Lansdown D, Ma CB. The influence of tibial and femoral bone morphology on knee kinematics in the anterior cruciate ligament injured knee. Clin Sports Med. 2018;37(1):127–36.

52. Wordeman SC, Quatman CE, Kaeding CC, Hewett TE. In vivo evidence for tibial plateau slope as a risk factor for anterior cruciate ligament injury: a systematic review and meta-analysis. Am J Sports Med. 2012;40(7):1673–81.

53. Rahnemai-Azar AA, Abebe ES, Johnson P, Labrum J, Fu FH, Irrgang JJ, Samuelsson K, Musahl V. Increased lateral tibial slope predicts high-grade rotatory knee laxity pre-operatively in ACL reconstruction. Knee Surg Sports Traumatol Arthrosc. 2017;25(4):1170–6.

54. Burnham JM, Pfeiffer T, Shin JJ, Herbst E, Fu FH. Bony morphologic factors affecting injury risk, rotatory stability, outcomes, and re-tear rate after anterior cruciate ligament reconstruction. Ann Joint. 2017;2:44.

55. Kim SE, Pozzi A, Kowaleski MP, Lewis DD. Tibial osteotomies for cranial cruciate ligament insufficiency in dogs. Vet Surg. 2008;37(2):111–25.
56. Slocum B, Devine T. Cranial tibial wedge osteotomy: a technique for eliminating cranial tibial thrust in cranial cruciate ligament repair. J Am Vet Med Assoc. 1984;184:564–9.
57. Agneskirchner JD, Hurschler C, Stukenborg-Colsman C, Imhoff AB, Lobenhoffer P. Effect of high tibial flexion osteotomy on cartilage pressure and joint kinematics: a biomechanical study in human cadaveric knees. Winner of the AGA-DonJoy Award 2004. Arch Orthop Trauma Surg. 2004;124:575–84.
58. Liu W, Maitland ME. Influence of anthropometric and mechanical variations on functional instability in the ACL-deficient knee. Ann Biomed Eng. 2003;31(10):1153–61.
59. Shelburne KB, Kim HJ, Sterett WI, Pandy MG. Effect of posterior tibial slope on knee biomechanics during functional activity. J Orthop Res. 2011;29:223–31.
60. Giffin JR, Vogrin TM, Zantop T, Woo SL, Harner CD. Effects of increasing tibial slope on the biomechanics of the knee. Am J Sports Med. 2004;32:376–82.
61. Fening SD, Kovacic J, Kambic H, McLean S, Scott J, Miniaci A. The effects of modified posterior tibial slope on anterior cruciate ligament strain and knee kinematics: a human cadaveric study. J Knee Surg. 2008;21:205–11.
62. Martineau PA, Fening SD, Miniaci A. Anterior opening wedge high tibial osteotomy: the effect of increasing posterior tibial slope on ligament strain. Can J Surg. 2010;53:261–7.
63. Nelitz M, Seitz AM, Bauer J, Reichel H, Ignatius A, Durselen L. Increasing posterior tibial slope does not raise anterior cruciate ligament strain but decreases tibial rotation ability. Clin Biomech (Bristol, Avon). 2013;28:285–90.
64. McLean SG, Oh YK, Palmer ML, Lucey SM, Lucarelli DG, Ashton-Miller JA, et al. The relationship between anterior tibial acceleration, tibial slope, and ACL strain during a simulated jump landing task. J Bone Joint Surg Am. 2011;93:1310–7.
65. Bernhardson AS, Aman ZS, Dornan GJ, Kemler BR, Storaci HW, Brady AW, Nakama GY, LaPrade RF. Tibial slope and its effect on force in anterior cruciate ligament grafts: anterior cruciate ligament force increases linearly as posterior tibial slope increases. Am J Sports Med. 2019;47(2):296–302.
66. Yamaguchi KT, Cheung EC, Markolf KL, Boguszewski DV, Mathew J, Lama CJ, McAllister DR, Petrigliano FA. Effects of anterior closing wedge tibial osteotomy on anterior cruciate ligament force and knee kinematics. Am J Sports Med. 2018;46(2):370–7.
67. Dejour D, Saffarini M, Demey G, Baverel L. Tibial slope correction combined with second revision ACL produces good knee stability and prevents graft rupture. Knee Surg Sports Traumatol Arthrosc. 2015;23(10):2846–52.
68. Dejour D, La Barbera G, Pasqualotto S, Valoroso M, Nover L, Reynolds R, Saffarini M. Sagittal plane corrections around the knee. J Knee Surg. 2017;30(8):736–45.
69. Hees T, Petersen W. Anterior closing-wedge osteotomy for posterior slope correction. Arthrosc Tech. 2018;7(11):e1079–87.
70. Sonnery-Cottet B, Mogos S, Thaunat M, et al. Proximal tibial anterior closing wedge osteotomy in repeat revision of anterior cruciate ligament reconstruction. Am J Sports Med. 2014;42(8):1873–80.
71. Dejour D, Kuhn A, Dejour H. Tibial deflexion osteotomy and chronic anterior laxity: a series of 22 cases. Rev Chir Orthop Reparatrice Appar Mot. 1998;84(02):28–9.
72. Lecuire F, Lerat JL, Bousquet G, Dejour H, Trillat A. The treatment of genu recurvatum (author's transl). Rev Chir Orthop Reparatrice Appar Mot. 1980;66:95–103.
73. Giffin JR, Stabile KJ, Zantop T, Vogrin TM, Woo SL, Harner CD. Importance of tibial slope for stability of the posterior cruciate ligament deficient knee. Am J Sports Med. 2007;35:1443–9.
74. Petrigliano FA, Suero EM, Voos JE, Pearle AD, Allen AA. The effect of proximal tibial slope on dynamic stability testing of the posterior cruciate ligament- and posterolateral corner-deficient knee. Am J Sports Med. 2012;40:1322–8.
75. Singerman R, Dean JC, Pagan HD, Goldberg VM. Decreased posterior tibial slope increases strain in the posterior cruciate ligament following total knee arthroplasty. J Arthroplasty. 1996;11(1):99–103.

76. Bernhardson AS, Aman ZS, DePhillipo NN, Dornan GJ, Storaci HW, Brady AW, Nakama G, LaPrade RF. Tibial slope and its effect on graft force in posterior cruciate ligament reconstructions. Am J Sports Med. 2019;47(5):1168–74.
77. Bernhardson AS, DePhillipo NN, Daney BT, Kennedy MI, Aman ZS, LaPrade RF. Posterior tibial slope and risk of posterior cruciate ligament injury. Am J Sports Med. 2019;47(2):312–7.
78. Gwinner C, Weiler A, Roider M, Schaefer FM, Jung TM. Tibial slope strongly influences knee stability after posterior cruciate ligament reconstruction: a prospective 5- to 15-year follow-up. Am J Sports Med. 2017;45(2):355–61.
79. Vicenzi G, Moroni A, Ceccarelli F, Binazzi R, Vaccari V. Tibial osteotomy in the treatment of genu recurvatum in the adult. Ital J Orthop Traumatol. 1986;12(4):427–32.
80. Moroni A, Pezzuto V, Pompili M, Zinghi G. Proximal osteotomy of the tibia for the treatment of genu recurvatum in adults. J Bone Joint Surg Am. 1992;74:577–86.
81. Balestro J, Lustig S, Servien E. Anterior opening wedge osteotomy of the tibia assessment for the treatment of genu recurvatum. Société Française de Chirurgie Orthopédique et Traumatologique. 2008.
82. Jung YB, Lee YS, Jung HJ, Nam CH, Yang JJ. Correction of bony genu recurvatum combined with ligamentous instability of the knee: three case reports. Knee Surg Sports Traumatol Arthrosc. 2008;16(2):185–7.
83. van Raaij TM, de Waal Malefijt J. Anterior opening wedge osteotomy of the proximal tibia for anterior knee pain in idiopathic hyperextension knees. Int Orthop. 2006;30:248–52.
84. Kim TW, Lee S, Yoon JR, Han HS, Lee MC. Proximal tibial anterior open-wedge oblique osteotomy: a novel technique to correct genu recurvatum. Knee. 2017;24(02):345–53.

Outcomes of Surgery for Coronal Instability

Robert Duerr and Robert A. Magnussen

7.1 Introduction

Chronic instability of the knee can pose a difficult challenge for both patients and orthopedic surgeons because multiple factors contribute to the restoration of a stable, functional joint. Patients with long-standing ligamentous laxity may develop progressively worsening degenerative changes that can lead to bony deformity and malalignment of the lower extremity, further exacerbating the initial instability. Additionally, patients with underlying malalignment may be at increased risk for overload syndromes, arthritis, and failure after ligament reconstruction alone. Recognizing and appropriately treating malalignment in combination with knee instability is an important step toward a successful outcome. While there is extensive literature evaluating the use of osteotomies for the treatment of osteoarthritis, there are limited reports on the functional outcomes after osteotomy for instability [1]. The purpose of this chapter is to discuss the role for osteotomies in the treatment of patients with coronal plane knee instability and review surgical outcomes.

7.2 Limb Alignment

It is first important to understand normal limb alignment and how it is assessed for preoperative planning. Limb alignment is measured on full-length standing anteroposterior (AP) radiographs of the entire lower limb, centered at the knee. The surgeon needs to be aware of the limitations of this technique, especially in patients with ligament injury or instability that may not allow them to bear full weight. Foot position and limb rotation can also affect coronal plane alignment, and orthopedists

R. Duerr · R. A. Magnussen (✉)
Department of Orthopaedics, OSU Sports Medicine Research Institute, The Ohio State University, Columbus, OH, USA
e-mail: robert.duerr@osumc.edu

© Springer Nature Switzerland AG 2020
S. Oussedik, S. Lustig (eds.), *Osteotomy About the Knee*,
https://doi.org/10.1007/978-3-030-49055-3_7

should consider standardizing the technique to obtain these images, as previously described [2]. The hip-knee-ankle (HKA) angle or mechanical axis of the limb is the most commonly referenced value for coronal plane alignment. Normal is generally considered within 3° of neutral. A recent review of 250 asymptomatic volunteers demonstrated 32% of males, and 17% of females were in constitutional varus (>3° of varus) [3]. Tibial slope is also an important factor in managing these patients, and an appropriate lateral knee X-ray should be obtained to assess slope. The effects and treatment of abnormal tibial slope and sagittal plane instability are addressed elsewhere in this book.

While constitutional varus or valgus is not itself a pathologic condition, it may predispose patients to further problems when a significant ligamentous injury occurs. These injuries often lead to worsening clinical symptoms of instability as the neural ligamentous input and proprioception is lost, leading to poor dynamic control, which over time may exacerbate the malalignment [4, 5]. For example, lateral collateral ligament (LCL) or posterolateral corner (PLC) injuries can lead to varus thrust and eventual medial compartment degeneration and varus deformity [6, 7]. Similarly, medial collateral ligament (MCL) injury may lead to opening of the medial compartment and worsening valgus malalignment [8].

7.3   Lateral or Posterolateral Instability

The posterolateral corner (PLC), or posterolateral ligament complex, consists primarily of the lateral collateral ligament, popliteus tendon, and popliteofibular ligament. Secondary stabilizers include the lateral capsular thickening, coronary ligament, lateral gastrocnemius tendon, fabellofibular ligament, long head of the biceps femoris tendon, and the iliotibial band [9]. The PLC provides the primary restraint to varus forces at the knee and external rotation of the tibia relative to the femur. In cruciate-deficient knees, the PLC also functions as a secondary stabilizer to anterior and posterior tibial translation [9]. Instability of the PLC most often occurs as a result of acute trauma, such as a direct blow to the anteromedial knee or with a hyperextension-varus noncontact sports injury [10]. Unfortunately, these injuries can go undiagnosed, and patients present in the chronic setting with continued instability, hyperextension-varus thrust gait, and varus malalignment of the lower extremity. Valgus-producing high tibial osteotomy (HTO) is indicated in these patients prior to or in conjunction with any procedure to address the PLC, as any isolated ligament repair or reconstruction would be subject to increased stress and early failure [9–11].

Additionally, patients with chronic anterior cruciate ligament (ACL) deficiency can similarly present with a varus thrust gait and posterolateral instability and often require HTO to optimize outcomes [12]. Noyes et al. described several distinct situations in which secondary malalignment can occur due to chronic ACL instability: termed primary, double, and triple varus (Table 7.2) [12]. Following anterior cruciate ligament (ACL) rupture, there is increased anterior translation and internal rotation of the tibia which necessitates recruitment of secondary stabilizers (e.g., medial meniscus) and can lead to increased mean contact stress in the medial compartment [13]. Over time, patients with chronic ACL injury can develop varus deformity owing to progressive degeneration of the medial compartment, preexisting varus malalignment, and/or initial injury to the medial compartment cartilage or meniscus with medial compartment narrowing, termed "primary varus" [12]. In varus-angulated knees, the lateral collateral ligament (LCL) and lateral soft tissue restraints may become slack, allowing for increased lateral joint opening, known as "double varus." Further progression leads to hyperextension-varus recurvatum deformity as the popliteus and posterolateral capsule become deficient, which is termed "triple varus" [12]. Acute combined injury to the ACL and posterolateral corner with constitutional varus alignment can result in a situation similar to triple varus. Additional injury to the posterior cruciate ligament (PCL) further exacerbates the hyperextension and varus deformities [5]. In each of these situations, joint realignment provides bony stability to either treat the instability and/or augment ligamentous reconstruction and improve overall joint function and soft tissue balance [5].

Such cases, with posterolateral and combined instabilities, can be some of the most challenging for orthopedic surgeons. These patients are often relatively young and active and have had one or more previous surgical procedures. It is important to set realistic expectations for these patients, and most authors advocate a return to light recreational athletic activities only [14, 15]. Many of the studies include a nonhomogenous population with varying amounts of tibiofemoral arthritis, differences in the condition of the medial menisci, varying degrees of malalignment, and differences in the amount of lateral and posterolateral ligament deficiency [12]. It is important to have a methodical evaluation to diagnose all of the anatomic abnormalities and appropriately counsel each individual patient [12]. Additionally, patients often require preoperative rehabilitation due to gait abnormalities and muscular weakness or imbalance. Having a physician-therapist team approach is recommended to assist patients continually throughout the prolonged rehabilitation course to optimize patient outcomes [12]. For the purposes of this chapter, we will focus on reports describing outcomes of osteotomy in patients with posterolateral deficiencies and combined ACL with posterolateral deficiencies. The outcomes and complications from these studies are summarized in Tables 7.1 and 7.2.

In 2000, Noyes et al. [12] described their outcomes in a prospective evaluation of 23 patients with double varus and 18 with triple varus who underwent lateral closing-wedge HTO and either concurrent or staged ACL reconstruction. All patients with triple varus also underwent PLC reconstruction with either proximal advancement of the posterolateral complex (12 patients) or allograft reconstruction (6 patients). The majority of patients (32/41) sustained the original knee injury during sports, and all except two had undergone at least one operative procedure before the HTO. The time from the original injury to the HTO was a mean of 98 months (range: 4–255 months) and 48 months (range: 4–76 months) in the double varus and triple varus groups, respectively. The goal of the lateral closing-wedge HTO was to align the weight-bearing axis of the limb to pass through the 62% coordinate of the width of the tibial plateau. An osteotomy of the fibular neck was also performed.

Table 7.1 Summary of outcomes for treatment of lateral or posterolateral instability

Author(s), year	Mean follow-up (range)	Satisfaction	Patient reported outcome scores	Subjective instability	Coronal alignment	Laxity measurements	Return to sports	Conclusions
Noyes et al., 2000	4.5 years (2–12)	1 normal 14 very good 14 good 10 fair 2 poor	CKS Pre: 63 FU: 82	85% report elimination of giving way	33/41 acceptable- mean WB line 61% (47–75%) 2 slight varus (40–45%) 5 marked varus (16–38%) 1 excess valgus (81%)	ACLR: 19 functional 11 partial function 15 failure PLCR: 13 functional 4 partial function 1 failure	9 preop and 14 at last FU able to run without limitation 14 preop and 27 at last FU able to participate in sports—encouraged to return to light recreational activities only	All triple varus knees should have staged ACL/PLCR after HTO Double varus knees if >12 mm lateral opening performs staged ACLR
Badhe and Forster, 2002	2.8 years (0.5–5.5 years)	8 good 4 fair 2 poor	CKS Pre: 53 (40–58) FU: 74 (58–82)	Pre: 100% FU: 2/14 (14.3%)	Pre: −5° (−3 to −11°) FU: 6° (−4 to 11°)		93% participated in recreational activities, but no patients returned to competitive sports	Double varus knees treated successfully with simultaneous HTO and ACLR Triple varus knees did better with OWHTO vs. CWHTO OWHTO alone may be reasonable treatment for triple varus
Goradia and Van Allen, 2002	1.5 years	Excellent			Pre: slight varus FU: slight valgus	Pre: 5 mm of lateral opening with varus stress at 30° FU: normal	Patient resumed jogging and all recreational activities at 6 months	HTO alone can successfully treat isolated lateral instability with varus malalignment Use of a dynamic external fixator allowed them to "dial in" correction with serial postop radiographs

Study	FU	Satisfaction	Scores	Stability	Alignment (WB line)	Laxity	Return to work	Conclusion
Naudie et al., 2004	4.7 years (1.8–6.9)	15/16 (93%) satisfied and would have operation again	*Tegner* Pre: 3.25 FU: 5.25	Pre: 100% FU: 44% somewhat 56% significantly improved	Pre: mean WB line 18% FU: mean WB line 46%	Not reported	2 sedentary patients able to return to work 1 patient able to return to play semiprofessional hockey after HTO alone	Medial OW HTO can obtain good functional and radiographic results in patients with posterolateral instability and hyperextension-varus thrust
Arthur et al., 2007	3.1 years (1.6–5.4)	Not reported	*CKS* Pre: 43.3 (recon) 61.5 (non-recon) FU: 47.8 (recon) 68.1 (non-recon)	8/21 stable after HTO alone	Pre: mean WB line 26.7% (9.2–38.8%) FU: 57.5% (50.7–65.9%)	Not reported	Not reported	Initial medial OW HTO can be used to successfully treat 38% of patients with chronic PLC injury and varus Patients with multi-ligament, high-energy injuries, and lower baseline functional scores were more likely to require a second-stage ligament reconstruction
Helito et al., 2018	2.4 years (2–3.4)	Not reported	*KOOS* FU: 79.2 (72–88.4) *Lysholm* FU: 83 (63–90) *IKDC* FU: 67.8 (56.3–75.8)	Pre: 100% FU: 0%	Pre: $-9.6° \pm 1.8°$ FU: $1.2° \pm 1.9°$	4/5 with minimal residual laxity with grade 1 lateral opening at 30°	All returned to work	Single-stage medial OW HTO with PLCR (with or without cruciate ligament reconstruction) can produce satisfactory outcomes with a low rate of complications This approach is recommended for young, higher functioning, and with high-grade posterolateral instability

ACLR anterior cruciate ligament reconstruction, *CKS* Cincinnati knee score, *PLCR* posterolateral corner reconstruction, *FU* follow-up

Table 7.2 Summary of outcomes for treatment of lateral or posterolateral instability

Author(s), year	Reoperations	Complications
Noyes et al., 2000	*14 knees (11 double varus, 3 triple varus)* 2 revision HTO due to excessive valgus after WB 1 loss of fixation 2 painful fibula nonunion requiring resection 3 early increase AP displacement—refixation of ACL at the tibia 4 ACL revisions 3 partial or total resection of painful meniscal allografts	No evidence of infection, peroneal nerve palsy, patella infera, or knee motion limitations at follow-up 33% failed ACLR 6% failed PLCR 17% recurrence of varus 3% valgus overcorrection
Badhe and Forster, 2002	1 deep infection requiring debridement 1 nonunion requiring revision with Ilizarov ring fixator	14% persistent instability (1 deep infection, 1 untreated ACL) 7% nonunion 7% recurrence of varus 7% valgus overcorrection
Goradia and Van Allen, 2002	None	Superficial infection of proximal pin site treated with oral cephalexin for 5 days
Naudie et al., 2004	5 delayed ligament reconstructions 3 PCLR 1 PCLR + ACLR 1 PCLR + PLC advancement + hardware removal 2 hardware removals 1 revision TTO after traumatic displacement	8 total reoperations (3 symptomatic hardware requiring removal) 1 delayed union treated with prolonged protected weight-bearing that healed uneventfully
Arthur et al., 2007	5 patients (24%) 4 removal of painful hardware 1 debridement for infection	1 major—deep infection requiring debridement and removal of PLC allograft—underwent treatment of the infection and eventual revision PLCR 4 minor—painful hardware
Helito et al., 2018	None reported	1 superficial wound infection requiring oral antibiotics

HTO high tibial osteotomy, *WB* weight-bearing

Patients were followed for an average of 4.5 years (range 2–12). Preoperatively, all patients with double varus knees had an abnormal increase in lateral joint opening (mean, 4 mm). At final follow-up, no patient had >2 mm increase in lateral joint opening. The authors suspected that the HTO is allowed for a physiologic remodeling and shortening of the posterolateral structures. All patients with triple varus had an abnormal increase in lateral joint opening (mean, 8 mm) and an increase in external tibial rotation (mean, 9°) and also underwent PLC reconstruction. At follow-up,

14 knees (77%) had <3 mm increase in lateral joint opening and <5° increase in external tibial rotation; 3 patients had between 3 and 5 mm of increase lateral opening or 6–10° increase in external rotation, while 1 patient had a failure of the PLC reconstruction with >5 mm increase in lateral opening or more than 10° increase in external tibial rotation. Based on KT-2000 arthrometry testing and pivot shift test, 15 (33%) of the ACL reconstructions had failed. 10 of the 15 failures were revision ACL reconstructions. It is also important to note that 73% of knees had total or near-total meniscectomy and 63% had marked articular cartilage damage in the medial compartment. At final follow-up, Cincinnati knee scores (CKS) were significantly improved, a reduction of pain was found in 71% of patients, and stability was improved with a subjective elimination of giving way in 85% of the patients. Overall, 15 (37%) rated their knee as normal or very good, whereas 10 patients (25%) rated the knee as fair, and 2 (5%) rated the knee as poor. Twenty-seven patients (66%) had returned to athletics without symptoms. Most were participating in light swimming or bicycling activities only, at the recommendation of the authors.

From this study, they concluded that all triple varus knees should be treated with a staged reconstruction of the ACL and PLC after HTO. In the double varus knee, if there is excessive lateral joint opening of >12 mm at the periphery of the lateral compartment (assessed by the arthroscopic gap test), the ACL should be reconstructed at a second stage, to allow for adaptive shortening of the posterolateral tissues after HTO.

In 2002, Badhe and Forster [15] reported on 14 patients with combined ligament deficiencies with varus alignment treated with ligament reconstruction and HTO. These patients were treated at a mean of 8.3 years (range: 1–20 years) from the initial injury. Six sustained the injury while playing sports and eight in a motor vehicle accident (MVA). The delay in surgery was due predominantly to misdiagnosis of the injury and its severity. All five patients with a double varus knee underwent a closing-wedge HTO and ACL reconstruction as a primary surgery. Six out of nine triple varus knees underwent primary HTO and PLC ligament reconstruction using Ligament Advanced Reconstruction System—LARS synthetic ligament (Arc-sur-Tille, France). Three of these patients also underwent concomitant PCL, and two underwent concomitant ACL reconstructions. The remaining three underwent primary HTO without ligament reconstruction.

At a mean follow-up of 2.8 years (range: 0.5–5.5), 86% of patients had a stable knee. One patient with instability had a severe infection of the posterolateral reconstruction which resulted in complete disruption of the lateral structures and was awaiting revision at the time of publication. The other patient with instability had an injury of the ACL, PCL, and PLC and was treated with HTO, PCL, and PLC reconstructions and was using a brace at 4.5 years of follow-up. One patient also had a nonunion of the opening-wedge HTO requiring revision with an Ilizarov ring fixator. This patient ultimately healed with stable knee function. At final follow-up one patient also had recurrence of the varus deformity, and one was found to be overcorrected into 11° of valgus. Though this study population was small and heterogeneous, improved CKS were reported with a mean preoperative score of 53 (range: 40–58) to 74 (range: 58–82) at final follow-up. In triple varus knees, better scores were found when a medial opening-wedge HTO was performed with PLC reconstruction (mean CKS improvement from 55 to 77) versus a lateral closing-wedge HTO and PLC reconstruction (mean CKS improvement from 49 to 65). The three patients treated with HTO alone had a mean improvement in CKS from 57 to 76 [15].

The authors acknowledge that due to the small number and heterogeneous group of patients, definitive conclusions cannot be drawn. However, they noted that double varus knees treated with simultaneous HTO and ACL reconstruction did well in this series. Triple varus knees treated with opening-wedge HTO did better than closing-wedge HTO, with the advantage of not disturbing the proximal tibiofibular joint. If the posterolateral structures are lax and not completely disrupted, an opening-wedge HTO alone without ligament reconstruction can stabilize the knee—though this was not quantified in their series [15].

In a case report, Goradia and Van Allen [6] described the successful treatment of a 22-year-old female with varus malalignment and isolated lateral laxity. She had a remote injury to the knee while falling from a horse 5 years prior to presentation. She had undergone two previous arthroscopic debridements of the medial meniscus. At presentation, she had 5 mm of increased lateral joint line opening at 30° of knee flexion and a varus thrust during the stance phase of her gait that worsened with jogging. Radiographs demonstrated slight varus malalignment. Patient underwent knee arthroscopy, which was noted to be unremarkable, and a proximal medial corticotomy with placement of a medial distraction external fixator. The corticotomy was held in compression for 6 days, followed by gradual distraction of 1 mm per day for 10 days until the mechanical axis was at the lateral tibial spine. Radiographs at 6 months postoperatively demonstrated maintenance of the mechanical axis correction, the knee was stable to varus stress, and patient resumed jogging and all recreational activities. At 18 months patient continued to be asymptomatic with all recreational activities. The authors concluded that the use of a dynamic external fixator permitted them to "dial in" the amount of correction based on serial radiographs. Reduction of the adductor moment corrected the varus thrust, decreasing tension on the lateral ligaments, which eliminated the patient's symptoms and the need for a lateral reconstruction.

In 2004, Naudi et al. reported the results from the Fowler Kennedy Sport Medicine Clinic in 16 patients (17 knees) who underwent medial opening-wedge HTO for posterolateral instability and hyperextension-varus thrust. The etiology of instability was an isolated PCL injury in four patients, a combined PCL and PLC injury in three, combined ACL, PCL, and PLC in four, and capsuloligamentous laxity in five patients. They specifically excluded patients with a primary diagnosis of medial compartment osteoarthritis, anterior instability, or those treated with a combined ACL reconstruction and HTO. Patients were initially treated with medial opening-wedge HTO, and three underwent concomitant tibial tubercle osteotomy (TTO) due to a proximal tibial correction of >1 cm. Because patients were being treated for instability alone, the goal with HTO was to shift the weight-bearing line to 50% of the width of the tibial plateau, or a neutral mechanical axis. Additionally, they increased the posterior tibial slope in all patients from an average of 6° (range: 0–11°) to an average of 8° (range: 6–21°) with the goal intraoperatively to increase the tibial slope enough to correct any hyperextension deformity to neutral. Five patients went on to have a subsequent PCL reconstruction, one of whom also underwent posterolateral ligament advancement and removal of hardware and one also had ACL reconstruction.

At a mean follow-up of 4.7 years (range: 1.8–6.9 years), all patients had significant improvement in Tegner scores. All patients had improvement in knee stability, with 44% felt that the instability had somewhat improved and 56% felt the instability significantly improved. All but one patient were satisfied with the operation and would undergo the procedure again under the same circumstances. This patient was dissatisfied because he fell after his initial surgery and displaced his TTO, requiring reoperation. One patient, a 23-year-old hockey player who sustained a combined PCL and PLC injury on an all-terrain vehicle, was able to return to play hockey at a semiprofessional level following osteotomy alone. In total, there were eight reoperations following osteotomy. The procedures included five patients who had delayed ligament reconstruction and one revision of the TTO as detailed above. Additionally, two patients required removal of painful hardware. One patient also had a delayed union of the osteotomy, which healed with prolonged course of protected weight-bearing. While they did not report on recurrence of varus or overcorrection into valgus, based on the results presented in the paper, one patient had a mechanical axis at 26.7% of the tibia, likely remaining in varus, while one patient had a mechanical axis of 82% and was likely overcorrected into valgus. These authors concluded that medial opening-wedge HTO can produce good functional and radiographic results in select patients with posterolateral instability and hyperextension-varus thrust. Mechanical axis realignment and sagittal plane correction are fundamental considerations when treating patients with complex knee instabilities [16].

In 2007, Arthur et al. [11] presented a prospective evaluation of 21 patients with chronic posterolateral instability and varus malalignment treated with initial HTO. Six patients had isolated PLC deficiency, six had combined ACL and PLC deficiency, six had PCL and PLC deficiency, two patients had ACL, PCL, and PLC deficiency, and one patient had an isolated PLC ligamentous injury with a medial tibial plateau fracture. The authors' approach for these patients was to first perform the HTO and then, after the osteotomy healed and the patient completed appropriate rehab, assess whether a second-stage ligament reconstruction was needed. All patients underwent medial opening-wedge HTO with the goal to correct the mechanical axis to pass through the downslope of the lateral tibial spine. In patients with concurrent ACL deficiency, a plate with an anterior sagittal plane slope was used in an attempt to decrease the posterior tibial slope. Conversely, in patients with concurrent PCL deficiency, plates with a posterior sagittal plane slope were used in an attempt to increase the tibial slope. Patients presented on an average of 5.5 years (range: 3 months to 22 years) after the initial injury. Ten patients had sustained a sports injury, nine were involved in a MVA, and two were injured in a work-related fall.

At a mean follow-up of 37 months (range: 19–65 months) after the initial HTO, 8 of 21 (38%) patients felt stable enough with the osteotomy alone. The remaining

13 patients underwent ligament reconstruction at a mean of 13.8 months after the initial operation. They found that only four out of ten (40%) of patients with a low-velocity sports injury required ligament reconstruction, whereas seven out of nine (78%) of patients involved in high-velocity MVA, and both patients with a work-related fall required second-stage ligament reconstruction. Further, 10 out of 14 patients (71%) with multi-ligament injuries required second-stage ligament reconstruction versus only 2 out of 6 patients (33%) with isolated PLC injuries. Modified CKS in the patients who required second-stage ligament reconstruction were an average of 43.3 (range: 8–83) at baseline and averaged 47.8 (range: 16–77) prior to the second surgery. These patients unfortunately were not further followed to determine if their scores improved after the ligament reconstruction. In patients who did not require a second-stage reconstruction, the modified CKS averaged 61.5 (range: 21–90) at baseline and improved to an average of 68.1 (range: 40–100) at follow-up, which was not significantly different than baseline scores.

The authors recommend a staged surgical approach for patients with chronic posterolateral instability and varus alignment, noting that 38% of the patients in this study did not require a second-stage ligament reconstruction. They also recommend a medial opening-wedge osteotomy technique due to theoretical advantage of tightening the posterior capsule and oblique popliteal ligament complex [17]. Additionally, they have demonstrated in a cadaveric study that medial opening-wedge HTO increases varus and external rotation stability [18]. While they did not demonstrate significant changes of the slope in this study, the medial opening-wedge technique does allow for the potential of improving sagittal plane deformity in associated ACL or PCL deficiency. They found that the most common factor in determining the need for a second-stage ligament reconstruction was the severity of the initial knee injury as measured by the overall patient function on the modified CKS, concurrent injuries, and multi-ligament injury patterns. One of the two patients with an isolated PLC injury who did require the second-stage PLC reconstruction was a highly competitive professional soccer player with high demands for side-to-side knee stability. The other patient was involved in a high-speed MVA and had a history of previous failed PLC reconstruction prior to the osteotomy.

The authors acknowledged that the heterogeneous group and small number of patients limits the conclusions that can be made but determined that using a staged approach with an initial opening-wedge HTO followed by a period of convalescence to determine subsequent clinical and functional stability is a reasonable approach for treating these patients. Patients with a multi-ligament injury, or history of high-energy injury pattern, and lower baseline functional scores were more likely to require a second-stage PLC and other cruciate ligament reconstructions.

In 2019, Helito et al. [7] reported on five patients with chronic PLC injuries and varus malalignment treated with a single-stage HTO and PLC reconstruction. Two patients had combined ACL and PLC injuries, one patient had combined PCL and PLC injuries, one patient had ACL, PCL, and PLC, and one patient had isolated PLC injury. All patients were treated with a medial opening-wedge HTO to correct the mechanical axis of the limb to the center of the knee. Reconstruction of the PLC was done using hamstring autograft with a single femoral tunnel and both fibular and tibial tunnels to reconstruct the lateral collateral ligament, popliteofibular ligament, and popliteus tendon. ACL or PCL reconstructions were performed arthroscopically using contralateral hamstring autograft for ACL and contralateral quadriceps tendon with bone plug for PCL reconstructions. The mean time between the initial injury and surgery was 40 months (range: 36–54). Three patients were injured in MVA, one patient during sports, and one from a fall from height.

Preoperative outcome scores were not reported, though at a mean follow-up of 29.4 months (range: 24–41) the mean postoperative scores for KOOS, Lysholm, and IKDC were 79.2 (range: 72–88.4), 83 (range: 63–90), and 67.8 (range: 56.3–78.2), respectively. Based on the results of the Lysholm score, one patient was considered to have a poor result (score < 65), two patients fair (score 65–83), and two patients with a good result (score between 84 and 90). They reported that all patients were able to return to work. One patient had a complication with a superficial wound infection requiring antibiotics.

Although there were very few patients in this study, the authors did report successful treatment of posterolateral instability and varus alignment with a single-stage medial opening-wedge HTO and PLC reconstruction with or without cruciate reconstruction. They advocate this approach in young and highly functioning patients with more pronounced posterolateral instability because these patients may not have satisfactory outcomes with osteotomy alone.

In summary, two studies (Badhe and Forster and Arthur et al.) reported that HTO alone can be used to successfully treat patients with chronic posterolateral instability and varus alignment. While Badhe and Forster did not use a staged surgical approach in their study, nor quantify the grade of posterolateral instability, patients with a multi-ligament injury were more likely to undergo ligamentous reconstruction (five of seven patients versus one of two patients with isolated PLC instability) at the time of osteotomy. Arthur et al., who did use a staged approach, similarly reported that multi-ligament injuries were more likely to require ligament reconstruction versus isolated PLC injuries (71% versus 33%, respectively). The patients presented by Noyes et al. differed in that all patients had chronic ACL deficiency as the primary diagnosis leading to varying degrees of posterolateral instability, or initially undiagnosed PLC injury, which lead to the posterolateral instability. All patients in their study underwent ligament reconstruction, though, in patients with combined ACL and PLC deficiency, Noyes et al. also advocate for a staged approach with an initial HTO followed by second-stage ligament reconstruction. None of the patients in their study were treated with HTO alone, though all patients with posterolateral instability had a multi-ligament injury. Advantages of a medial opening-wedge HTO include the following: preservation of the proximal tibiofibular joint, corrects medial laxity, can be used for larger varus deformities (>12°), and prevents patella baja. Historically, this technique has had a higher nonunion rate, but with better patient selection and newer locking plate technology, the risk of nonunion has decreased.

7.4   Treatment of Medial Laxity and Valgus Deformity

Medial collateral ligament (MCL) injuries are common, and most are successfully treated with conservative management alone. In patients with valgus malalignment, the MCL is subject to increased loads and has been demonstrated to carry as much as 81% of ligamentous load during valgus loading in biomechanical studies [8]. Patients with valgus alignment and MCL injuries can develop a distinct medial thrust during the single-leg stance phase of gait, and patients generally describe this medial thrust as instability. MCL repair or reconstruction alone in these patients is at high risk for failure [8], and correction of the axial alignment may be necessary.

Varus-producing osteotomy in patients with valgus malalignment for the treatment of lateral compartment arthritis or unloading of concomitant meniscus or cartilage procedures is relatively common with good results reported in the literature [19–21]. However, in the treatment of medial knee laxity, there are only two articles published in the same issue of Orthopedic Clinics of North America in 1994 that report outcomes of osteotomy for medial knee instability [8, 22].

Cameron and Saha [8] reported on a group of 35 patients treated with osteotomy for knee instability. Fourteen of the patients had chronic medial collateral ligament (MCL) insufficiency and valgus malalignment treated with medial closing-wedge distal femur osteotomy (DFO). Six patients had a complete knee dislocation, and eight had combined ACL and MCL injuries. 19 of the original 35 patients had undergone 2 or more previous surgical procedures prior to the osteotomy. The average preoperative anatomical axis was 17° of valgus and was corrected to an average of 0°. They reported an improvement in the gait pattern in all but one patient, who had a persistent antalgic gait. They noted that the objective change in instability by comparing pre- and post-osteotomy stress radiographs was minimal and recommended for a staged MCL reconstruction after osteotomy in symptomatic patients [8].

Paley et al. [22] reported on a group of 23 limbs in 17 patients with chronic laxity of 1 or both collateral ligaments and bony deformity. The causes of underlying deformity were Blount's disease (7), bone dysplasia (4), pseudoachondroplasia (2), brachydactyly (1), growth arrest (3), iatrogenic after Coventry osteotomy (1), rickets (1), and tibial plateau fracture malunion (1). These patients had an average age of 21 years (range: 5–50 years) with a mean follow-up of 1 year (range: 6–36 months). Patients were treated with realignment osteotomy and distraction osteogenesis with the goal to tighten the collateral ligaments. Fifteen procedures were for isolated LCL, 1 isolated MCL, and 7 combined MCL and LCL laxities. The surgical correction was obtained by various osteotomy techniques using a ring external fixator:

(a) Two limbs underwent osteotomy of the junction of the mid and distal third of the fibula with distal transport of the proximal portion of the fibula to tighten the LCL.

(b) Thirteen limbs underwent transverse osteotomy of the tibia with lengthening of the tibia and fixation of the fibula to the distal tibia segment to transport the fibular head distally, tightening the LCL.

(c) One limb underwent a medial opening-wedge HTO proximal to the insertion of the MCL to tighten the MCL.

(d) One limb underwent focal dome rotational osteotomy to tighten the MCL and lengthen the tibia.

(e) Six limbs underwent an oblique osteotomy of the proximal tibia from proximal to the MCL insertion with tibia lengthening to tighten both the MCL and LCL.

They reported 19 excellent, 2 fair, and 2 poor results. The patients with a fair result included one who suffered a buckle fracture after removal of the fixator leading to a varus deformity. The second patient with fair result underwent correction of tibial varus and LCL laxity; however, she had untreated varus of the femur, and the LCL laxity recurred by 3-year follow-up. The two poor results were in patients with significant postoperative pain. One patient had iatrogenic tibia valgus after a Coventry osteotomy, and despite correction of this valgus by the authors, the patient reported continued pain. The second patient underwent fibular osteotomy, which was complicated by osteomyelitis and a transient peroneal nerve palsy requiring nerve decompression and debridement of the pin site. Both problems are resolved; however, the patient developed reflex sympathetic dystrophy (RSD) and had persistent pain at follow-up. One other patient developed RSD, though it resolved after removal of the apparatus. They felt it may have been due to stretch of the peroneal nerve, but they observed no instances of peroneal nerve palsies. All other patients reported improved gait postoperatively. All patients with obvious preoperative lateral or medial thrust had no thrust in follow-up. Only one patient complained of clinically noticeable instability postoperatively.

While this cohort of patients may not translate to a typical joint realignment practice today, Paley et al. discuss several important points to consider. Mechanical axis deviation (MAD) is usually attributable to femoral or tibial osseous deformities or both. It is less often recognized as a function of ligamentous laxity between the tibia and femur, and the closer an osseous angulation of the femur or tibia is to the knee, the greater the MAD produced per degree of angulation. Therefore, angulation due to collateral ligament laxity produces a greater amount of MAD per degree of angulation, so even small degrees of ligamentous laxity can produce large amounts of MAD. This ligamentous laxity must be considered when correcting lower extremity malalignment. Early authors have recommended overcorrection of the tibia to compensate for the varus due to LCL laxity [23]. However, others have found that if the angle between the joint surfaces was greater than 7°, the amount of overcorrection required to close the lateral joint may be so large that the knee becomes overloaded laterally [24]. Others recommend not considering the lateral ligament laxity in the correction, as it would correct spontaneously once the limb is realigned with slight overcorrection into 3° of valgus [25]. Early attempts at repair or reconstruction of the posterolateral soft tissues often failed or stretched with time. Paley advocates for gradual distraction, which allows for overtightening of the lateral ligament complex to compensate for some gradual stretching over time. They found that tightening of the collateral ligaments did not significantly increase the risks of realignment by osteotomy and feel that this is a safe procedure resulting in a greater correction for the same amount of surgery.

7.5 Conclusions

Patients presenting with coronal plane instability in association with varus or valgus deformity are a challenging population to treat. In most cases, isolated ligament repair or reconstruction is insufficient due to stretching of the soft tissues as a result of increased load. There are data to support both a staged approach with completion of the osteotomy followed by delayed ligamentous reconstruction as well as single-stage osteotomy combined with ligament reconstruction. Medial opening-wedge HTO is recommended for larger (>8 mm) corrections and corrections associated with posterior or posterolateral laxity and hyperextension-varus thrust in which surgeons should preserve the proximal tibiofibular joint to maintain the PLC. If a staged approach is chosen, subsequent ligament reconstruction may or may not be necessary depending on the patient's symptoms following osteotomy. Patients with higher-energy injuries and those with multiple ligament injuries are more likely to require ligament reconstruction.

References

1. Cantin O, Magnussen RA, Corbi F, Servien E, Neyret P, Lustig S. The role of high tibial osteotomy in the treatment of knee laxity: a comprehensive review. Knee Surg Sports Traumatol Arthrosc. 2015;23(10):3026–37. https://doi.org/10.1007/s00167-015-3752-z.
2. Paley D, Tetsworth K. Mechanical axis deviation of the lower limbs. Preoperative planning of uniapical angular deformities of the tibia or femur. Clin Orthop Relat Res. 1992;280:48–64. http://www.ncbi.nlm.nih.gov/pubmed/1611764. Accessed 27 May 2019.
3. Bellemans J, Colyn W, Vandenneucker H, Victor J. Is neutral mechanical alignment normal for all patients? The concept of constitutional varus. Clin Orthop Relat Res. 2012;470:45–53. https://doi.org/10.1007/s11999-011-1936-5.
4. Lephart SM, Pincivero DM, Rozzi SL. Proprioception of the ankle and knee. Sports Med. 1998;25(3):149–55. https://doi.org/10.2165/00007256-199825030-00002.
5. Phisitkul P, Wolf BR, Amendola A. Role of high tibial and distal femoral osteotomies in the treatment of lateral-posterolateral and medial instabilities of the knee. Sports Med Arthrosc Rev. 2006;14(2):96–104.
6. Goradia VK, Van Allen J. Chronic lateral knee instability treated with a high tibial osteotomy. Arthroscopy. 2002;18(7):807–11. https://doi.org/10.1053/jars.2002.35270.
7. Helito CP, Sobrado MF, Giglio PN, et al. Posterolateral reconstruction combined with one-stage tibial valgus osteotomy: technical considerations and functional results. Knee. 2019;26(2):500–7. https://doi.org/10.1016/j.knee.2018.12.001.
8. Cameron JC, Saha S. Management of medial collateral ligament laxity. Orthop Clin North Am. 1994;25(3):527–32. http://www.ncbi.nlm.nih.gov/pubmed/8028893. Accessed 25 Apr 2019.
9. Chahla J, Moatshe G, Dean CS, Laprade RF. Posterolateral corner of the knee: current concepts. Arch Bone Jt Surg. 2016;97(9):97–103.
10. LaPrade RF, Terry GC. Injuries to the posterolateral aspect of the knee. Am J Sports Med. 1997;25(4):433–8. https://doi.org/10.1177/036354659702500403.
11. Arthur A, LaPrade RF, Agel J. Proximal tibial opening wedge osteotomy as the initial treatment for chronic posterolateral corner deficiency in the varus knee: a prospective clinical study. Am J Sports Med. 2007;35(11):1844–50. https://doi.org/10.1177/0363546507304717.
12. Noyes FR, Barber-westin SD, Hewett TE. High tibial osteotomy and ligament reconstruction for varus angulated anterior cruciate ligament-deficient knees. Am J Sports Med. 2000;28(3):282–96.

13. Simon D, Mascarenhas R, Saltzman BM, Rollins M, Bach BR, MacDonald P. The relationship between anterior cruciate ligament injury and osteoarthritis of the knee. Adv Orthop. 2015;2015:1–11. https://doi.org/10.1155/2015/928301.
14. Dean CS, Liechti DJ, Chahla J, Moatshe G, LaPrade RF. Clinical outcomes of high tibial osteotomy for knee instability: a systematic review. Orthop J Sports Med. 2016;4(3):1–9. https://doi.org/10.1177/2325967116633419.
15. Badhe NP, Forster IW. High tibial osteotomy in knee instability: the rationale of treatment and early results. Knee Surg Sports Traumatol Arthrosc. 2002;10(1):38–43. https://doi.org/10.1007/s001670100244.
16. Naudie DDR, Amendola A, Fowler PJ. Opening wedge high tibial osteotomy for symptomatic hyperextension-varus thrust. Am J Sports Med. 2004;32(1):60–70. https://doi.org/10.1177/0363546503258907.
17. LaPrade RF, Morgan PM, Wentorf FA, Johansen S, Engebretsen L. The anatomy of the posterior aspect of the knee: an anatomic study. J Bone Joint Surg Am. 2007;89(4):758–64. https://doi.org/10.2106/JBJS.F.00120.
18. LaPrade RF, Engebretsen L, Johansen S, Wentorf FA, Kurtenbach C. The effect of a proximal tibial medial opening wedge osteotomy on posterolateral knee instability: a biomechanical study. Am J Sports Med. 2008;36(5):956–60. https://doi.org/10.1177/0363546507312380.
19. Harris JD, Hussey K, Saltzman BM, et al. Cartilage repair with or without meniscal transplantation and osteotomy for lateral compartment chondral defects of the knee: case series with minimum 2-year follow-up. Orthop J Sport Med. 2014;2(10):2325967114551528. https://doi.org/10.1177/2325967114551528.
20. Kim YC, Yang J-H, Kim HJ, et al. Distal femoral varus osteotomy for valgus arthritis of the knees: systematic review of open versus closed wedge osteotomy. Knee Surg Relat Res. 2018;30(1):3–16. https://doi.org/10.5792/ksrr.16.064.
21. Wang J-W, Hsu C-C. Distal femoral varus osteotomy for osteoarthritis of the knee. J Bone Joint Surg Am. 2005;87(1):127–33. https://doi.org/10.2106/JBJS.C.01559.
22. Paley D, Bhatnagar J, Herzenberg JE, Bhave A. New procedures for tightening knee collateral ligaments in conjunction with knee realignment osteotomy. Orthop Clin North Am. 1994;25(3):533–55. http://www.ncbi.nlm.nih.gov/pubmed/8028894. Accessed 25 Apr 2019.
23. Aglietti P, Rinonapoli E, Stringa G, Taviani A. Tibial osteotomy for the varus osteoarthritic knee. Clin Orthop Relat Res. 1983;176:239–51. http://www.ncbi.nlm.nih.gov/pubmed/6851332. Accessed 11 June 2019.
24. Hernigou P, Medevielle D, Debeyre J, Goutallier D. Proximal tibial osteotomy for osteoarthritis with varus deformity. A ten to thirteen-year follow-up study. J Bone Joint Surg Am. 1987;69(3):332–54. http://www.ncbi.nlm.nih.gov/pubmed/3818700. Accessed 11 June 2019.
25. Hetsroni I, Lyman S, Pearle AD, Marx RG. The effect of lateral opening wedge distal femoral osteotomy on medial knee opening: clinical and biomechanical factors. Knee Surg Sports Traumatol Arthrosc. 2014;22(7):1659–65. https://doi.org/10.1007/s00167-013-2405-3.

Part III

Surgical Technique

Medial Open-Wedge High Tibial Osteotomy

Philipp Lobenhoffer

High tibial osteotomy (HTO) has become a widely accepted technique for treatment of tibial varus malalignment and medial osteoarthritis of the knee [1–3]. Osteotomy of the proximal tibia may be performed by a subtractive technique (closed wedge), by a barrel-vault (dome) osteotomy, or by an additive technique (open wedge). In the past, the closed-wedge technique with removal of a bone wedge from a lateral approach and fixation with staples, a plate or a tension-band system, has gained most popularity. Disadvantages of this technique are the risk for peroneal nerve injuries [4], the need of fibula osteotomy or separation of the proximal tibiofibular joint, and the detachment of the extensor muscles. Large corrections cause marked shortening of the leg and an offset of the proximal tibia, which may compromise later placement of the tibial component of a total knee replacement. Open-wedge osteotomy from the medial side can be performed without any muscle detachment, the correction can be "fine-tuned" during the procedure, and no leg shortening occurs. Open-wedge osteotomy received increased interest with the development of plate fixators that enable the surgeon to fix the correction safely as well as to avoid bone grafting in most cases [5, 6].

8.1 Indications

The technique described is indicated for degeneration and osteoarthritis of the medial knee joint in patients with constitutional varus of the tibia. Patients with normal anatomy of the tibia may still have varus deformity of the leg by medial osteoarthritis and wear. They may be also treated by HTO but the success rate will

P. Lobenhoffer (✉)
Orthopaedic and Trauma Surgery, Go:h Gelenkchirurgie Orthopädie Hannover,
Hannover, Germany
e-mail: philipp.lobenhoffer@g-o-hannover.de

© Springer Nature Switzerland AG 2020
S. Oussedik, S. Lustig (eds.), *Osteotomy About the Knee*,
https://doi.org/10.1007/978-3-030-49055-3_8

be limited [3, 7]; patients with constitutional femoral varus deformity should be treated with a femur osteotomy [8]. Age and weight of the patient are no exclusion factors for HTO [9]. A limited flexion contracture may be accepted if a sagittal correction of the tibial slope is included in the surgical plan. Open-wedge osteotomy should not be used if leg lengthening is contraindicated and if the medial soft tissue coverage is compromised. Patella pain is not a contraindication; however, in cases of patella infera, a special type of osteotomy described later should be used [10]. An intact lateral compartment of the knee is an obligatory prerequisite for this technique. The patient should not have lateral joint line pain, and no radiographic signs of lateral osteoarthritis should be present. Nicotine use is a relative contraindication, because bone healing and bone formation may be compromised [9]. Primary cancellous bone grafting may be discussed in this situation.

8.2 Clinical Examination

Clinical examination should focus on range of motion of the knee, ligamentous stability, and leg length. Joint line pain is regularly found on the medial side. Patella tracking is registered and patella pain should be carefully evaluated. Pain on the lateral side of the knee is a warning sign and may indicate degeneration of the lateral compartment of the knee. Deficiency of the anterior or posterior cruciate ligament is no contraindication against this type of osteotomy, because joint stability can be improved by adjustment of the tibial slope. The medial collateral ligament is usually intact in constitutional varus malalignment.

8.3 Imaging

Imaging should include weight-bearing radiographs of the knee in two planes, a patella skyline view and a flexed-knee posteroanterior weight-bearing radiograph. A long-leg weight-bearing radiograph of the involved leg is necessary for deformity analysis and preoperative planning. In cases of ligament instability, stress radiographs should be performed to study the medial and lateral joint line opening, because significant ligament instability must be considered in the preoperative planning. Magnetic resonance tomography may be used to study the joint status but is not obligatory. In questionable indications, a technetium scintigraphy may be helpful to identify the area of maximum pathology (hot spot) of the knee, usually indicating the source of pain.

8.4 Planning

A formal deformity analysis on a long-leg film is mandatory [1, 2, 11]. This analysis should indicate pathological values for the medial proximal tibia angle (MPTA). Preoperative planning of the correction is performed as second step. We recommend to plan the exact amount of separation of the two planes of the osteotomy in millimeters on a long-leg radiograph either digitally or manually.

First step: The center of the femoral head and the center of the ankle joint are marked on the radiograph. A template with circles of varying diameter is used to find the center of the femoral head. The bisector of the transverse width of the talus under the joint line is used as center of the ankle joint.

Second step: The knee baseline is drawn parallel to the subchondral sclerosis of the two tibial plateaus. The weight-bearing line through the knee joint is now drawn connecting the center of the femoral head and the center of the ankle. The line will cut the knee baseline in the medial compartment of the knee, depending on the degree of varus the patient has.

Third step: The projected postoperative intersection of the weight-bearing line with the knee baseline is marked. Because the osteotomy aims to shift the weight-bearing line laterally, this intersection will be located at a point 50–62% of the total width of the proximal tibia from medial to lateral, depending on the individual treatment strategy of the surgeon. In our routine, we aim for a correction of the weight-bearing line to the lateral spine which equals a point at 55% of the entire width of the tibia [12].

Fourth step: The projected postoperative weight-bearing line is now drawn by connecting the center of the femoral head with the new intersection point mentioned previously. This line is continued to the area of the ankle joint.

Fifth step: The hinge point of the open-wedge osteotomy is marked on the radiograph. We use a hinge point on the lateral cortex at the upper border of the proximal tibiofibular joint. Two lines of the same length are drawn from this hinge point to the old and then to the new ankle joint center. The angle between these lines is the correction angle of the open-wedge osteotomy. The osteotomy planes can now be marked on the radiograph. We perform an oblique ascending osteotomy and start the cut at the transition between the convex upper and the concave lower part of the proximal tibia, which usually represents the upper border of the pes anserinus tendons. When the two planes with the correction angle between are marked, the opening of the osteotomy in millimeters can be read at the medial cortex. In digital planning, the radiograph should be calibrated, and a correction factor is used to compensate for magnification of the picture. Caution should be used when significant discongruency of the medial and lateral opening is encountered in the weight-bearing long-leg radiograph (JLCA angle pathological). In this situation, a correction formula must be used to avoid overcorrection in HTO [1, 13].

8.5   Technique

This procedure can be performed under spinal or general anesthesia. We routinely do not use a tourniquet and drape the entire leg and hemipelvis free. This allows the surgeon to control the entire extremity visually during the procedure or to harvest a bone graft from the pelvis, if necessary. A small buttress is mounted to the operating table to support the heel in 90° flexion of the knee. A side post is placed against the thigh to stabilize the leg laterally in knee flexion. If this setup is used, only one surgical assistant is required. Intravenous antibiotic prophylaxis is used (2 g of cefazolin). A fluoroscope is mandatory for this procedure and is placed on the ipsilateral side. The surgeon should check that correct visualization of the hip, knee, and ankle is possible in the AP plane before the leg is draped (Fig. 8.1).

After the leg is prepared and draped, the anatomic landmarks are marked with a surgical marker. Points of interest are the superior border of the pes anserinus, the tibial tuberosity, and the medial joint line. A longitudinal skin incision of 5-cm length is placed in the anteromedial area of the tibia. The incision starts 1 cm below

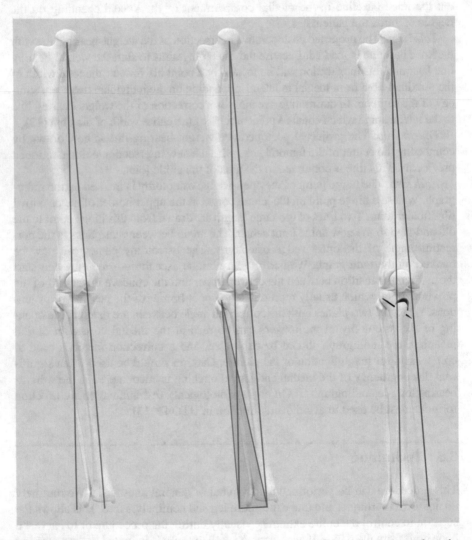

Fig. 8.1 Principles of planning an open-wedge osteotomy of the tibia. A line is drawn from the center of the hip to the point, where the center of the ankle joint is planned after the procedure. The hinge point of the osteotomy is marked (usually at the upper border of the proximal tibiofibular joint). Two lines are drawn from the hinge point to the old and the new center of the ankle joint. The angle between these two lines is the correction angle for the open-wedge osteotomy. The planned osteotomy is marked at the proximal tibia, and the opening is measured at the medial tibia cortex

the joint level. More extensive approaches are possible but not necessary. The implant is designed for percutaneous application (MIPO), and the distal screws are placed by a separate stab incision.

The upper border of the pes tendons is identified. The bursa between pes and medial collateral ligament (MCL) is opened. The interval behind the patellar tendon is identified, and the insertion area of the tendon is marked. The long fibers of the medial collateral ligament are mobilized from the tibia, and a release is performed by inserting a scalpel under the distal part of the ligament and detaching the fibers gradually. As many fibers are detached as to allow the insertion of a blunt retractor behind the posteromedial cortex of the tibia.

The leg is now extended and the fluoroscope is placed over the knee. Slight adjustments of the flexion angle are made until the fluoroscope shows an exact anteroposterior projection of the lateral tibial plateau (no double projection of the joint line). The rotatory position of the tibia is now modified until exact neutral rotation is achieved (patella anterior, fibula one-third superimposed by the tibia). In this position, two Kirschner wires with drill tips (K-wires, 2.3–2.5 mm) are drilled from medial to lateral to mark to osteotomy plane. These K-wires are controlled fluoroscopically until they end exactly at the level of the lateral cortex of the tibia. The wires start at the upper border of the pes anserinus and end at the upper border of the proximal tibiofibular joint. The two wires should be absolutely parallel in the AP plane, i.e., completely superimposed on the anteroposterior fluoroscopy image (Fig. 8.2).

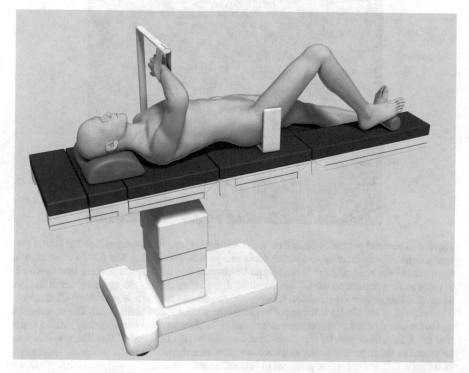

Fig. 8.2 The patient is positioned on a standard radiolucent table. A side post and a heel support are fixed to the table. The leg is draped up to the pelvic crest. No tourniquet is used

The width of the proximal tibia at the level of the osteotomy is now measured. The easiest method is to use a third K-wire of the same length as the two wires inserted into the tibia. The third wire is held parallel to the wire inserted into the bone with the tip in contact with the tibial cortex. The difference in free length between the two K-wires equals the total width of the tibia at the level of the oste-otomy. Usually the posterior width of the tibia is 5–10 mm more than the anterior width. The measurements are marked on a sterile paper with a surgical marker. The depth of the osteotomy is 5–10 mm less than the total width of the tibia, depending on the bone quality.

The insertion depth of the oscillating saw and the chisels should be marked on the instruments with a surgical marker. The saw cut is planned distal of the K-wires to rule out any possibility of deviation of the saw into the joint (Fig. 8.3). By starting the osteotomy relatively low, the tibial tuberosity would be cut in many patients. However, we use a biplanar L-shaped osteotomy with a 100°-angulated anterior cut behind the tuberosity. With this modification, the position of the tuberosity does not

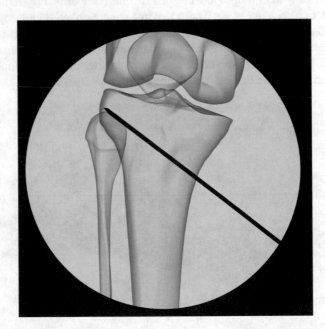

Fig. 8.3 The tibial plateau is visualized under the fluoroscope in ap.-projection. The lateral pla-teau should be in an exact ap.-projection (only one joint line is visible). The patella is oriented in the center of the knee, and the fibula should be covered one-third by the tibia. A first K-wire is inserted as far posterior on the tibia as possible. The starting point is the upper border of the pes anserinus. This reflects the transition between the convex and the concave part of the tibial cortex. The endpoint of the K-wire is the upper border of the proximal tibiofibular joint. The wire should end in the lateral cortex. A second wire is inserted under fluoroscopic control exactly parallel to the first one 1.5 cm more anterior (the distance reflects the width of the saw blade). The saw will then be guided by the two wires giving an osteotomy plane exactly parallel to the individual tibial slope of the patient. The width of the proximal tibia is measured with a third K-wire, and the depth of the osteotomy (5–10 mm less than the distance measured) is marked on the saw blade

Fig. 8.4 The posterior two-thirds of the tibia are cut with an oscillating saw. The saw is inserted under the two K-wires, and a special retractor is used to protect the posterior soft tissues. The osteotomy is performed at a slow pace, and heat is avoided by continuous irrigation with cold fluid

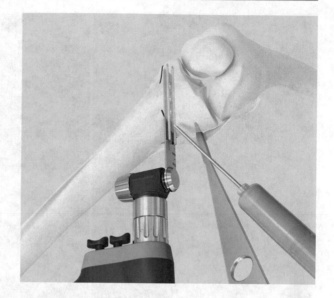

interfere with the osteotomy, and the anterior second osteotomy plane induces a higher rotational stability and an anterior restraint against extension. The angulation point of the osteotomy is at approximately 70% of the posterior-anterior diameter of the medial tibia, and the anterior cut should exit the tibia behind the insertion of the patellar tendon. The anterior cut can be marked with an electrocautery on the bone (Figs. 8.4, 8.5, and 8.6).

High tibial osteotomy has an inherent risk of damage to the popliteal artery and vein by saw blades or chisels. We have developed a retractor, which may be inserted from a fascia incision posterior to the MCL directly on the periosteum of the tibia. This retractor is beveled and radiolucent and allows protection of the posterior structures.

At this point, the retractor is inserted, and the position is adjusted under fluoroscopic control. The osteotomy is now created with an oscillating saw. Battery-driven motors and saw blades of 90-mm length are employed. In contrast to total joint replacement, the success of the procedure depends mainly on the biologic healing of the osteotomy planes. All efforts must be undertaken to avoid damages to the local bone stock and the periosteum. The saw is advanced at a slow pace and the blade continuously irrigated with cold fluid. The saw is withdrawn periodically to allow for better irrigation, and all debris is flushed out of the osteotomy plane. It usually takes several minutes to create the osteotomy, and the depth is carefully controlled to leave 5–10 mm of the bone on the lateral side. It is important to cut the posteromedial and posterolateral crest of the tibia completely. When the saw is carefully pressed against the posterior bone with a low power setting, the loss of resistance can be easily felt when the bone is divided. The saw can then be stopped without contact to the retractor.

For the anterior cut, a smaller and thinner saw blade is used. The tibia is divided completely behind the tuberosity, taking care to orient the cut exactly in the frontal

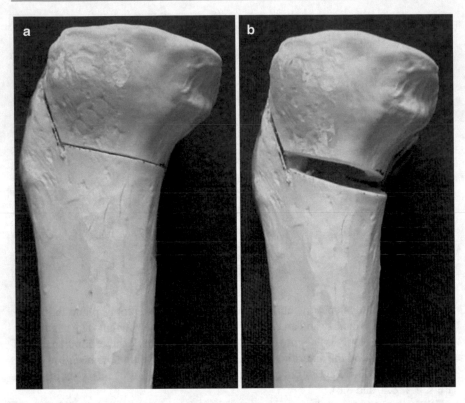

Fig. 8.5 The biplanar osteotomy technique greatly improves stability against sagittal angulation and rotation. Healing of this bone area behind the tuberosity was observed as early as 3 weeks after surgery

Fig. 8.6 The second osteotomy is angulated 100° against the first cut and is performed with a thinner blade. In contrast to the first osteotomy, this cut goes through the opposite cortex

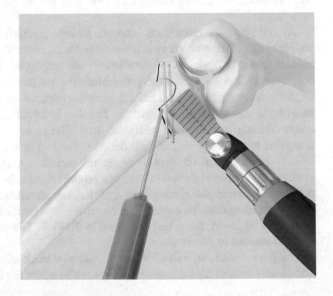

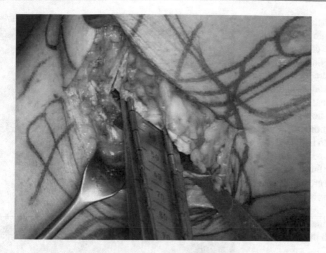

Fig. 8.7 Flat chisels are now introduced sequentially into the posterior part of the osteotomy. The first chisel is driven in as deep as the osteotomy was cut with the saw. The next chisels are each inserted 1 cm less deep. The second chisel and the next chisels thereafter are tapped in with light hammer blows, with constant monitoring of the osteotomy site. The osteotomy should open gradually in the transverse and in the ascending parts. The angle of 100° between the transverse and the ascending parts of the bone cut is seen in the anterior part of the wound

plane of the tibia. In cases with patella baja or preoperative patella pain, this anterior osteotomy may be directed inferior thus avoiding any change in patella position. The tuberosity fragment should be fixed with a bicortical lag screw in this case to avoid tilt of the fragment.

The saw is now withdrawn, and a flat chisel is inserted in the transverse part of the osteotomy. This chisel glides into the saw slot under the K-wires and is inserted to the lateral extent of the saw cut. A second chisel is now inserted between the first chisel and the K-wires. This chisel is now tapped into the osteotomy with light blows of a hammer, slightly less deep than the first chisel (Fig. 8.7). The surgeon should take some time for this step to allow the bone to adapt to the gradual opening of the osteotomy. The opening of the transverse and anterior oblique osteotomy planes should be monitored carefully. There should be a continuous and smooth separation of the two planes. A third and fourth chisel can now be inserted between the first two chisels. Again, these chisels are tapped into the osteotomy with light blows of a hammer over the course of 1–2 min. An opening of the gap of 6 mm should now be achieved. A wedge is now inserted in the anterior part of the gap and the chisels withdrawn.

An osteotomy spreader is placed on the most posteromedial cortical aspect of the osteotomy. Further opening is now performed by opening of the spreader in full extension of the knee. The opening of the osteotomy is measured with a caliper (Fig. 8.8). The correction is checked visually and fluoroscopically. A long metal alignment rod is placed over the leg. Using fluoroscopic screening, the center of the femoral head is aligned with the center of the ankle, and the intersection with the knee as well as the orientation of the new joint line in the frontal plane is observed.

Fig. 8.8 When the
planned opening has been
achieved, the chisels are
exchanged by a bone
spreader inserted exactly
on the posteromedial crest
of the proximal tibia. The
alignment is now checked
with the alignment rod.
The metal rod is placed
over the hip and ankle
center under fluoroscopy.
The planned crossing point
should be reached at the
knee joint. The orientation
of the joint line can also be
checked with this
instrument

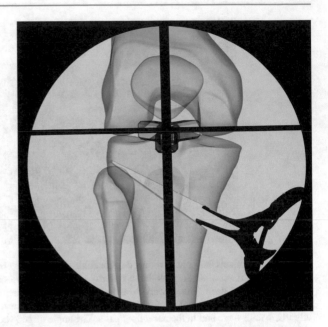

If no alignment rod is available, the cable of the electrocautery device can be used
for this purpose. Modification of the correction is easy by opening or closing the
spreader gradually.

Besides the correction in the anteroposterior plane, the change in the sagittal
plane must be closely monitored. The tibial slope is an important parameter for knee
extension. In patients with preoperative full knee extension, the tibial slope usually
should not be altered. Because of the anatomy of the proximal tibia, this means that
the osteotomy planes should have opened asymmetrically when looked at from the
medial side (one-third more in the back than in the front) and the surgeon should be
able to extend the patient's knee completely at this step of the procedure. The opening of the osteotomy can be modified at this time by repositioning of the spreader,
by using an additional wedge in the anterior part of the osteotomy, or by shifting the
wedge more anterior or posterior. If the patient had an extension deficit preoperatively, reduction of the tibial slope can be used to improve extension. The osteotomy
should then be opened markedly more in the back and less in the front, and the
effect on knee extension should be carefully monitored intraoperatively. A hard bol-
ster under the heel is very helpful.

An extension osteotomy may also be used in patients with a high natural tibial
slope and anterior knee instability. Slope reduction will shift the tibia backward on
weight-bearing and will reduce the anterior translation. If the patient has a symptomatic posterior knee instability and hyperextension of the knee, the opposite
effect can be helpful to reduce the posterior drawer and hyperextension. The tibial
slope can be increased by lifting the anterior part of the osteotomy more than that of
the posterior part until the knee has no hyperextension during the procedure. The

increased tibial slope also induces an anterior shift of the tibia in stance and gait, thus counteracting the posterior drawer of these patients. In many cases, modification of the slope is only possible if the surgeon removes some bone in the ascending cut by inserting the saw repeatedly into the cut.

When the correction fulfills all criteria, the osteotomy can be fixed. A locking-screw fixation plate can be employed to this effect. This plate is pre-contoured for the proximal medial tibia and carries four locked screws for the proximal fragment and four locked screws for the distal fragment (Fig. 8.9). The directions of the screws are adapted to the anatomy of the proximal tibia, and the plate is designed for medial placement on the tibia, thus giving proximal screw lengths of 50–85 mm. The proximal long screws are self-tapping, and in the interest of precise placement, predrilling is required with a special plate-mounted drill sleeve. The lengths of the proximal screws can be measured by the drill bit or with the AO/ASIF measuring device after the drill sleeve is removed. The three most distal screws are usually 26 mm long. Because they are placed in the hard bone of the tibial shaft, only mono-cortical fixation is needed here. The plate is mounted with three drill sleeves in the upper three holes. An insertion tool eases the mounting of the drill sleeves.

It is important to understand that this implant is placed subcutaneously above the MCL and the pes anserinus. In the elder plate versions, two 3-mm distance bolts are used to keep the plate in due distance from the soft tissues during application, thus avoiding compression of the pes anserinus or the medial collateral ligament by the plate. The newest plate version is pre-contoured and does need distance holders. A subcutaneous tunnel is created distally to enable the plate to glide under the skin on the periosteum of the tibia. The subcutaneous layer is also dissected proximally as

Fig. 8.9 The Tomofix implant is now inserted into a subcutaneous pouch. It usually centers itself automatically on the proximal tibia. The Tomofix plate is specifically configured for use in this osteotomy technique. Four locked screws are placed in the proximal fragment, and their position is predetermined to achieve maximum length. Four locked screws are used in the distal fragment. The screws in the shaft are inserted by a stab skin incision

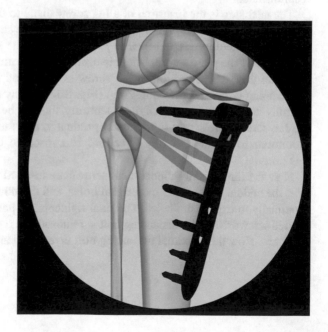

much as it is necessary to push the plate upward to the desired height near the joint line.

The leg is now extended and the fluoroscope is placed over the knee. An exact anteroposterior projection is obtained using the guidelines mentioned. The longitudinal part of the plate is pushed under the skin distally, and the transverse part is now pushed upward toward the joint line. Usually, the plate ends 10 mm under the joint line, and firm contact with the tibia should be obtained. A 2-mm inner drill sleeve is inserted into the middle drill sleeve mounted on the plate, and a K-wire is drilled into the proximal tibia under fluoroscopic control while pressure is applied to the plate. This K-wire should be placed in the proximal tibia with sufficient clearance to the joint but still allowing the placement of the fourth ascending screw into the proximal fragment of the osteotomy. The surgeon should keep in mind that the direction of this K-wire indicates the future position of the three proximal screws. These screws should be parallel to the joint line for optimum fit of the plate. The longitudinal part of the plate should be oriented parallel to the tibia and well centered over the tibial shaft. The surgical assistant must control the position of the plate end by palpation until the two first proximal screws are inserted (Fig. 8.13). If the placement of the plate is suboptimal, the K-wire is removed and replaced after correction.

The first screw is predrilled, the drill sleeve is removed, and a measuring device is used to determine the length of the screw. Bicortical fixation is not necessary. The screw is advanced initially with the power drill and then tightened with a torque-limited screwdriver to guarantee the correct insertional torque. The two other proximal screws are inserted in the same manner. Fluoroscopic control of the positions is recommended.

The next step is the insertion of a lag screw distal to the osteotomy. This conventional lag screw will pretension the plate and cause compression on the lateral side of the osteotomy. The screw is predrilled with the special drill sleeve. The lower part of the plate's combi-hole is used to avoid damage to the threads in the proximal part. The direction of the screw is distal and lateral. After drilling, a self-tapping cortical screw is inserted (Fig. 8.13). If any distraction has occurred laterally during the opening of the osteotomy, this can be reversed by insertion of the lag screw. The screw is tightened gradually, and the osteotomy is carefully monitored to avoid loss of correction. Fluoroscopic control is advocated at this time.

Now the three distal monocortical screws are inserted. A stab incision is made over the middle of the three most distal holes, and the skin is retracted distally and proximally to expose the holes. The final tightening is performed with the torque-limited screwdriver. The distancing bolt is removed and replaced with a monocortical screw. Now the proximal distancing bolt is removed and replaced with the drill sleeve. A self-tapping screw is inserted after predrilling and length measurement. The lag screw is removed, and the drill sleeve is mounted to the proximal part of this hole. Both cortical surfaces are drilled, and a screw with adequate length for bicortical fixation is inserted in this hole.

The spreader is now removed, and a final fluoroscopic control of the osteotomy is achieved in anteroposterior and lateral projection,. The clearance of the pes anserinus and the medial collateral ligament are checked. These structures should move freely under the plate. No formal repair of the medial collateral ligament fibers is required, but the distal ligament fibers should be repositioned over the osteotomy gap. A small collagen sponge is placed over the anterior osteotomy cleft to seal the gap and to avoid postoperative hematoma formation. A low-pressure drain is inserted. The osteotomy site should be filled with blood clots at this moment, and these clots must not be aspirated, nor should the osteotomy be flushed empty. The subcutaneous layer is closed with interrupted thin resorbable sutures, and the skin is closed with interrupted sutures. A padded elastic compression drape is applied over the entire leg, and a cryocompression unit is placed over the knee.

8.6 Complications

8.6.1 Intra-Articular Fractures

Fractures into the joint have been described during open-wedge procedures (Type 3 [14]). When the osteotomy is not opened gradually with chisels but forces are applied directly on the medial cortex, cracks may occur into the lateral tibial plateau with frank separation of the fragments. The spreading tool should be removed from the osteotomy in this situation. When the osteotomy is closed, the fracture should reduce and a clamp can be used to fix the reduction. Two or three percutaneous small fragment cortical screws are now inserted from the lateral side under fluoroscopic control parallel to the joint line, close to the subchondral sclerosis zone. The osteotomy is now carefully checked to assure that the bone cut is deep enough, leaving not more than 5- to 10-mm lateral bone in all areas. Chisels are now introduced and the osteotomy plane is opened again as described. The plate fixator can then be applied in the way described.

8.6.2 Fracture of the Lateral Hinge

Fractures of the lateral cortical hinge with separation of the two fragments (Type 1 [14]) may occur especially in young patients with hard bone. If this scenario occurs, the plate is first fixed to the proximal tibia, and then the lag screw is applied in a posterolateral direction in the first hole of the distal fragment. By tightening this lag screw carefully under fluoroscopic control, the distal fragment moves medially, and due to the oblique osteotomy plane, the lateral hinge will come under compression, and the planes will approximate again. Care must be taken not to tighten this screw too much; otherwise, the correction might be partially lost. The implant is so stable that when all screws are applied correctly, no change in the rehabilitation program is necessary.

8.6.3   Distal Fractures of the Hinge

A fracture line aiming distally from the hinge area (Type 2) causes significant instability of the osteotomy. The surgeon may use a screw crossing the lateral osteotomy line or even a small plate to stabilize such a fracture. If a distal fracture is identified later, the patient should be informed that healing will take longer [14].

8.6.4   Hematoma Formation

Because of the exposed cancellous bone, significant hematoma may develop in the lower leg after surgery, especially when the patient starts walking. The calf will be warm and redness may appear over the shin. Significant edema is also present. Treatment should include rest, ice, manual lymph drainage, and the use of a pneumatic calf pump. Since we seal the osteotomy site with a collagen sponge and restrict mobilization in the first 48 h, the incidence of hematoma has decreased significantly. The use of tranexamic acid may be considered [15, 16].

8.6.5   Inadvertent Change of the Tibial Slope

Whereas the correction in the frontal plane may be controlled clinically and fluoroscopically during the procedure, it is more difficult to monitor the position of the proximal fragment in the sagittal plane. The medial osteotomy gap should be carefully inspected during the procedure. The two planes should be oriented according to the surgical plan. The anterior opening (positive slope) can be increased by using a second osteotomy spreader or a wedge in the anterior part of the osteotomy. The posterior opening (negative slope) can be increased by extending the leg and placing the spreader in the very posterior part of the osteotomy. Active change of the tibial slope may be considered in three situations. In cases of extension deficit, decreasing the slope will improve knee extension. In cases of hyperextension of the knee, an increase of the tibial slope may limit hyperextension and thus stabilize the knee. In cases of chronic posterior knee instability, increasing the slope will improve stability of the knee in extension, because the femur slides back and the tibia slides anterior [1, 2, 17].

8.7   Rehabilitation

The patient is allowed to walk on the operated leg with partial weight-bearing the day after surgery using two crutches. Flexion of the knee is trained actively. If significant swelling of the lower leg develops, manual lymph drainage is performed, and an intermittent pneumatic compression unit is used for the first days. The patient leaves the hospital as soon as the wounds are dry and when walking with crutches is safe. He is allowed to load the leg adapted to the pain level, and no formal weight-restriction protocol is used anymore. Many patients are able to walk without crutches on flat ground after 3–4 weeks. Four weeks after surgery, the patient is examined in the outpatient department, and radiographs of the knee in two planes are obtained. Range of motion should be normal at this time, the patient should be pain-free, and the radiographs should demonstrate partial healing of the osteotomy and no lysis zones or instability signs. The patient is allowed to progress to all activities of daily living, which usually takes 1–4 more weeks. Occasionally, pain may develop in the hip or the ankle joint because of changes in the weight-bearing line. The patient is counseled that the full effect of the osteotomy will not be experienced until 3–5 months after surgery. No further routine radiographic controls are scheduled, and the patient returns to the care of the referring physician. The plate may not be removed before healing of the osteotomy gap, usually not earlier than 12–18 months after surgery, but can also be left in place if the patient does not request implant removal (Figs. 8.10, 8.11, 8.12, and 8.13).

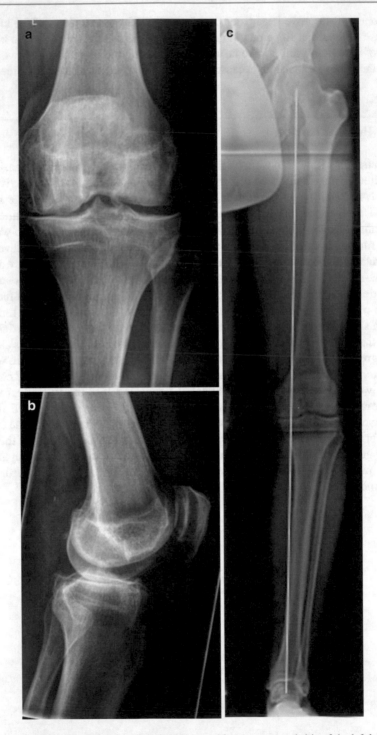

Fig. 8.10 (a–c) Radiographs of a 70-year-old man with varus osteoarthritis of the left knee after medial meniscectomy. Deformity analysis reveals a constitutional varus of the tibia (MPTA 83°)

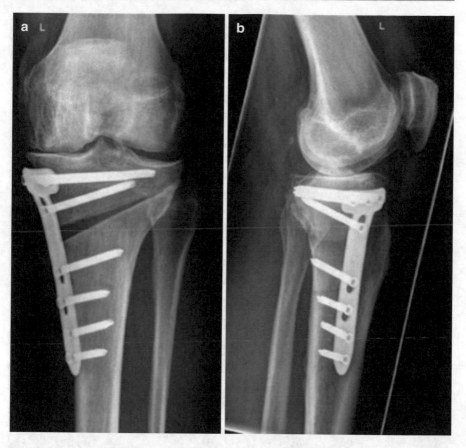

Fig. 8.11 (**a, b**) Postoperative radiographs after 10-mm biplanar open-wedge correction. Full weight-bearing and unrestricted ADL were achieved after 6 weeks

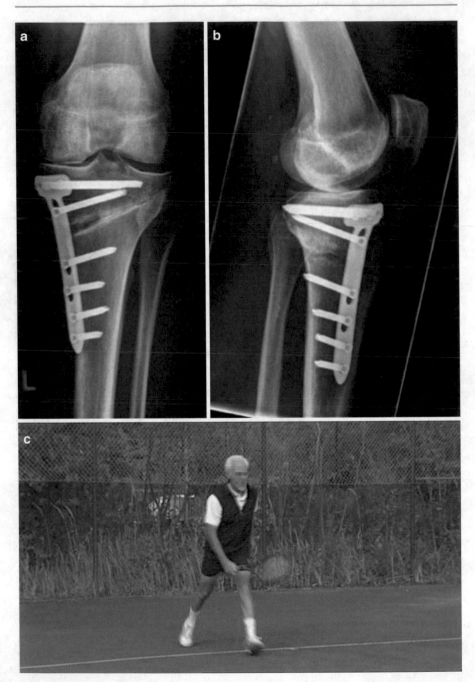

Fig. 8.12 (**a, b**) Anteroposterior and lateral radiographs after 5 months. Note the solid bone formation in the central and posterior parts of the osteotomy. (**c**) The patient was able to play tennis for 3 h per week without pain

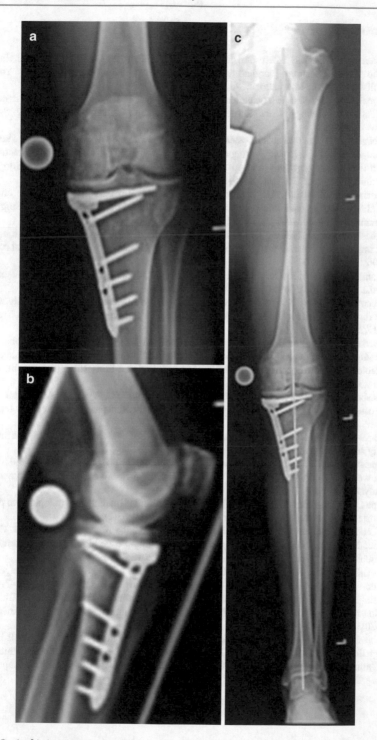

Fig. 8.13 (**a, b**) Anteroposterior and lateral radiographs 9 years after HTO. The patient is completely pain-free and is not restricted in his activities. (**c**) Long-leg radiograph 9 years after HTO. The alignment has not changed

References

1. Lobenhoffer HP, Van Heerwaarden R, Staubli A, Jakob R. Osteotomy around the knee. Indications – planning – surgical techniques using plate fixators. Stuttgart, New York: AO Publishing Thieme International; 2008, 277p.
2. Lobenhoffer HP, Van Heerwaarden R, Agneskirchner JD. Kniegelenknahe Osteotomien. Indikation – Planung – Operationstechniken mit Plattenfixateuren. Thieme Verlag: Stuttgart, New York; 2014.
3. Lobenhoffer P. The rationale of osteotomy around the knee. J Knee Surg. 2017;30(5):386–92.
4. Aydogdu S, Cullu E, Arac N, Varolgunes N, Sur H. Prolonged peroneal nerve dysfunction after high tibial osteotomy: pre- and postoperative electrophysiological study. Knee Surg Sports Traumatol Arthrosc. 2000;8(5):305–8.
5. Floerkemeier S, Staubli AE, Schroeter S, Goldhahn S, Lobenhoffer P. Outcome after high tibial open-wedge osteotomy: a retrospective evaluation of 533 patients. Knee Surg Sports Traumatol Arthrosc. 2013;21(1):170–80.
6. Agneskirchner JD, Freiling D, Hurschler C, Lobenhoffer P. Primary stability of four different implants for opening wedge high tibial osteotomy. Knee Surg Sports Traumatol Arthrosc. 2006;14(3):291–300.
7. Bonnin M, Chambat P. [Current status of valgus angle, tibial head closing wedge osteotomy in media gonarthrosis]. Orthopade. 2004;33(2):135–42.
8. Lobenhoffer P, Kley K, Freiling D, van Heerwaarden R. [Medial closed wedge osteotomy of the distal femur in biplanar technique and a specific plate fixator]. Oper Orthop Traumatol 2017;29(4):306–19.
9. Floerkemeier S, Staubli AE, Schroeter S, Goldhahn S, Lobenhoffer P. Does obesity and nicotine abuse influence the outcome and complication rate after open-wedge high tibial osteotomy? A retrospective evaluation of five hundred and thirty three patients. Int Orthop. 2014;38(1):55–60.
10. Gaasbeek RD, Sonneveld H, van Heerwaarden RJ, Jacobs WC, Wymenga AB. Distal tuberosity osteotomy in open wedge high tibial osteotomy can prevent patella infera: a new technique. Knee. 2004;11(6):457–61.
11. Schroter S, Elson DW, Ateschrang A, Ihle C, Stockle U, Dickschas J, et al. Lower limb deformity analysis and the planning of an osteotomy. J Knee Surg. 2017;30(5):393–408.
12. Agneskirchner JD, Hurschler C, Wrann CD, Lobenhoffer P. The effects of valgus medial opening wedge high tibial osteotomy on articular cartilage pressure of the knee: a biomechanical study. Arthroscopy. 2007;23(8):852–61.
13. Pape D, Seil R, Adam F, Rupp S, Kohn D, Lobenhoffer P. [Imaging and preoperative planning of osteotomy of tibial head osteotomy]. Orthopade. 2004;33(2):122–34.
14. Takeuchi R, Ishikawa H, Kumagai K, Yamaguchi Y, Chiba N, Akamatsu Y, et al. Fractures around the lateral cortical hinge after a medial opening-wedge high tibial osteotomy: a new classification of lateral hinge fracture. Arthroscopy. 2012;28(1):85–94.
15. Kim KI, Kim HJ, Kim GB, Bae SH. Tranexamic acid is effective for blood management in open-wedge high tibial osteotomy. Orthop Traumatol Surg Res. 2018;104(7):1003–7.
16. Steinhaus ME, Buksbaum J, Eisenman A, Kohli M, Fragomen AT, Rozbruch SR. Tranexamic acid reduces postoperative blood loss in distal femoral osteotomy. J Knee Surg. 2020;33(5):440–4.
17. Agneskirchner JD, Hurschler C, Stukenborg-Colsman C, Imhoff AB, Lobenhoffer P. Effect of high tibial flexion osteotomy on cartilage pressure and joint kinematics: a biomechanical study in human cadaveric knees. Winner of the AGA-DonJoy Award 2004. Arch Orthop Trauma Surg. 2004;124(9):575–84.

Lateral Closing-Wedge High Tibial Osteotomy

Philipp von Roth and Clemens Gwinner

9.1 Introduction (Indication/Contraindication)

Since the development of internal fixed-angle plate fixators, the medial opening high tibial osteotomy has become the most widely used procedure for the treatment of unicompartimental, medial osteoarthritis with an underlying bony varus alignment of the tibia [1]. Even though surgical techniques continue to evolve, there still is considerable controversy concerning the possibility of subsequent postoperative leg lengthening and reduction of the patella height (i.e., patella baja) [2–4]. In addition, medial opening-wedge osteotomies might lead to higher tension of the patella tendon and medial collateral ligament, which in turn increases the intra-articular pressure and may negatively influence clinical outcome [5].

Despite recognition of the aforementioned, lateral closing-wedge high tibial osteotomy is viewed as a less attractive alternative. However, it should belong to the surgical repertoire of an individually tailored correction osteotomy of varus malalignments of the proximal tibia.

Symptomatic varus arthritis of the knee and post-traumatic varus deformities are the main indications for a lateral closing-wedge high tibial osteotomy. Some authors also advocate the relief of the medial femorotibial compartment in combination with cartilage reconstructions as a reasonable indication.

In line with medial opening-wedge osteotomies, outcome depends on proper patient selection in terms of cartilage deterioration and range of motion. Even though there is little consensus on patient selection, some broad criteria can be described. Consequently, contraindications include:

P. von Roth (✉)
Sporthopaedicum, Straubing, Germany
e-mail: roth@sporthopaedicum.de

C. Gwinner
Department of Orthopaedic Surgery, Charité Universitätsmedizin Berlin, Berlin, Germany
e-mail: clemens.gwinner@charite.de

© Springer Nature Switzerland AG 2020
S. Oussedik, S. Lustig (eds.), *Osteotomy About the Knee*,
https://doi.org/10.1007/978-3-030-49055-3_9

- Concomitant chondromalacia > III° according to the ICRS classification in the lateral femorotibial compartment.
- Extrusion or insufficiency of the lateral meniscus.
- An extension deficit of more than 10°, which cannot be adequately reduced arthroscopically (e.g. by notchplasty, resection of eminence osteophytes).
- Risk factors for delayed bone healing including neuropathies, rheumatic diseases, immunosuppressive drugs and heavy smoking [6].

9.2 Patient Preparation, Radiologic Analysis and Planning

The clinical examination should include a thorough analysis of the leg geometry in the frontal and sagittal planes, leg length and torsion ratios in both thighs and lower legs. In addition, the ranges of motion of the hip, knee and ankle joints need to be determined. Moreover, ligament stability should be evaluated, and the patellofemoral tracking should be assessed. Additional intra-articular pathologies such as meniscus lesions or a concomitant plica syndrome must be detected, as they need to be addressed intraoperatively (e.g. arthroscopically).

The standard set of radiographs should contain weight-bearing full leg and lateral radiographs of the respective knee. Rosenberg views with the knee in 45° of flexion can be used to further evaluate the lateral compartment joint space. An additional MRI examination can be useful for identifying accompanying pathologies. Notably, the whole-leg images need to confirm that the deformity is located in the proximal tibia. If the deformity is in the femur, it should be corrected by a femoral osteotomy.

Notwithstanding the contributions of soft tissue restraints on knee kinematics, there is an emerging consensus that the tibial slope has an analogous impact on sagittal stability, centre of rotation and loading of the cruciate ligaments. In a landmark cadaveric study, Agneskirchner and Lobenhoffer revealed that alterations of the sagittal tibial alignment can be used to counteract insufficiencies of the cruciate ligaments [7]. Hence, assessment of the tibial slope should be an integral part of the preoperative workup.

Most authors intend to transfer the mechanical axis from the impaired medial compartment to a point slightly lateral of the knee's midline in order to decrease abnormal joint loading and subsequently delay further osteoarthritic changes. This originates from the research of Fujisawa et al., and the alignment target has been later referred as Fujisawa's point [8]. Consequently, the weight-bearing line should pass roughly 62.5% of the tibial plateau width when measured from medial to lateral. Commonly, this marking point is projected just lateral to the lateral tibial eminence.

In order to determine the amount of tibial correction on the long-leg AP radiograph, the ideal postoperative weight-bearing line (WBL) needs to be assessed, which should ideally cross the joint level at the desired Fujisawa point (Fig. 9.1). In a next step, a second line is drawn from the medial hinge of the osteotomy through the centre of the talus. Finally, a third line is applied from the osteotomy's hinge at

Fig. 9.1 A meticulous planning is the basis for a success surgical treatment. The figure shows the relevant lines that have to be drawn to define the angle of correction in order to calculate the size of the lateral wedge

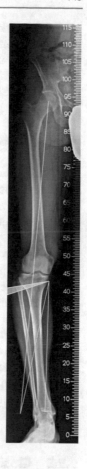

the intersection of the postoperative WBL at level of the ankle joint. The angle between the second and the third line represents the correction angle and can now be transformed to the proximal tibia. The respective distance between both lines on the lateral cortex indicates the amount of the lateral closing-wedge osteotomy.

9.3 Surgical Technique

9.3.1 Patient Positioning and Approach

Both spinal and general anaesthesia are suitable options. The patient is placed in a supine position, and the operating table ideally has motor-adjustable upper and lower-leg plates. A tourniquet can be used upon the surgeon's preference.

After preoperative antibiotic administration, team-time-out, disinfection and sterile draping, a routine arthroscopy is performed using a standard high lateral portal to verify the indication for a high tibial osteotomy. Further arthroscopic measures can be performed according to the existing intra-articular pathology [9]. Next, bony landmarks such as the patella, tibial tuberosity and fibula head need to be identified, then, an approximately 6-cm-long and almost horizontal skin incision starting 1 cm above the anterior tibial tuberosity towards a point 1 cm below the fibular head. The lower-leg fascia is then dissected, and the insertion of the tibialis anterior is released as a Z-plasty.

9.3.2 Osteotomy of the Fibula

The fibula osteotomy can be realised via the existing approach at the neck of the fibula (advantage, same approach; disadvantage, higher risk for peroneal nerve injury) or via an additional approach at the transition from the middle to the distal third of the fibula (advantage, lower risk for nerve injury; disadvantage, additional approach).

If the first mentioned variant is the preferred location for the osteotomy, the neck of the fibular head has to be presented. Next, the periosteum should be elevated at the level of the osteotomy by using a blunt elevator. It is mandatory to stay close to the fibular bone in order to protect the peroneal nerve. Some authors advocate dissecting and presenting the peroneal nerve in all of the cases. Depending on the degree of correction, the size of the bone resection has to be made, and the osteotomy is then conducted with the oscillating saw using a short 0.6-mm saw blade.

In the latter variant, a longitudinal short fasciotomy and predominantly blunt preparation on the fibula are performed. Under the protection of Hohmann retractors, the osteotomy is then conducted with the oscillating saw, again using a short 0.6-mm saw blade.

9.3.3 Closing-Wedge Osteotomy of the Tibia

After the above-mentioned Z-plasty of the tibialis anterior muscle, the tibial is prepared by sharply dissecting the origin of the tibialis anterior muscle, leaving a fascial bridge of about 0.5–1 cm. The preparation is continued dorsally to the dorsolateral edge of the tibia. A precise haemostasis with the electrocautery is obligatory to minimise the risk of a subsequent compartment syndrome. In the area of the ventrolateral edge of the tibia, the anterior tibial muscle is prepared with a blunt elevator. The subperiosteal detachment of the posterior soft tissues from the tibia with the curved elevator with the knee in a slightly flexed position is performed, and the insertion of a Hohmann retractor takes place at the planned level of the osteotomy.

Next, the tibial tuberosity must be visualised, and the lateral margin of the patella tendon is identified. The tibial tuberosity should now be chiselled from proximal to distal for a few millimetres in the sense of two-plane osteotomy while protecting the patellar tendon. Alternatively, the ascending osteotomy can be performed with a short 0.6-mm saw blade.

The height of the tibial osteotomy and the correction angle are now determined by the use of an image intensifier. First, a 1.8-mm Kirschner wire is drilled under image intensifier control at right angles to the tibia axis. The direction can increase medially in case of an isolated valgus correction. For an additional rotational correction, a right angle to the mechanical tibial axis must be maintained. A second Kirschner wire is then inserted at the defined correction angle ascending from distal lateral to proximal medial. In cases of an isolated valgising osteotomy, a medial cortical bridge should be maintained; in case of additional supra-tuberosity torsion correction, a complete transverse osteotomy must be performed. The planned correction angle can be checked by a sterile goniometer at the two ends of the Kirschner wires or by image intensifier control in exact orthograde projection.

The next step is to check the soft tissue release. In particular, reliable subperiosteal exposure must be ensured dorsally and ventrally in order to be able to recover the osteotomy wedge completely and without any problems. The soft tissues are protected with Hohmann retractors. The osteotomy is performed with the oscillating saw using a 0.6-mm saw blade. Care should be taken that the saw blade is guided precisely along and distal to the proximal Kirschner wire. It is advisable to leave a saw blade in situ as an indicator of the sagittal plane of the saw cut. The second osteotomy is then performed along the second Kirschner wire and parallel to the first saw blade. The cortical bone must be completely divided both ventrally and dorsally, carefully protecting the neurovascular and muscular structures dorsally as well as the tuberosity and patellar tendon ventrally. Once the osteotomy has been completed, the bone wedge is gently mobilised and extracted.

9.3.4   Fixation

If the medial tibial head cortex has been deliberately preserved, it can now be weakened by drilling with a 2.0-mm drill to avoid uncontrolled fracturing.

The lower leg is then gently and patiently valgised manually. The correction can be temporarily transfixated with Kirschner wires or lag screws. Guiding jigs and reduction clamps are also available from several manufacturers. Now the anatomical axis between the hip centre and the centre of the upper ankle can be checked by using the cable of the electrocautery under the image intensifier. If the correction is satisfactory, the osteosynthesis material can be inserted. Depending on the author, fixation is performed with staples, screws, specific plates or conventional internal fixed-angle plate fixators [10–14].

9.4   Complications

In addition to general complications such as neurovascular injuries, wound disturbance, infection and remaining pain, the patient must be informed about the specific complications of this procedure. Critics of lateral closed-wedge osteotomy usually call the damage of the peroneal nerve the main complication. The literature reports a percentage ranging from 3% to 12% [15].

As mentioned earlier, some authors advocate dissecting and presenting the peroneal nerve in all of the cases. Performing the fibular osteotomy via a second approach at the middle to distal third of the fibular may further decrease the incidence for peroneal nerve palsy [16].

Another possible complication is an over- or undercorrection due to an insufficient preoperative analysis, adequate planning of the correction and/or incorrect surgical implementation [6].

According to the literature, the risk of non-union is about 1% [15].

The accidental fracturing of the medial tibial head corticalis should also be stated as a possible complication [17]. In this case, an internal fixed-angle plate fixators should be considered.

Sherman and Cabanela recommend in order to minimise the risk of intra-articular fracture that the apex of the osteotomy cut should end within 5 mm of the far cortex leaving the proximal fragment 15 mm thick at a minimum [15].

Finally, there is a risk for developing a compartment syndrome. The use of a drain should decrease this risk [15].

If there is a clinical suspicion of compartment syndrome and/or an intra-compartmental increase in pressure, an immediate fasciotomy of the tibialis anterior loge must be performed, possibly also of the other lower-leg compartments.

9.5 Postoperative Care

A possible compartment syndrome should be monitored for the first 24 h. Due to the higher risk for a compartment syndrome in case of a closing-wedge osteotomy with an additional rotation correction, a monitoring for 3 days is recommended [6]. A radiograph of the knee in two planes should be taken before and after mobilisation (e.g. day 1 and day 7 after surgery).

The mobilisation of the patient can be realised from the first postoperative day on forearm crutches under partial load of 20 kg without movement restriction. No external splinting or orthosis is necessary. Active and passive physiotherapeutic exercise and also lymphatic drainage can be applied as required. A weight- and risk-adapted thromboembolic prophylaxis should be initiated according to the national guidelines.

In the fifth postoperative week, another radiograph of the knee in two planes should be taken for monitoring the healing process. Afterwards, the load of the operated limb can be increased with 20 kg weekly. Implant removal is possible from the 12th postoperative month.

9.6 Summary

Closing-wedge lateral osteotomy of the proximal tibia is an effective treatment for the medial compartment gonarthrosis. Advantages over an opening-wedge technique include the ability to reduce tibial slope, allowing compression across the broad surfaces of the osteotomised tibia, promoting union. Possible disadvantages include a greater distortion to the epiphyseal/diaphyseal relationship, complicating subsequent total knee arthroplasty if required. However, it remains useful procedure in the knee surgeon's armamentarium.

References

 1. Niemeyer P, Schmal H, Hauschild O, von Heyden J, Sudkamp NP, Kostler W. Open-wedge osteotomy using an internal plate fixator in patients with medial-compartment gonarthritis and varus malalignment: 3-year results with regard to preoperative arthroscopic and radiographic findings. Arthroscopy. 2010;26(12):1607–16.
 2. Kim JH, Kim HJ, Lee DH. Leg length change after opening wedge and closing wedge high tibial osteotomy: a meta-analysis. PLoS One. 2017;12(7):e0181328.
 3. Kim JI, Kim BH, Lee KW, Lee O, Han HS, Lee S, et al. Lower limb length discrepancy after high tibial osteotomy: prospective randomized controlled trial of lateral closing versus medial opening wedge osteotomy. Am J Sports Med. 2016;44(12):3095–102.
 4. Smith TO, Sexton D, Mitchell P, Hing CB. Opening- or closing-wedged high tibial osteotomy: a meta-analysis of clinical and radiological outcomes. Knee. 2011;18(6):361–8.
 5. Agneskirchner JD, Hurschler C, Wrann CD, Lobenhoffer P. The effects of valgus medial opening wedge high tibial osteotomy on articular cartilage pressure of the knee: a biomechanical study. Arthroscopy. 2007;23(8):852–61.
 6. Strecker W, Muller M, Urschel C. [High tibial closed wedge valgus osteotomy]. Oper Orthop Traumatol 2014;26(2):196–205.
 7. Agneskirchner JD, Hurschler C, Stukenborg-Colsman C, Imhoff AB, Lobenhoffer P. Effect of high tibial flexion osteotomy on cartilage pressure and joint kinematics: a biomechanical study in human cadaveric knees. Winner of the AGA-DonJoy Award 2004. Arch Orthop Trauma Surg. 2004;124(9):575–84.
 8. Fujisawa Y, Masuhara K, Shiomi S. The effect of high tibial osteotomy on osteoarthritis of the knee. An arthroscopic study of 54 knee joints. Orthop Clin North Am. 1979;10(3):585–608.
 9. Strecker W, Dickschas J, Harrer J, Muller M. [Arthroscopy prior to osteotomy in cases of unicondylar osteoarthritis]. Orthopade 2009;38(3):263–8.
10. Zuegel NP, Braun WG, Kundel KP, Rueter AE. Stabilization of high tibial osteotomy with staples. Arch Orthop Trauma Surg. 1996;115(5):290–4.
11. Hee HT, Low CK, Seow KH, Tan SK. Comparing staple fixation to buttress plate fixation in high tibial osteotomy. Ann Acad Med Singap. 1996;25(2):233–5.
12. van Raaij TM, Brouwer RW. Proximal tibial valgus osteotomy: lateral closing wedge. JBJS Essent Surg Tech. 2015;5(4):e26.
13. Bae DK, Mun MS, Kwon OS. A newly designed miniplate staple for high tibial osteotomy. Bull Hosp Jt Dis. 1997;56(3):167–70.
14. Takeuchi R, Ishikawa H, Miyasaka Y, Sasaki Y, Kuniya T, Tsukahara S. A novel closed-wedge high tibial osteotomy procedure to treat osteoarthritis of the knee: hybrid technique and rehabilitation measures. Arthrosc Tech. 2014;3(4):e431–7.
15. Sherman C, Cabanela ME. Closing wedge osteotomy of the tibia and the femur in the treatment of gonarthrosis. Int Orthop. 2010;34(2):173–84.
16. Wootton JR, Ashworth MJ, MacLaren CA. Neurological complications of high tibial osteotomy—the fibular osteotomy as a causative factor: a clinical and anatomical study. Ann R Coll Surg Engl. 1995;77(1):31–4.
17. van Raaij TM, Brouwer RW, de Vlieger R, Reijman M, Verhaar JA. Opposite cortical fracture in high tibial osteotomy: lateral closing compared to the medial opening-wedge technique. Acta Orthop. 2008;79(4):508–14.

Lateral Opening-Wedge Distal Femoral Osteotomy

10

S. Cerciello, K. Corona, and P. Neyret

10.1 Introduction

The alignment of the lower limb is important for correct function and to prevent complications such as cartilage degeneration of the knee and ankle [1]. The normal physiologic anatomic knee alignment is within 5–8° of valgus, while the mechanical axis of the lower limb is approximately 178° in men and 176° and 174° in Asian and Caucasian women, respectively [2]. When the axis is beyond this threshold, there is increased load on lateral compartment, with further cartilage wear, overstress on medial ligamentous structures, and alterations in gait which are even more relevant in patients with body mass index >25 [3, 4]. Moreover, the anatomic damage increases with the degree of valgus deformity [1]. Valgus malalignment, which is less common than varus, may result from trauma, from previous lateral meniscectomy, or from other conditions affecting growth plate morphology [5]. When dealing with these situations, it is crucial to locate the deformity itself. Varus knee is almost always the consequence of bony deformity on the tibia, while valgus knee may be caused by femoral (hypoplasia of the lateral condyle) or tibial (lateral meniscectomy or lateral tibial plateau fractures) deformities. Osteotomies are challenging procedures, which are indicated in relatively young patients. By restoring correct

S. Cerciello (✉)
Casa di Cura Villa Betania, Rome, Italy

Marrelli Hospital, Crotone, Italy

K. Corona
Department of Medicine and Health Sciences "Vincenzo Tiberio", University of Molise, Campobasso, Italy

P. Neyret
Infirmerie Protestante, Lyon Caluire, France

© Springer Nature Switzerland AG 2020
S. Oussedik, S. Lustig (eds.), *Osteotomy About the Knee*,
https://doi.org/10.1007/978-3-030-49055-3_10

lower-limb axis, they delay progression of knee arthritis, allowing a return to physical activity [6–8]. The procedure is technically demanding, and several complications such as stiffness and patellofemoral arthrosis have been reported [9]; nonetheless, it yields satisfactory long-term clinical and functional results [10–12]. It seems logical to address bony deformity where it happens; therefore tibial varization osteotomy is indicated for tibial deformity and femoral osteotomy for femoral deformity. However, due to the physiologic joint line obliquity, femoral osteotomy is indicated even for tibial severe deformities (beyond 12°). In these cases, tibial osteotomy would result in increased joint line obliquity and lateral subluxation of the tibia [13]. In addition, it should be highlighted that distal femoral osteotomy (DFO) only corrects limb malalignment in extension and not in flexion. Whether an opening- or a closing-wedge osteotomy yields superior outcomes remains to be determined, as current literature supports both procedures.

10.2 Indications and Contraindications

Indications for a distal femoral varization osteotomy are valgus femur from either femoral or tibial deformity, mild to moderate cartilage degeneration of the lateral compartment, focal cartilage lesions of the lateral femoral condyle, and lateral meniscal transplantation. It should be highlighted that the correction threshold for a lateral opening-wedge osteotomy should be limited up to 10–15°, while for medial closing wedge osteotomy, it should be up to 20–25°. Relative contraindications include severe patellofemoral osteoarthritis, smoking (especially for open wedge), high body mass index, ligamentous instability, and age over 55 years. Absolute contraindications include severe medial or tricompartmental osteoarthritis, symptomatic medial compartment disease, inflammatory arthritis, flexion contracture >15°, knee flexion <90°, and severe osteoporosis. The theoretical advantages of the opening-wedge technique over the medial closing-wedge technique include a single bone cut with less potential errors, avoidance of the medial vascular structures, and better control of the amount of correction [14]. Relative disadvantages include potential for delayed union or nonunion and irritation of the sensitive lateral knee structures by hardware or surgical trauma.

10.3 Planning

Preoperative planning is crucial to predict all surgical steps and calculate desired correction. Imaging is mainly based on traditional X-rays. Long-leg standing weight-bearing, 45° flexion postero-anterior (Rosenberg) views of both knees and lateral knee radiographs are required.

The Rosenberg view is helpful to evaluate the lateral and medial compartment cartilage wear and to evaluate deformity associated with cruciate deficiency, because the cartilage wear is typically located in the posterior tibial plateau [15]. Based on these views, the following parameters are calculated: axis of the lower limb, tibial and femoral mechanical axes, patellar height, and the inclination of the joint line. Additional exams may include magnetic resonance imaging (MRI) to assess the status of the cartilage and the subchondral bone or the presence of bone edema.

The osteotomy should aim at a postoperative neutral alignment, such that the mechanical axis line passes through the center of the knee [16]. However such a goal usually ends up with loss of correction and recurrence of lateral cartilage degeneration; therefore some authors recommend slight overcorrection [17]. The final axis should aim at a point just medial to the medial tibial spine to unload the diseased lateral compartment while avoiding overload of the medial side of the joint [18]. This trend has been confirmed in a recent biomechanical analysis that showed better unloading of the lateral compartment and better restoration of the normal biomechanics in overcorrected knees compared with normo-correction to neutral alignment [19]. The authors concluded that overcorrecting the osteotomy of 5° respect to the normal anatomic alignment normalizes contact pressure and contact areas in the lateral compartment [19]. Similarly, other authors reported good clinical outcomes with overcorrection (mechanical axis goal at 40–41% of tibial plateau) due to lateral compartment unloading and medial muscles' force neutralization [20, 21].

The amount of correction is calculated based on the angle formed between the mechanical axis of the femur and tibia. The calculated angle of correction in degrees determines the amount of wedge opening. The geometric triangle method is commonly used, measuring the distance on a size-calibrated radiograph [22]. Al-Saati et al. proposed more sophisticated algorithm with individual goals [23]. If the osteotomy is performed to correct the sequelae of a hypercorrect valgization osteotomy, the goal should be similar to those of the initial procedure: a final valgus of around 3°. If it is performed to protect the degeneration of the lateral compartment (e.g., in the sequelae of a lateral meniscectomy), then the goal should be a neutral axis. If the valgus is consequent to a malunion of the lateral tibial plateau, then a neutral alignment or slight overcorrection of the mechanical axis into the medial compartment should be planned. In any case, the correction must consider the alignment of the contralateral leg and the possible complication related to major corrections.

10.4   Surgical Technique

The surgical technique differs if a locking plate or a 95° blade plate is used. The patient is supine, and the sterile field should include the entire limb from the iliac crest in order to assess the axis per operatively. Intraoperative fluoroscopy is mandatory to assess the level and direction of the osteotomy, the axis, and the correction, and therefore the index limb should be raised to not overlap the contralateral limb. The limb is held in slight flexion (around 45°) to minimize the risk of iatrogenic neurovascular injury and to decrease tension on the neurovascular bundle and increase their distance from the posterior cortex. A sterile tourniquet can be used.

When a *95° blade plate* is used (Fig. 10.1), a 10–12 cm incision is made on the lateral distal femur from the lateral epicondyle proximally along the axis of the

Fig. 10.1 95° blade plate
has the advantage of
automatic correction of the
deformity of 5° when
inserted parallel to the
joint line

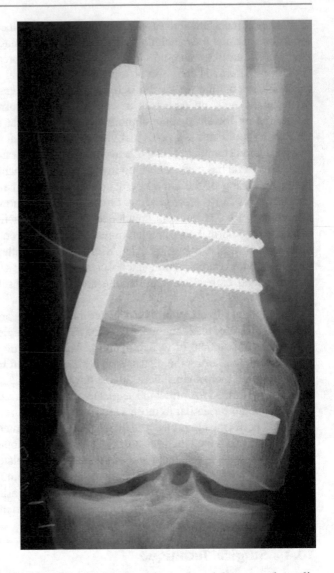

thigh (Fig. 10.2). The iliotibial band is identified and incised, and the vastus lateralis
is elevated and dissected off the lateral intermuscular septum to expose the femoral
shaft. During this manoeuver, great care should be taken to coagulate arterial
branches of the profunda femoris.

The patella tendon is identified and a limited lateral arthrotomy is performed.
This is strongly advised to visualize the orientation of the trochlea and the condyles. Two guide pins are inserted into the joint: one at the femorotibial joint line
and another in the patella femoral joint (Fig. 10.3). The guide pins help orienting
the surgeon to accurately place the blade plate. A mark on the cortex above and
below the anticipated osteotomy helps assess any potential rotation of the femur

Fig. 10.2 A 10–12 cm incision is made on the lateral distal femur from the lateral epicondyle proximally along the axis of the thigh

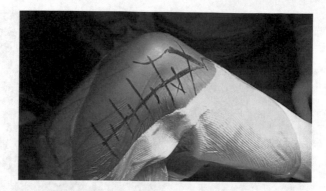

Fig. 10.3 Two guide pins are inserted into the joint: one at the femorotibial joint line and another in the patella femoral joint to guide the surgeon for blade plate insertion

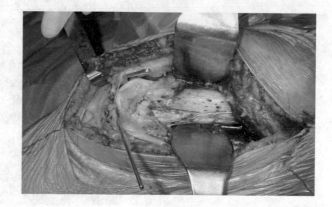

(Fig. 10.4). The osteotomy is horizontal, just proximal to the lateral part of the trochlea. It is performed with an oscillating saw and then completed with sharp thin osteotomes. The medial cortex should be preserved but can be weakened using a 3.2 mm drill bit. An additional anterior coronal osteotomy may be added, to increase stability. Progressive opening of the osteotomy with dedicated devices or osteotomes is not mandatory since it is the impaction of the blade plate that will progressively open up the osteotomy once in contact with the diaphysis. The blade is then introduced into the epiphyseal region around 30 mm proximal to the joint line, anteriorly and proximally to the femoral insertion of the lateral collateral ligament. The angle of insertion depends on the level of the deformity. If the deformity is situated at the diaphyseal level, the blade should be introduced obliquely to the joint line (Fig. 10.5). To obtain a varization of 10°, the angle should be set at 75° (85–10°; complementary angle to the anatomical distal femoral angle (95°)—angle of correction). If the deformity is situated at the metaphyseal level, which is the most common situation, the blade is introduced parallel to the joint line (Fig. 10.6). In this last case, an automatic correction to the normal anatomical femoral valgus of 5° is automatically obtained. In others words, if the femur is normal, no correction would be obtained when the blade plate is introduced parallel to the joint line. The position of the blade can be checked using the

Fig. 10.4 A mark on the cortex above and below the anticipated osteotomy helps assess any potential rotation of the femur

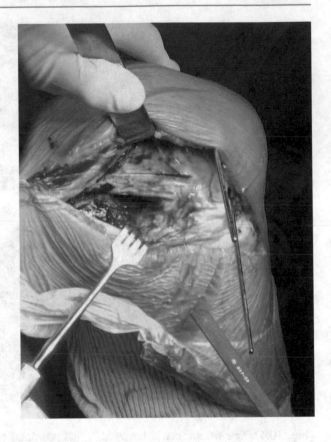

image intensifier. The angle of correction can now be measured on a printout by drawing a line tangent to the medial and lateral condyle and another line tangent to the blade. Progressive impaction of the plate allows opening of the osteotomy. Temporary fixation with one proximal screw (in the proximal part of the oval hole) helps to control the correction and gives additional stability. Managing the impaction and the positioning of the screws can help in fine adjusting the amount of opening. If the blade plate is impacted with the screw left in place, the correction will be halted. On the contrary, if an additional screw is placed in the distal part of the screw hole and the former screw is taken out, the correction can be augmented. Final fixation of the blade plate is achieved with four 4.5 mm-diameter cortical screws (Fig. 10.7). The osteotomy defect should be filled with iliac crest autograft or cancellous allograft if the opening is >8 mm. In case of corrections <8 mm and especially in nonsmoker patients, the defect can be left empty. The soft tissues and skin are closed over a drain, which is introduced underneath the fascia lata.

Fig. 10.5 If the deformity is situated at the diaphyseal region, the blade should be introduced obliquely to the joint line

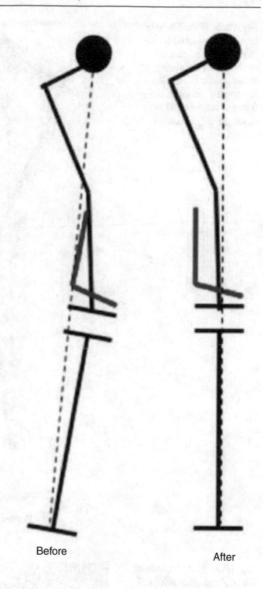

Before   After

When a *locking plate* is used (Fig. 10.8), a smaller approach of around 8–10 cm can be used. It is then possible to elevate the very distal part of the vastus lateralis while the plate slides under the vastus lateralis, and screw insertion is performed through the skin and muscle. In any case, clear visualization of the metaphysis and distal diaphysis is preferable. An arthrotomy is optional and indicated to assess and treat intra-articular pathology. The lateral aspect of the femur is thoroughly exposed, and a longitudinal mark on the cortex is performed to avoid any mal-torsion. Under fluoroscopic control, the starting point for the osteotomy is identified approximately 3 cm above the lateral femoral epicondyle, and a guide pin is angled medially and

Fig. 10.6 If the blade is introduced parallel to the joint line (as in case of metaphyseal deformities), an automatic correction to the normal anatomical femoral valgus of 5° is automatically obtained

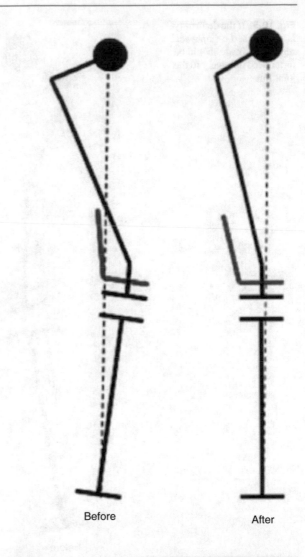

Before

After

Fig. 10.7 Final fixation of the blade plate is achieved with four 4.5 mm-diameter cortical screws

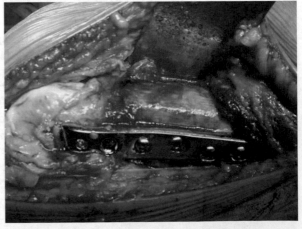

Fig. 10.8 Locking plate has the advantage of smaller incision with reduced soft tissue damage

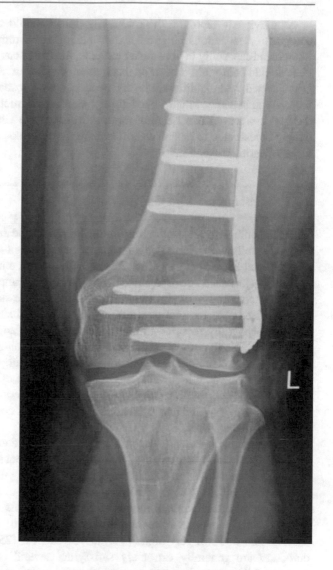

distally toward the medial femoral condyle just above the level of the medial epicondyle. It should be highlighted that the line must pass above the articular surface of the trochlea to avoid any cartilage damage. After fluoroscopic check, the osteotomy is performed with an oscillating saw and completed with sharp thin osteotomes, taking care to maintain approximately 1 cm of medial bone bridge for osteotomy stability. As previously described, an additional anterior coronal plane osteotomy helps control the rotation and stabilize the construct per operatively and increases the surface area for healing. Once the osteotomy is mobile, it is opened free hand or with dedicated devices. When the desired correction is achieved and confirmed clinically and fluoroscopically, a lateral fluoroscopy check is performed to ensure that no flexion or extension of the osteotomy is present. Several plates are available on the market; in any case, the osteotomy should be fixed with at least six screws.

As previously reported, the osteotomy defect should be filled with iliac crest autograft or cancellous allograft if the opening is >8 mm. In case of corrections <8 mm and especially in nonsmoker patients, the defect can be left empty. A locking plate should be used in case of an unstable medial cortex. After final check, a drain is positioned, and the different layers are closed with absorbable sutures. The leg is then placed in a knee brace locked in full extension for mobilization/ambulation for the first 6 weeks. Knee range-of-motion exercises are allowed after surgery. The patient is restricted to partial weight-bearing for 6 weeks, followed by progressive weight-bearing thereafter.

10.5   Outcomes and Complications

Lateral opening-wedge femoral osteotomies yield good functional results even at long-term follow-up. Zarrouk et al. reported a significant improvement in terms of International Knee Society (IKS) score, modified KSS, and Functional Score in 22 patients [24]. Ekeland et al. reported significant improvement in KOOS score and in each sub-score at 1-year FU; the score remained at the same level for all patients with survived osteotomy at final follow-up [25]. Good survival rate at 5-year follow-up is generally reported in literature with values ranging from 74% to 100% [24, 26–30]. Saithna et al. reported that 16 of 21 patients who had undergone opening-wedge osteotomies (76%) underwent further surgery, the most common of which was removal of hardware (locking plate) because of irritation of the iliotibial band [28]. They also reported two cases of loss of correction, one infection, and one nonunion. The 5-year survival with the endpoint of conversion to arthroplasty was 79%.

Dewilde et al. reported that 4 of 19 patients who had an opening-wedge osteotomy underwent hardware removal, one patient underwent fracture fixation, and two patients were converted to TKA [29]. Survivorship at 7 years with revision surgery or conversion to TKA as the endpoint was 82%. Das et al. reported one delayed union that prolonged rehabilitation and seven patients who required hardware removal. Survivorship at 74 months with the endpoint of TKA was 83% [30]. The survival rate was still very high (74%) at 10 years FU [25]. Although the reported outcomes are generally extremely satisfying, several complications have been reported. Minor complications such as iliotibial irritation from the lateral plate are common and affect up to 50% of patients [25]. Nonunion rate is lower; Ekeland et al. reported that 75% of their 24 osteotomies healed in 3 months and the rest within 6 months [25]. Postoperative infection is another possible complication with a comprehensive rate of superficial infection from 1% to 9% and deep infection from 0.5% to 4.7% [31].

Medial hinge fracture is another complication of medial opening-wedge osteotomy. It usually occurs if the pin is positioned too close to the joint or if the surgeon does not leave enough bone on the medial hinge. The most severe complication is the injury to the popliteal neurovascular bundle; however, its rate is very low.

10.6   Summary

Distal femoral opening-wedge osteotomy is a reliable option in the treatment of varus knees resulting from tibial or femoral deformities. Actual indications include values knees resulting either from femoral or tibial deformity, mild to moderate cartilage degeneration of the lateral compartment, focal cartilage lesions of the lateral femoral condyle, and lateral meniscal transplantation. Absolute contraindications include severe medial or tricompartmental osteoarthritis, symptomatic medial compartment disease, inflammatory arthritis, flexion contracture >15°, knee flexion <90°, and severe osteoporosis. If these indications and contraindications are followed and surgery is carried out respecting all the steps, satisfactory outcomes even at long-term FU can be expected.

References

1. Sharma L, Song J, Felson DT, et al. The role of knee alignment in disease progression and functional decline in knee osteoarthritis. JAMA. 2001;286:188–95.
2. Luo CF. Reference axes for reconstruction of the knee. Knee. 2004;11:251. https://doi.org/10.1016/j.knee.2004.03.003.
3. Gugenheim JJ Jr, Brinker MR. Bone realignment with use of temporary external fixation for distal femoral valgus and varus deformities. J Bone Joint Surg Am. 2003;85-A:1229–37.
4. Brouwer GM, van Tol AW, Bergink AP, et al. Association between valgus and varus alignment and the development and progression of radiographic osteoarthritis of the knee. Arthritis Rheum. 2007;56(04):1204–11.
5. Healy WL, Anglen JO, Wasilewski SA, Krackow KA. Distal femoral varus osteotomy. J Bone Joint Surg Am. 1988;70:102–9.
6. Drexler M, Gross A, Dwyer T, Safir O, Backstein D, Chaudhry H, Goulding A, Kosashvili Y. Distal femoral varus osteotomy combined with tibial plateau fresh osteochondral allograft for post-traumatic osteoarthritis of the knee. Knee Surg Sports Traumatol Arthrosc. 2015;23:1317–23.
7. Gardiner A, Richmond JC. Periarticular osteotomies for degenerative joint disease of the knee. Sports Med Arthrosc Rev. 2013;21:38–46.
8. Gao L, Madry H, Chugaev DV, Denti M, Frolov A, Burtsev M, Magnitskaya N, Mukhanov V, Neyret P, Solomin LN, Sorokin E, Staubli AE, Stone KR, Vilenskiy V, Zayats V, Pape D, Korolev A. Advances in modern osteotomies around the knee: report on the Association of Sports Traumatology, Arthroscopy, Orthopaedic surgery, Rehabilitation (ASTAOR) Moscow International Osteotomy Congress 2017. J Exp Orthop. 2019;6(1):9. https://doi.org/10.1186/s40634-019-0177-5.
9. Wang J-W, Hsu C-C. Distal femoral varus osteotomy for osteoarthritis of the knee. J Bone Jt Surg Am. 2005;87:127–33.
10. Saithna A, Kundra R, Modi CS, Getgood A, Spalding T. Distal femoral varus osteotomy for lateral compartment osteoarthritis in the valgus knee. A systematic review of the literature. Open Orthop J. 2012;6:313–9.
11. Haviv B, Bronak S, Thein R, Thein R. The results of corrective osteotomy for valgus arthritic knees. Knee Surg Sports Traumatol Arthrosc. 2013;21:49–56.
12. Sternheim A, Garbedian S, Backstein D. Distal femoral varus osteotomy: unloading the lateral compartment: long-term follow-up of 45 medial closing wedge osteotomies. Orthopedics. 2011;34:e488–90.
13. Hanssen AD, Stuart MJ, Scott RD, Scuderi GR. Surgical options for the middle-aged patient with osteoarthritis of the knee joint. Instr Course Lect. 2001;50:499–511.

14. Görtz S, Bugbee W. Valgus malalignment: diagnosis, osteotomy techniques, clinical outcomes. Philadelphia, PA: Elsevier Saunders; 2008. p. 896–904.
15. Rosso F, Margheritini F. Distal femoral osteotomy. Curr Rev Musculoskelet Med. 2014;7:302–11.
16. Paccola CAJ, Fogagnolo F. Open-wedge high tibial osteotomy: a technical trick to avoid loss of reduction of the opposite cortex. Knee Surg Sports Traumatol Arthrosc. 2005;13:19–22.
17. Dejour D. L'ostéotomie tibiale de varisation résultats: a propos de 118 cas. In: Neyret P, Dejour H, editors. 7émes Journées Lyonnaises de Chirurgie du Genou Sauramps; 1991:169–80.
18. Collins B, Getgood A, Alomar AZ, et al. A case series of lateral opening wedge high tibial osteotomy for valgus malalignment. Knee Surg Sports Traumatol Arthrosc. 2013;21(01):152–60.
19. Quirno M, Campbell KA, Singh B, et al. Distal femoral varus osteotomy for unloading valgus knee malalignment: a biomechanical analysis. Knee Surg Sports Traumatol Arthrosc. 2017;25:863–8.
20. Forkel P, Achtnich A, Petersen W. Midterm results following medial closed wedge distal femoral osteotomy stabilized with a locking internal fixation device. Knee Surg Sports Traumatol Arthrosc. 2015;23:2061–7.
21. Mitchell JJ, Dean CS, Chahla J, et al. Varus-producing lateral distal femoral opening-wedge osteotomy. Arthrosc Tech. 2016;5:e799–807.
22. Puddu G, Cipolla M, Cerullo G, Franco V, Giannì E. Which osteotomy for a valgus knee? Int Orthop. 2010;34:239–47.
23. Al-Saati MF, Magnussen RA, Demey G, Lustig S, Servien E, Neyret P. Lateral opening-wedge high tibial osteotomy. Tech Knee Surg. 2011;10(3):178–85.
24. Zarrouk A, Bouzidi R, Karray B, et al. Distal femoral varus osteotomy outcome: is associated femoropatellar osteoarthritis consequential? Orthop Traumatol Surg Res. 2010;96:632–6.
25. Ekeland A, Nerhus TK, Dimmen S, Heir S. Good functional results of distal femoral opening-wedge osteotomy of knees with lateral osteoarthritis. Knee Surg Sports Traumatol Arthrosc. 2016;24:1702–9.
26. Thein R, Bronak S, Thein R, Haviv B. Distal femoral osteotomy for valgus arthritic knees. J Orthop Sci. 2012;17:745–9.
27. Saragaglia D, Chedal-Bornu B. Computer-assisted osteotomy for valgus knees: medium-term results of 29 cases. Orthop Traumatol Surg Res. 2014;100:527–30.
28. Saithna A, Kundra R, Getgood A, Spalding T. Opening wedge distal femoral varus osteotomy for lateral compartment osteoarthritis in the valgus knee. Knee. 2014;21:172–5.
29. Dewilde TR, Dauw J, Vandenneucker H, Bellemans J. Opening wedge distal femoral varus osteotomy using the Puddu plate and calcium phosphate bone cement. Knee Surg Sports Traumatol Arthrosc. 2013;21:249–54.
30. Das D, Sijbesma T, Hoekstra HJ, Van Leuven W. Distal femoral opening-wedge osteotomy for lateral compartment osteoarthritis of the knee. Open Access Surg. 2008;1:25–9.
31. Anagnostakos K, Mosser P, Kohn D. Infections after high tibial osteotomy. Knee Surg Sports Traumatol Arthrosc. 2013;21:161–9.

Medial Closing-Wedge Distal Femoral Osteotomy: Surgical Technique

11

Filip R. Hendrikx and Peter Verdonk

11.1 Introduction

Medial closing-wedge distal femoral osteotomy is a well-established procedure in correcting symptomatic valgus deformities with existing or imminent lateral compartment degeneration. This can be the result of constitutional valgus alignment, osteochondral disease, or decompensation after lateral meniscus insufficiency. The goal of a correcting osteotomy is to decrease or slow down the process of lateral compartment degeneration by altering the mechanical alignment. A distal femoral osteotomy (DFO) is often indicated when idiopathic valgus alignment is caused by lateral femoral condyle hypoplasia or femoral valgus deformity.

It should be noted that axial correction osteotomies are joint-preserving procedures and should therefore be executed before the lateral compartment is too far gone. Moreover, the medial compartment cartilage and its soft tissue structures should be of sufficient quality as they will suffer extra loading after varization.

11.2 Indications/Contraindications

11.2.1 Indications

- Constitutional valgus alignment of the femur (meaning a medial distal femoral mechanical angle of more than 93° as measured on full-leg standing X-ray) and:
  - Decompensation after (sub)total lateral meniscectomy
  - Chondral or osteochondral disease of the lateral compartment
  - Isolated lateral compartment osteoarthritis (OA) grades 1–3 (grade 4 in Schuss X-ray view in certain indications)
  - Higher activity level

F. R. Hendrikx · P. Verdonk (✉)
ORTHOCA, Monica Hospitals, Deurne, Belgium

11.2.2 Contraindications

• Inflammatory arthritis
• Medial and patellofemoral OA
• Flexion contracture >15°
• Flexion <90°
• Obesity

11.2.3 Relative Contraindications

• Smoking
• Age >60

11.3 Pre-op Planning

Imaging studies are fundamental in preoperative planning, starting with low threshold plain X-rays. They include four views for assessment of all compartments: standing AP, lateral, Merchant, and Rosenberg view. Standing full-leg X-rays are essential for evaluation and quantification of joint malalignment. Different angles are calculated to estimate the amount of correction needed.

The mechanical axis is a straight line that crosses the center of the femoral head and the ankle joint. It crosses the tibial eminence or even somewhat the medial compartment in neutral alignment, while valgus alignment displays a mechanical axis through the lateral compartment.

The hip-knee-ankle (HKA) (Fig. 11.1b) describes the overall valgus angle, measured between the mechanical axes of the femur and tibia.

The mechanical proximal tibial angle (mPTA) (Fig. 11.1c) and mechanical distal femoral angle (mDFA) (Fig. 11.1d) are then measured in order to evaluate whether malalignment is of femoral, tibial, or combined origin and thus where to perform the corrective osteotomy. It is the authors' surgical concept that a DFO is only indicated if the valgus is situated at the femoral level visualized by a medial mDFA of 93° or more as previously discussed in the inclusion criteria.

An MRI is used to evaluate subchondral bone, ligamentous integrity, and cartilage lesions in the other compartments. Bone marrow edema can be seen on T2-weighted images as a sign of stress overload. An arthroscopy grants a direct view on the cartilage and meniscus and can be carried out as a combined procedure.

Patients who qualify for a DFO should always be tested first with a 3-month period of lateral compartment unloader bracing. Surgery should only be performed when a significant reduction of symptoms is achieved during bracing.

Previously published studies are not consistent about the amount of correction needed. Some recent findings suggest overcorrection rather than correction to neutral position to reduce stress on the lateral compartment [1]. The authors of this work however advocate correction to neutral alignment.

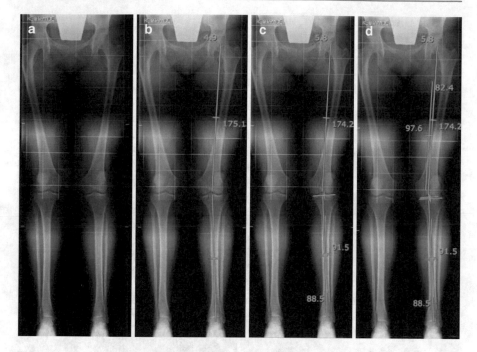

Fig. 11.1 Preoperative planning. (**a**) Full-leg standing radiograph. (**b**) 4.9° of valgus alignment. (**c**) mPTA of 88.5°. (**d**) mDFA of 97.6°

11.4   Implants

A TomoFix medial distal femoral (MDF) compression plate that fits the medial distal femur is used and fixed with self-tapping screws. Locking screws are used distal to the osteotomy. For compression, an eccentric 4.5 mm cortical screw is inserted just proximal to the osteotomy, which will later be replaced with a bicortical locking screw. Monocortical locking screws are then used in the remaining proximal holes.

11.5   Surgical Technique

11.5.1 Positioning

The patient is placed in supine position with side and foot support. A tourniquet can be used. The lower leg is individually packed in sterile drapes. Fluoroscopy is present in the OR and should be able to display the hip, knee, and ankle.

11.5.2 Surgery

A paramedian skin incision (Fig. 11.2a, b) is chosen to avoid wound complications in potential subsequent surgery if the patient should ever need one, e.g., total knee arthroplasty (TKA) [2]. The incision starts from the superomedial edge of the patella, extending to about 10 cm proximally. The subcutis is dissected to the level of the fascia, which is then opened to expose the medial vastus obliquus (VMO) muscle.

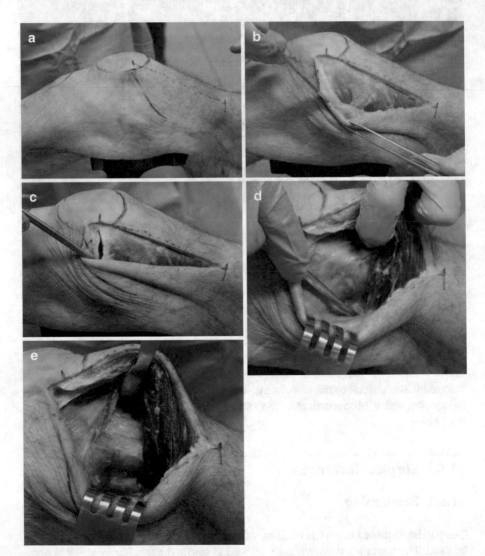

Fig. 11.2 Surgical approach. (**a**) Surface landmarks. (**b**) Paramedian skin incision from the superomedial edge of the patella extending to 10 cm proximally. (**c**) Subvastus approach with incision of distal insertion of VMO. (**d**) Stripping the VMO of the intermuscular septum. (**e**) Anterior retraction of the periosteum, exposing the medial cortex

The distal insertion of the VMO is partially dissected (Fig. 11.2c), and a subvastus approach is performed using blunt dissection (Fig. 11.2d). The VMO is released from the intermuscular septum and retracted anteriorly and laterally. A periosteal elevator is placed in the back and a Homann in the front of the femur to give a clear view on the medial femur (Fig. 11.2e). The small perforating vessels along the septum are coagulated. The retractors are then replaced to expose the medial cortex.

Two K-wires are introduced (Fig. 11.3a) under image intensifier on the medial side of the femur just proximal to the metaphysis and directed laterally and distally just proximal of the scar of the posterior lateral femoral condyle in the transition area of the lateral cortex and more spongeous bone of the lateral metaphysis at a precalculated distance and angle to guide the sawblade. Both represent the planned osteotomy cuts in the axial plane. The pins should be placed very precisely, with or without the help of patient-specific instruments like 3D-printed guides. The proximal cut (Fig. 11.3b) is made from the medial supracondylar area and runs obliquely

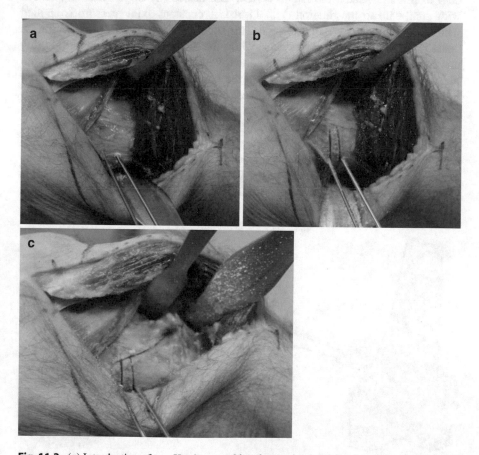

Fig. 11.3 (a) Introduction of two K-wires, marking the proximal and distal osteotomy planes. (b) Proximal and distal cut, using both K-wires for guidance of the sawblade. (c) Anterior proximal step cut

to just proximal of the lateral condyle. The distal cut is then made. A too proximal cortical bone cut will increase the risk of fracture; too distal cut could damage the lateral condyle. The osteotomy is oblique to provide more stability and more bone surface in comparison to a strictly transverse osteotomy. The length of the cut is measured with a marge of 5 mm from the lateral cortex. It is imperative not to break the lateral cortex. An intact lateral cortex functions as a hinge and protects the osteotomy from unwanted rotation. Importantly, stability of the osteotomy is additionally improved by an anterior and proximal step cut in the sagittal plane (Fig. 11.3c). A schematic representation of the K-wires and the osteotomy is given in Fig. 11.4.

The leg is manually supported during the entire surgical procedure, which is done in 45° of flexion. The bone fragment is carefully removed (Fig. 11.5a). In particular, the posterior cortex should be checked to make sure it is completely transected and free of debris. To weaken the lateral hinge, without breaking it, the lateral hinge is perforated three times with a 3.2 mm drill at different levels. A chisel can help to further weaken the lateral cortex. The osteotomy is progressively closed with great care to the rotation (Fig. 11.5b). A constant axial pressure is applied while supporting the knee in extension. This should not be rushed. Sufficient time is taken to allow the osteotomy to close while the hinge is under pressure. Ignoring this can lead to fracture of the lateral cortex, with subsequent loss of rotational stability. The plate is then positioned and fitted on the medial side of the distal femur in full extension (Fig. 11.5c). The cortices touch to prevent collapse and thus overcorrection. Compression is given to allow faster bone healing.

The final result is evaluated under fluoroscopy, using a radio-opaque cable wire that is spanned over the hip and ankle to display the mechanical axis. After correction, it should cross the tibial eminence. Overcorrection, however, should be avoided. Hemostasis and closure of the wound are performed when final result is satisfactory. A subvastus drain is left for 24 h postoperatively.

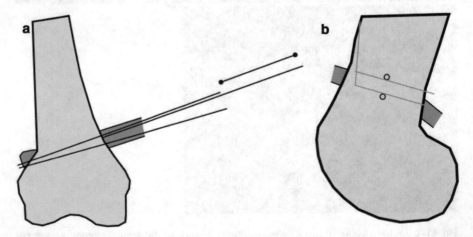

Fig. 11.4 (**a**) Frontal view of introduction of K-wires, marking the osteotomy plane. (**b**) Medial view of the proximal, distal, and anterior step cut

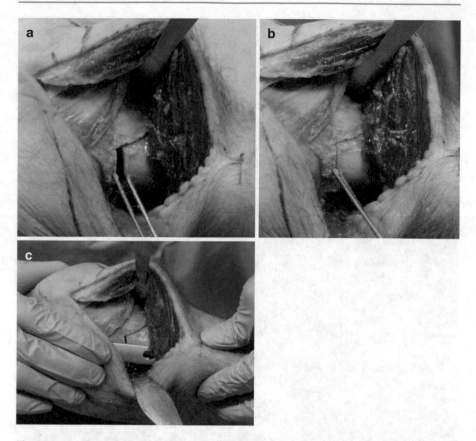

Fig. 11.5 (**a**) Extraction of the wedge. (**b**) Gradually closing of the medial cortex. (**c**) Positioning of the TomoFix plate

Example Case

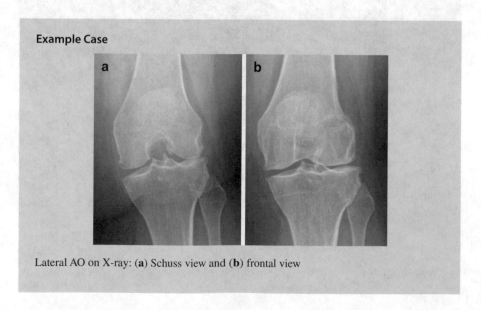

Lateral AO on X-ray: (**a**) Schuss view and (**b**) frontal view

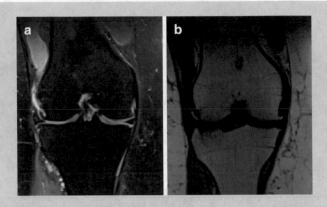

Lateral AO on MRI: (a) T2-weighted images and (b) T1

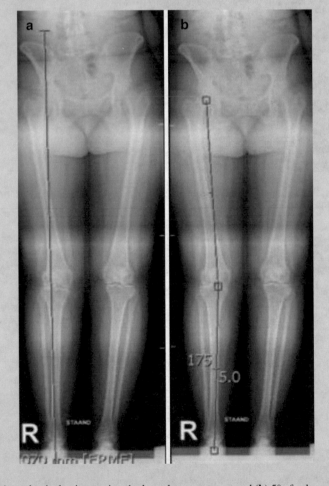

Pre-op (a) mechanical axis crossing the lateral compartment and (b) 5° of valgus alignment

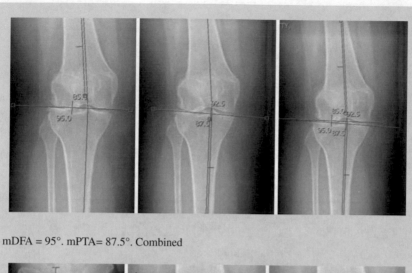

mDFA = 95°. mPTA= 87.5°. Combined

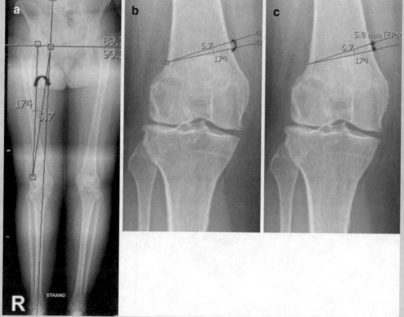

Pre-op planning: (**a**) 5.7° to correct on the femur (**b**) 5.7° on the distal femur is (**c**) 5.8 mm on the medial cortex

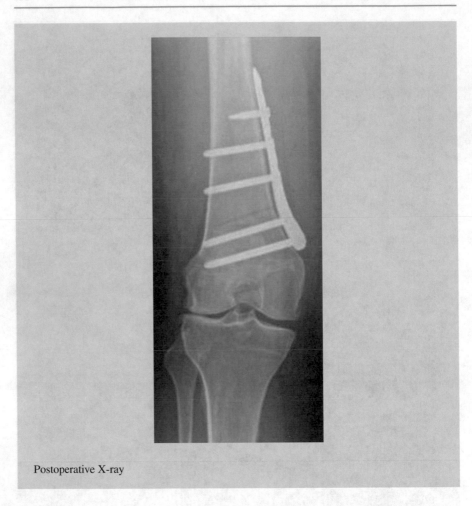

Postoperative X-ray

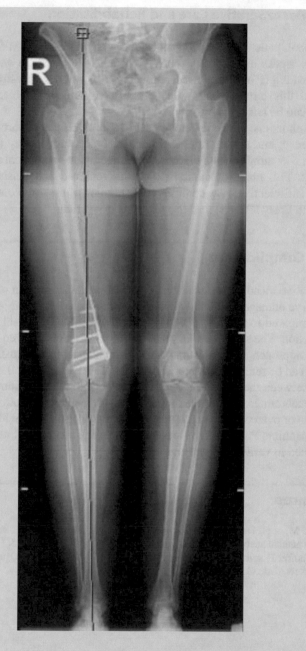

Postoperative standing full leg: mechanical axis crossing the tibial eminence

11.6 Postoperative Care and Rehabilitation

Per protocol, patients receive low molecular weight heparin (LMWH) for 30 days.

In 0–4 weeks after surgery, only toe touch is allowed. In weeks 5–8, partial weight-bearing (PWB) is allowed, still using two crutches. Obesity can be a reason to extend this term. After 8-week progressive full weight-bearing is allowed, crutches can be left out if possible.

The authors encourage patients to start light, nonimpact sports like swimming, aqua training, and cycling after 2–3 months. Full return to play (RTP) is allowed only after 6–9 months when surgeon, physiotherapist, and patient are satisfied with the result. Full range of motion (ROM) is achieved and muscular volume has regained sufficiently. X-ray confirms consolidation of the osteotomy and symptoms are absent. Early RTP can lead to symptoms of overload.

11.7 Complications

Postoperative bleeding and hematoma, as well as infection, can occur but are rare. Local nerve damage is seldomly observed using a medial closing-wedge technique when compared to a lateral opening wedge, where the peroneal nerve can suffer from traction. The same goes for plate irritation, which is not frequently seen using a medial approach, as there is no conflict with adjacent structures. If it does occur, the plate can be removed, but preferably only after 1 year. Lateral fixation can cause friction between the ITB and the plate. There is a low rate of nonunion in closing-wedge osteotomies. Loss of the hinge can occur, leading to rotation.

Under- or overcorrection can and should always be avoided with accurate preoperative planning. Preoperative measurements of the mechanical axis should always be executed to verify adequate axis correction.

References

1. Quirno M, et al. Distal femoral varus osteotomy for unloading valgus knee malalignment: a biomechanical analysis. Knee Surg Sports Traumatol Arthrosc. 2017;25(3):863–8.
2. Lobenhoffer P, van Heerwaarden RJ, Staubli AE, Jakob RP, editors. Osteotomies around the knee. New York: Georg Thieme Verlag Stuttgart; 2008.

Lateral Opening-Wedge High Tibial Osteotomy

12

Mattia Basilico, Tomas Pineda, Elliot Sappey-Marinier, and Sebastien Lustig

12.1 Introduction

In a knee with unicompartmental arthritis, limb alignment is altered, and more load is distributed to the affected compartment, causing further degenerative changes and angular deformity.

High tibial osteotomy (HTO) is a well-established procedure in the treatment of osteoarthritis of the knee. Osteotomies are performed to redistribute the weight-bearing load from a diseased compartment of the knee toward a compartment that has well-preserved articular cartilage.

The outcome of valgus producing HTO has been well documented. Numerous authors have demonstrated good long-term results utilizing either a lateral closing-wedge or a medial opening-wedge technique [1–7].

The use of HTO in the treatment of valgus deformities is much less common: as femoral valgus deformity is prevalent, numerous authors have recommended distal femoral osteotomy (DFO) [8–10]. Collins et al. reported 91% of survival at an average follow-up of 4.3 years of varus-producing HTO, indicating that the early results in these patients are comparable to the previously published results for HTO in patients with varus malalignment [11].

The advantage, however, of HTO for valgus deformity is that the joint is unloaded in both flexion and extension. In comparison, DFO unloads the joint only in extension [12].

M. Basilico
Fondazione Policlinico Universitario A. Gemelli IRCCS, Università Cattolica del Sacro Cuore, Rome, Italy

T. Pineda
Universidad de Chile, Santiago, RM, Chile

E. Sappey-Marinier (✉) · S. Lustig
Department of Orthopaedic Surgery, Croix-Rousse Hospital, Lyon, France

© Springer Nature Switzerland AG 2020
S. Oussedik, S. Lustig (eds.), *Osteotomy About the Knee*,
https://doi.org/10.1007/978-3-030-49055-3_12

12.2   Indications and Contraindications

Indications for proximal tibial osteotomy for valgus deformity have evolved over time. Typically, younger, healthier patients are candidates for this procedure, as it is hoped that activity levels can be maintained and that joint arthroplasty procedures can be postponed.

Initially Jackson and Waugh corrected all valgus deformities of the lower limb by tibial osteotomy but noted that significant joint line angulation can occur if the origin of the deformity is in the distal femur [13].

Coventry and Healy et al. suggested that distal femoral osteotomy should be performed if more than 10° of joint line obliquity or more than 12° of valgus was present [10–15]. This obliquity, if superior to 10°, can generate excessive stress on the patellofemoral joint, especially on the medial side.

Today, lateral opening-wedge high tibial osteotomy is suggested for patients with valgus deformities of the lower limb driven primarily by the tibia and is not indicated when the deformity is located in the distal femur, which is the most common situation. Generally, these are patients with posttraumatic deformity of the tibia and patients in whom a varus deformity was overcorrected with a lateral closing-wedge osteotomy.

The contraindications for this surgery include a flexion contracture >10°, ligamentous instability, and advanced osteoarthritis with complete joint space loss [16].

12.3   Preoperative Planning

A detailed history should be obtained, including patient expectations, current symptoms in the knee, and details of prior injuries and operative reports from any prior knee surgery. Physical examination should include a careful evaluation of knee range of motion, ligamentous stability, and an assessment of the location of previous surgical scars.

At the time of the consultation, minimum work-up includes single leg AP view, single leg lateral view at 30°, skyline view of the patella in 30° of flexion to examine patellofemolar joint, bilateral leg stance at 45° of flexion view (Schuss view) to evaluate tibiofemoral joint space narrowing that is frequently underestimated on the AP view, and full-length lower extremity films to measure alignment.

Appropriate preoperative planning is critical in obtaining good outcomes after lateral opening-wedge HTO.

The overall aim of this osteotomy is to correct the mechanical axis of the lower limb to a normal varus (0–3° of varus). In general, it is better to slightly overcorrect than undercorrect. During preoperative planning one can determine the desired angle of correction and the opening that will be needed to obtain this correction [17].

If the osteotomy is being performed to remedy overcorrection from a lateral closing-wedge osteotomy, the goal should be similar to the initial surgery: creation of an overall limb alignment of approximately 3° of valgus.

However, if the osteotomy is being performed for lateral compartment arthritis, a goal of neutral limb alignment may be indicated. These goals must be tempered by consideration of the alignment of the contralateral limb and limitations as the grade of correction can be safely obtained with an isolated tibial osteotomy, particularly in cases of large preoperative deformity [18].

12.4   Surgical Technique

12.4.1 Patient Positioning

The supine position is recommended for this operation with a bump under the ipsilateral buttock to obtain a better exposure of the iliac crest. An addition bump is placed distally to hold the knee in 90° of flexion.

A tourniquet is applied for a bloodless field.

The ipsilateral iliac crest is prepped and draped using square drapes because it requires an autologous bone graft from the ipsilateral anterior iliac crest. The C-arm should be available, as it is performed under fluoroscopic control.

12.4.2 Incision

A longitudinal or slightly oblique anterolateral incision is suggested, centered between the tibial tubercle and fibular head: it should be raised 1 cm above the anterior tibial tuberosity to 1 cm below the fibular head. If there is a previous scar, the incision should be performed on that previous scar.

The fascia of the anterior compartment is opened, leaving 1 cm of fascia attached to the tibial crest (Fig. 12.1a).

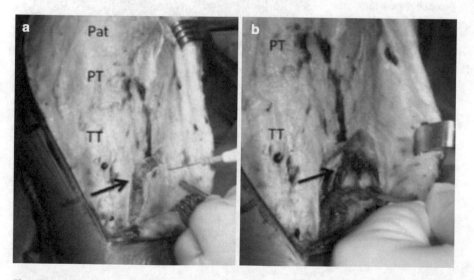

Fig. 12.1 Left leg undergoing lateral opening-wedge high tibial osteotomy. (**a**) The fascia of the tibialis anterior muscle is incised (arrow). (**b**) The muscles tibialis anterior and the extensor digitorum longus are elevated from the lateral tibial metaphysis (arrow) using a periosteal elevator. The patella (Pat), patellar tendon (PT), and tibial tubercle (TT) are marked in the picture

Afterward a periosteal elevator is used to elevate the tibialis anterior muscle and extensor digitorum longus from the lateral tibial metaphysis (Fig. 12.1b).

In this phase, it is important to perform an extensive elevation of muscles, to facilitate mobilization of common peroneal nerve.

12.4.3 Fibular Osteotomy

We prefer performing the fibular osteotomy in the neck. Firstly, it is necessary to identify and expose adequately the neck of fibula. A 3.2 mm drill bit is then used to make two holes in the fibular neck (Fig. 12.2), and the osteotomy is completed with an osteotome.

It is critical to protect the peroneal nerve during the entire procedure, using a periosteal elevator that should be always in contact with the bone. For this reason, the peroneal nerve should be identified and mobilized before starting the fibular osteotomy.

It is possible to perform the osteotomy in fibular diaphysis, but it should not be more distal than 10 cm below the tip of fibula to avoid the risk of denervating the extensor hallucis longus muscle.

Fig. 12.2 Intraoperative photographs of a left leg undergoing fibular osteotomy. Protecting the peroneal nerve with a periosteal elevator (arrow), two drill holes are placed in the fibula (fib)

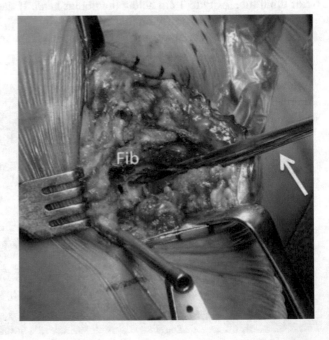

12.4.4 Tibial Osteotomy

During the tibial osteotomy, it is important to protect the posterior neurovascular structures and anteriorly the patellar tendon.

An elevator must be kept in contact with the posterior surface of tibial bone to avoid neurovascular injury, and a retractor is placed between the tibial tuberosity and the patellar tendon to protect it. The osteotomy should be performed starting just above the tibial tuberosity on the lateral tibial metaphysis. The cut is more horizontal than the medial opening-wedge osteotomy, direct proximally and medially to a point about 1 cm below the medial tibial plateau. The correct trajectory of the osteotomy is checked using two 2.5 mm threaded Kirschner wires under fluoroscopic control. They should be placed parallel to each other according to the orientation described above (Fig. 12.3).

The osteotomy is performed using an oscillating saw just below the two K-wires, always staying in contact with them, from the middle portion of the tibia proceeding to the anterior and posterior cortices. Care is taken so that the periosteal elevator and the retractor are in contact with the bone during the saw cut, to avoid neurovascular damage or tendon tears (Fig. 12.4). The medial cortical hinge must be protected during the osteotomy. We mobilize the medial cortical hinge using a 3.2 mm drill bit to weaken it. Then the cut is completed with an osteotome. We prefer to use three osteotomes to gradually open the osteotomy. The first osteotome is placed in the osteotomy just below the K-wire forward the opposite cortex. The second osteotome is placed just below it (Fig. 12.5a). The osteotomes must come into contact with the medial cortex without fracturing it. This correct positioning can be controlled using fluoroscopy *or* "feeling" the change in sound given by the impact of osteotomes with the medial cortex (Fig. 12.5b).

A third osteotome is placed between the first two osteotomes, opening the osteotomy site.

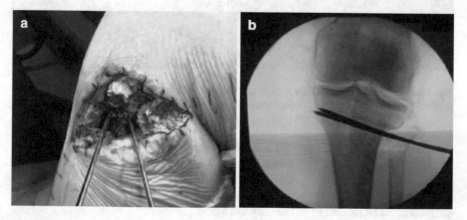

Fig. 12.3 (a) Two Kirschner wires are placed in the proximal tibial metaphysis to guide the osteotomy cut. (b) A fluoroscopic image exhibits the correct position of the wires

Fig. 12.4 Tibial osteotomy using an oscillating saw below the Kirschner wires. A periosteal elevator (arrow) positioned to protect the posterior neurovascular structures

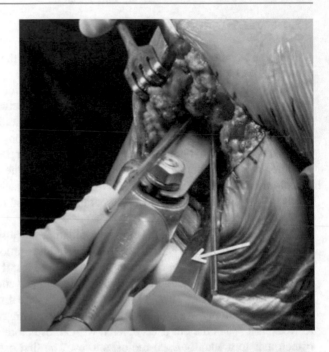

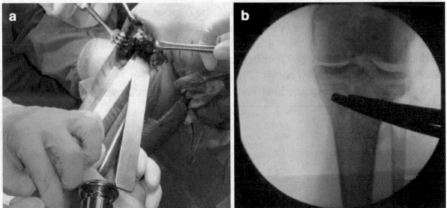

Fig. 12.5 (a) Two osteotomies are used to gradually open the osteotomy. (b) Fluoroscopy allows to check the correct placement of osteotomes against the tibial medial cortex before the opening

It should not be on contact with the opposite cortex, to avoid the risk of cortex fractures. More osteotomes could be used to achieve the desired correction (Fig. 12.6).

A common mistake is to open the osteotomy more anteriorly and posteriorly: the surgeon must be careful to not modify the slope.

Fig. 12.6 Additional osteotomies could be placed between the first two to progressively open the osteotomy

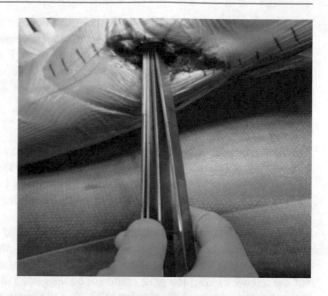

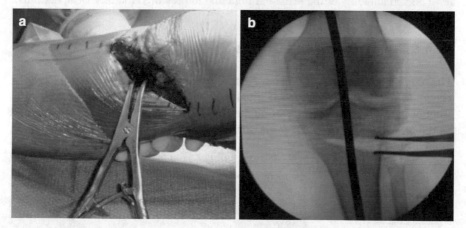

Fig. 12.7 (**a**) A lamina spreader is placed to maintain correction and the osteotomes are removed. (**b**) A metal bar centered over the femoral head and ankle is used to demonstrate the new mechanical axis of the limb under fluoroscopic control

The opening thus obtained can be maintained with a lamina spreader instead of osteotomes (Fig. 12.7a).

At this point we must check the limb alignment. This can be done utilizing three methods. The first is to check the alignment using a metal bar under fluoroscopic control (Fig. 12.7b). The bar is centered over the middle of the femoral head and the ankle. The fluoroscopy allows us to check the position at which the bar meets that tibial plateau and the integrity of the medial hinge.

The second method consists of measuring the degrees of opening of osteotomy; that should be the degrees decided upon in the preoperative planning. The final method is a visual check of the overall limb alignment: it is just a final check to identify any obvious mistakes.

12.4.5 Fixation

The fixation of the osteotomy should be rigid and stable to avoid loss of correction degrees. It is possible to use locking plates or staples for the osteosynthesis. In clinical practice we use two staples: the first placed obliquely between the tibial tuberosity and Gerdy's tubercle and the second more lateral vertically between the tibial epiphysis and diaphysis (Fig. 12.8).

We prefer to do this because the staples can be placed easily than the plate and require minimal bone proximal to the osteotomy. Furthermore, placing a plate requires a greater sacrifice of soft tissues, a larger incision, or additional incisions for the screws. Finally, the plate could not be suggested in these patients who often have altered anatomy of the proximal tibia due to previous fractures or operations.

12.4.6 Bone Grafting and Closure

The osteotomy can be filled with bone grafting or bone substitutes (calcium triphosphate). In all cases, we prefer to use tricortical bone graft harvest from the ipsilateral anterior iliac crest (Fig. 12.9). During the closure, the anterior muscle fascia should be repaired, taking care to cover the bone graft material and the staples. A suction drain is placed.

Fig. 12.8 Fixation is obtained by placement of two staples: the first staple is placed from the tibial tubercle (TT) to Gerdy's tubercle (GT). The second is placed posterolateral to the first in a vertical position

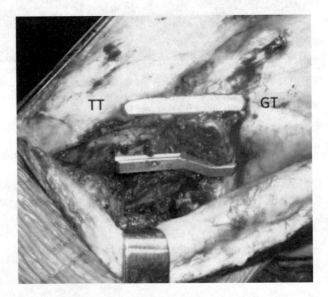

Fig. 12.9 After fixation, corticocancellous bone graft (arrow) from the anterior iliac crest is used to fill in the osteotomy site

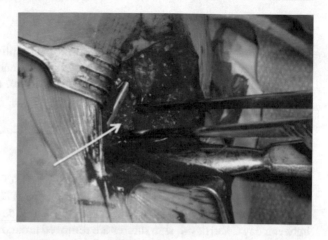

12.5   Complications

12.5.1 Peroneal Nerve Injury

The surgeon must be careful to not tear the peroneal nerve during the approach and to not stretch it during all the operation. The peroneal nerve should be identified and mobilized from the soft tissue. Furthermore, it is critical to protect it with a periosteal elevator and to avoid a vigorous lateral retraction.

12.5.2 Injury to Posterior Neurovascular Structures

As already explained, it is essential to protect the posterior neurovascular structures using a periosteal elevator in contact with the posterior cortex of the tibial metaphysis to avoid severe neurovascular injury.

12.5.3 Fracture of the Medial Cortical Hinge

Fracture of the medial cortical hinge can be observed in large correction. It results in deformity and loss of correction. To avoid it weakening of the medial hinge should be performed. When fracture of the medial cortical hinge occurs, it should be placed a plate over the tibial medial cortex via an additional medial approach.

12.5.4 Fracture of the Tibial Plateau

The fracture of the medial tibial plateau is a severe complication. Care must be taken to ensure that the medial hinge is about 1 cm from the tibial plateau to avoid this issue.

12.5.5 Compartment Syndrome

Compartment syndrome is a rare but redoubtable complication. It can be avoided by careful attention to hemostasis intraoperatively and postoperative control. Persistent and not-responsive-to-drugs pain should not be underestimated in an early diagnosis.

12.6 Postoperative Management

The postoperative guidelines after opening-wedge HTO is similar to that after a lateral closing-wedge HTO or medial opening-wedge HTO.

At our center, the hospital stay is between 4 and 7 days. The drain is removed between day 2 and day 4, skin sutures are removed around day 12, and thromboprophylaxis is utilized for 1 month. The limb is braced in approximately 10° of flexion after the surgery and is worn for 2 months. The patient is limited to partial weight-bearing with two crutches, and passive range of motion exercises start on postoperative day number 1, with flexion limited to 120° for the first 15 days. After that date flexion can be progressively advanced.

Driving a car is not allowed for 10 weeks and physical work for 3–4 months. Full return to normal activities generally requires 6 months.

12.7 Results

Between 2002 and 2009, we treated eight patients with lateral opening-wedge high tibial osteotomies. Three patients were treated after overcorrection of varus deformities with lateral closing-wedge osteotomies (Fig. 12.10), and five were treated for valgus deformities after lateral tibial plateau fractures (Fig. 12.11).

Postoperative alignment improved to a mean HKA of 183.9° (range, 181–187°). No complications were noted. Two patients required revision to TKA during the follow-up period (at 3 and 5 years postoperative) for progression of osteoarthritis.

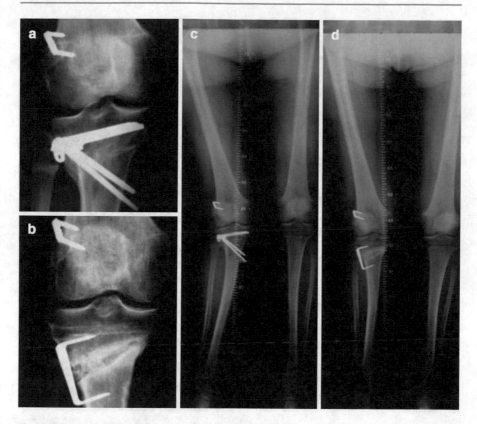

Fig. 12.10 Radiographs of a patient treated for overcorrection of a varus deformity. (**a, c**) Preoperative radiographs: after a prior lateral closing-wedge high tibial osteotomy, hip-knee-ankle (HKA) angle was 198°. (**b, d**) Postoperative radiographs: correction of the HKA to 187° with lateral opening-wedge osteotomy

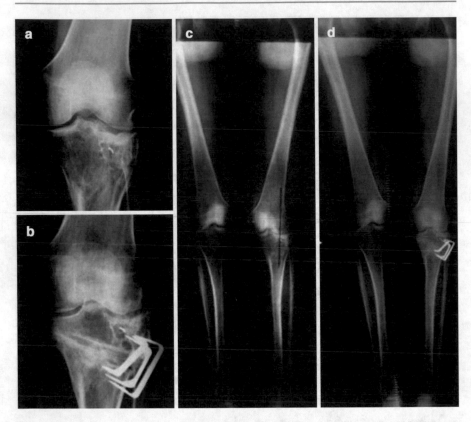

Fig. 12.11 Radiographs of a patient treated for posttraumatic arthritis of the lateral tibial plateau. (**a, c**) Preoperative radiographs: posttraumatic arthritis with a hip-knee-ankle (HKA) angle of 188°. (**b, d**) Postoperative radiographs: correction of the HKA to 181° after a lateral opening-wedge osteotomy

12.8 Conclusions

Lateral opening-wedge proximal tibial osteotomy is a useful but uncommon treatment for valgus deformities of the lower limb that are primarily tibial in origin. Mainly these deformities are consequence of proximal tibial fractures or varus deformity overcorrected with a lateral closing-wedge osteotomy.

Although the indication remains extremely rare, the results appear optimal.

Possible future improvements for this procedure include the utilization of alternative grafts to fill up the opening, thus preventing the extraction from the iliac crest, or the use of surgical navigation during the procedure.

References

1. Gstöttner M, Pedross F, Liebensteiner M, et al. Long-term outcome after high tibial osteotomy. Arch Orthop Trauma Surg. 2008;128:111–5.
2. Hui C, Salmon LJ, Kok A, et al. Long-term survival of high tibial osteotomy for medial compartment osteoarthritis of the knee. Am J Sports Med. 2010;39:64–70.
3. Demeo PJ, Johnson EM, Chiang PP, et al. Midterm follow-up of opening-wedge high tibial osteotomy. Am J Sports Med. 2010;38:2077–84.
4. Saragaglia D, Blaysat M, Inman D, et al. Outcome of opening wedge high tibial osteotomy augmented with a Biosorb((R)) wedge and fixed with a plate and screws in 124 patients with a mean of ten years follow-up. Int Orthop. 2011;35:1151–6.
5. Naudie D, Bourne RB, Rorabeck CH, Bourne TJ. Survivorship of the high tibial valgus osteotomy: a 10- to 22-year followup study. Clin Orthop Relat Res. 1999;367:18–27.
6. Sprenger TR, Doerzbacher JF. Tibial osteotomy for the treatment of varus gonarthrosis: survival and failure analysis the twenty-two years. J Bone Joint Surg Am. 2003;85A(3):469–74.
7. Tang WC, Henderson IJP. High tibial osteotomy: long term survival analysis and patients' perspective. Knee. 2005;12:410–3.
8. Edgerton BC, Mariani EM, Morrey BF. Distal femoral varus osteotomy for painful genu valgum. A five-to-11-year follow-up study. Clin Orthop Relat Res. 1993;(288):263–9.
9. Wang JW, Hsu CC. Distal femoral varus osteotomy for osteoarthritis of the knee. J Bone Joint Surg Am. 2005;87:127–33.
10. Healy WL, Anglen JO, Wasilewski SA, et al. Distal femoral varus osteotomy. J Bone Joint Surg Am. 1988;70:102–9.
11. Collins B, Getgood A, Abdulaziz A, Giffin R, Willits K, Fowler P, et al. A case series of lateral opening wedge high tibial osteotomy for valgus malalignment. Knee Surg Sports Traumatol Arthrosc. 2013;21:152–60.
12. Chambat P, Selmi TA, DeJour D, Denoyers J. Varus tibial osteotomy. Oper Tech Sports Med. 2000;8:44–7.
13. Jackson JP, Waugh W. Tibial osteotomy for osteoarthritis of the knee. J Bone Joint Surg Br. 1961;43-B:746–51.
14. Coventry MB. Osteotomy about the knee for degenerative and rheumatoid arthritis: indications, operative technique, and results. J Bone Joint Surg Am. 1973;55:23–48.
15. Coventry MB. Proximal tibial varus osteotomy for osteoarthritis of the lateral compartment of the knee. J Bone Joint Surg Am. 1987;69:32–8.
16. Marti RK, Verhagen RA, Kerkhoffs GM, et al. Proximal tibial varus osteotomy. Indications, technique, and five to twenty-one-year results. J Bone Joint Surg Am. 2001;83-A:164–70.
17. Neyret P, Demey G. Surgery of the knee. 1st ed. New York: Springer; 2014.
18. Al-Saati M, Magnussen R, Demey G, Lustig S, Servien E, Neyret P. Lateral opening-wedge high tibial osteotomy. Tech Knee Surg. 2011;10:178–85.

Medial Closing-Wedge High Tibial Osteotomy

13

Jean-Marie Fayard, Nicolas Jan, Padhraig O'Loughlin, and Benjamin Freychet

13.1 Introduction

Numerous factors have an established association with the development of osteoarthritis. These factors can be either traumatic, biological, or mechanical. Lateral femorotibial osteoarthritis is less common than medial osteoarthritis and represents just 12.5% of the uni-compartmental osteoarthritis [1]. In a typical knee, approximately 60% of the weight-bearing force is transmitted through the medial compartment and 40% through the lateral compartment. Valgus alignment leads to greater forces concentrated in the lateral compartment. The lateral femoral condyle and lateral tibial plateau have convex surfaces with congruency maintained by the integrity of the lateral meniscus. Altered biomechanics as a result of lateral meniscal injury can lead to progressive deterioration of the lateral compartment.

Management of gonarthrosis should utilize conservative (nonoperative) modalities initially, when feasible. This includes weight loss in overweight patients, physiotherapy with muscle strengthening, and medications such as analgesics (paracetamol and nonsteroidal anti-inflammatory drugs). Hyaluronic acid joint infiltration has been widely adopted although its efficacy has not been definitively established [2]. If conservative treatment is unsuccessful, surgery is generally the next step. While knee arthroplasty is known to provide effective pain relief and deliver long-term implant survivorship in older patients, young and active patients

J.-M. Fayard (✉) · B. Freychet
Ramsay Générale de Santé, Hôpital Privé Jean Mermoz, Centre Orthopédique Santy, Lyon, France

N. Jan
Centre Hospitalier de Dunkerque, Service Orthopédie Traumatologie, Dunkerque, France

P. O'Loughlin
Cork University Hospital, South Infirmary Victoria University Hospital, Mater Private Cork, Cork, Ireland

© Springer Nature Switzerland AG 2020
S. Oussedik, S. Lustig (eds.), *Osteotomy About the Knee*,
https://doi.org/10.1007/978-3-030-49055-3_13

have a 3- to 5-time increased risk of revision surgery [3]. Conservative surgery such as osteotomies represents a valuable alternative in those cases.

Patients who are physiologically young with uni-compartmental lateral knee osteoarthritis should be considered as suitable candidates for varus-producing osteotomies. To address this form of malalignment, the main options include distal femoral medial closing-wedge osteotomy, distal femoral lateral open-wedge osteotomy, or proximal tibial medial closing-wedge osteotomy. Early clinical studies on varus tibial osteotomies reported overcorrection leading to joint line obliquity and shear stresses generated by the femur on the tibia [4–7]. Due to these findings, recent studies were focused mainly on distal femoral varus osteotomies as a procedure that was perceived to be safer for valgus knees with tibiofemoral lateral compartment osteoarthritis.

If the anatomical valgus deformity is greater than 12°, Coventry [4] recommended a varus-producing distal femoral osteotomy. However, when a small correction is required, a high tibial medial closing-wedge osteotomy could be performed successfully. Since the first report by Jackson and Waugh in 1961 [5], the results of high tibial varus closing-wedge osteotomies have been reported in only five clinical studies up to 2019, according to the current authors' literature review.

The current authors describe the indications for closing-wedge high tibial varus osteotomies, technique, potential complications, their own experience with this technique, and results from the literature.

13.2   Indications and Contraindications

The indications for varus tibial osteotomies are:

- Symptomatic osteoarthritis of the lateral knee compartment (Ahlbäck scores 2–3) [8] and absence of OA signs in the medial compartment
- AND
- Valgus deformity <6° (hip knee angle: HKA) on the preoperative long-leg standing radiographs without tibia vara (mechanical medial proximal tibial angle, mMPTA)

The contraindications for varus tibial osteotomies are:

1. BMI > 30
2. Rheumatoid arthritis
3. Severe lateral femorotibial osteoarthritis with tibiofemoral subluxation (Ahlbäck grade 4)
4. Medial femorotibial osteoarthritis (Ahlbäck grade > 1)
5. Knee stiffness with greater than 10° of flexion contracture and/or less than 90° of knee flexion.

13.3 Preoperative Planning and Patient Selection

13.3.1 Clinical Examination

Physical examination should include analysis of physiological age, activity level, medical comorbidities, and BMI measurement. Clinical examination should be focused on knee range of motion, status of the deformity of the lower limb in supine and standing positions, and whether it is fixed or reducible. The examiner should examine for tenderness or pain in both femorotibial and patellofemoral compartments.

13.3.2 Radiological Planning

13.3.2.1 Radiographic Views
Full weight-bearing anteroposterior (Fig. 13.1) and lateral views in full extension and at 30° of flexion (Fig. 13.2) and also axial views are performed to evaluate the status of the tibiofemoral and patellofemoral compartments. The mechanical axis of

Fig. 13.1 Full weight-bearing anteroposterior view in extension showing lateral femorotibial joint space narrowing

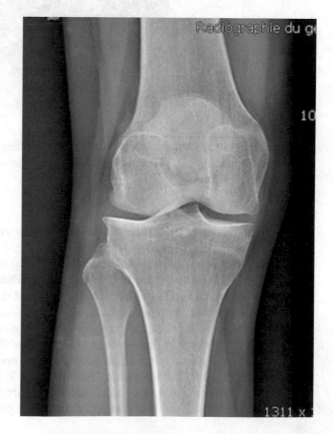

Fig. 13.2 Full weight-bearing anteroposterior view at 30° of flexion

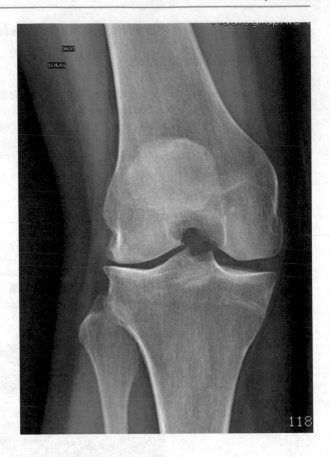

the lower limb is analyzed using bilateral long-leg standing radiographs (Fig. 13.3) or EOS scan. Both tibial and femoral mechanical axes are also evaluated to define the basis of the deformity.

13.3.2.2 Surgical Planning

Surgical planning may be performed on the preoperative long-leg radiographs using the Miniaci technique [9] to evaluate the height of the resected wedge (Fig. 13.4). The lower limb weight-bearing line joining the center of the hip (H) to the center of the ankle (A) is plotted (line 1, HA). The desired weight-bearing axis is constructed by plotting a line from the center of the femoral head through the desired weight-bearing point of the knee. Classically, the target point is positioned on the edge of the medial tibial spine. Then a line connecting the hip center and the target point and the desired center of the ankle (line 2, HA′) is drawn. A line connecting the lateral hinge of the osteotomy (O) and the center of the ankle joint (line 3, OA) and a line connecting the hinge and A′ (line 4, OA′) are drawn. The desired correction angle (α) is obtained by the angle formed by lines 3 and 4. The osteotomy site is drawn from the upper part of the proximal tibiofibular joint

Fig. 13.3 Bilateral long-leg standing radiographs

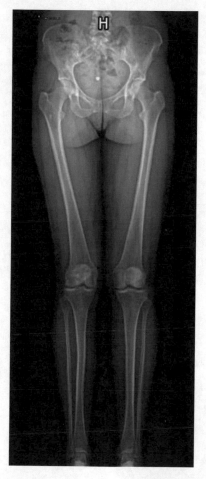

to the desired medial osteotomy start (4–5 cm distal to the medial tibial plateau). The amount of resection is determined by the correction angle on the lateral hinge (Fig. 13.5).

13.4   Surgical Technique

A general or neuraxial anesthetic is administered to the patients, and they are placed in a supine position on the operating table, with the knee flexed to 90°. The procedure is performed under fluoroscopic guidance. Special attention should be paid to adequate access for the image intensifier so as to facilitate intraoperative fluoroscopy of the hip and the ankle. A pneumatic tourniquet is applied to the proximal ipsilateral thigh. Arthroscopy is systematically performed at the beginning of the procedure to assess the condition of the cartilage of the patellofemoral and medial tibiofemoral compartments and also to treat any meniscal or cartilage pathology or to remove any loose bodies.

Fig. 13.4 Preoperative planning according to Miniaci technique

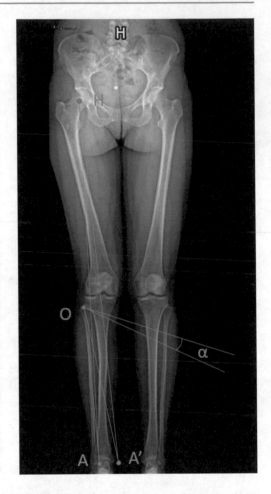

A standard anteromedial approach for HTVO is utilized. A 10–15 cm straight anterior midline incision is made, ending 2–3 cm medial to the tibial crest.

The pes anserinus tendons are exposed and then released from their tibial insertion. With the use of a sharp periosteal elevator, the posterior aspect of the tibia is exposed, and a retractor is carefully placed against the bone, to protect the neurovascular structures.

Two parallel Kirschner wires (K-wires) are introduced from the medial aspect of the tibia to the upper part of the proximal tibiofibular joint (Fig. 13.6). Correct K-wire positioning is facilitated by fluoroscopy, with the knee in full extension. The superficial layer of the medial collateral ligament (MCL) is cut at the level of the osteotomy site. Then the osteotomy is performed just below the K-wires with the knee at 90° of flexion (Fig. 13.7). A second cut is made at a pre-defined point, superior to the first one in accordance with the preoperative planning. The lateral cortex is not breached so as to preserve a lateral hinge. Then the K-wires are removed and a triangular bone wedge is resected (Fig. 13.8). Primary resection should be as

Fig. 13.5 Evaluation of
the wedge resection
according to Miniaci
technique

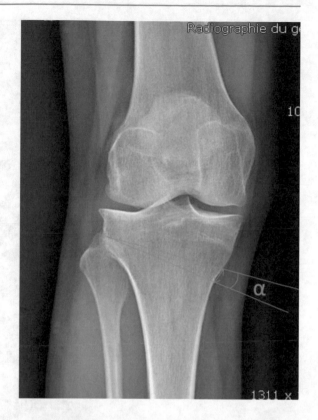

Fig. 13.6 Osteotomy
direction simulated by two
parallel Kirschner wires

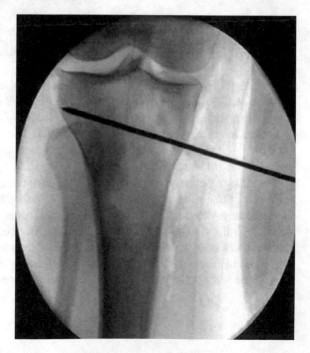

Fig. 13.7 Osteotomy is performed just below the K-wires

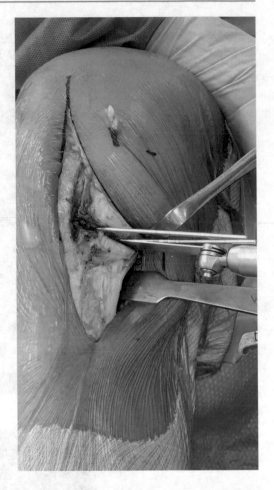

conservative as possible to avoid overcorrection. Applying a varus stress on the tibia achieves closure of the resection site. If a lateral hinge fracture occurs, it should be fixed with a surgical staple before definitive closure of the osteotomy site.

Evaluation of the correction achieved may be ascertained intraoperatively. The extent of correction is assessed with fluoroscopy and incorporating a rod joining the center of the hip to the center of the ankle (Fig. 13.9).

Acquiring a normal mechanical axis is the goal (i.e., the rod should pass through the medial tibial spine post-correction). In the early days of high tibial varus osteotomies, an overcorrection was the objective, leading to overloading of the tibiofemoral medial compartment and early failure. As a consequence of these findings, some authors stated that the optimal target for osteotomies of valgus knees should be normal mechanical alignment [7, 10]. A loading point just medial to the medial tibial spine was also proposed for HTVO in valgus knees [11].

Fig. 13.8 Resection of a triangular bone wedge

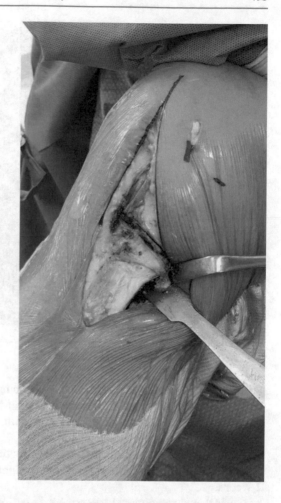

The primary resection has to be as minimal as possible (Fig. 13.10). The osteotomy is temporarily fixed with a surgical staple (Fig. 13.11a, b). The correction is assessed with fluoroscopy (Fig. 13.9). At this stage, no varus stress should be applied to avoid lateral collateral ligament (LCL) tensioning and pseudo-overcorrection (Fig. 13.12). If the correction is insufficient, an additional bone wedge is removed.

When the final desired correction is achieved, the staple is removed, and the osteotomy is fixed with a four-hole locking L-plate (NewClip Technics, Nantes, France) or a four-hole C-plate (Otis, SBM SAS, Lourdes, France) (Fig. 13.13).

At the end of the procedure, hemostasis is confirmed following deflation of the tourniquet. A drain is sited in the operative site posterior to the tibia for 24 h. The hamstring tendons are restored to their normal position which now overlies the plate, and the wound is carefully closed.

Fig. 13.9 Fluoroscopy assessment of the extent of correction

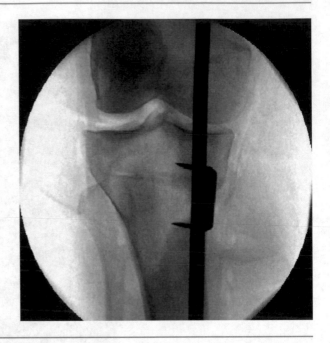

13.5 Postoperative Management

Postoperatively, the lower limb is protected in a functional brace, but early rehabilitation is allowed. Patients may partially weight-bear if the lateral hinge has been maintained. If the patient complains of knee pain, they are educated to modify their weight-bearing according to their symptoms.

In those cases of lateral hinge fracture, patients are non-weight-bearing for 6 weeks and then begin progressive weight-bearing over the subsequent 2 weeks.

Clinical and radiological assessment is performed at 6 weeks, 3 months, and 6 months, to evaluate bone healing of the osteotomy site.

A progressive return to nonimpact sports is usually permitted after 3 months. Patients are informed that a return to impact sports is not recommended.

13.6 Outcomes

The current authors report on a series of 30 patients who underwent medial closing-wedge tibial osteotomies at a mean of 12-year follow-up (range, 3.1–16.6 years). Two patients were lost to follow-up, and one could not be evaluated because of an unrelated cerebrovascular injury. All the osteotomies were healed at 3-month follow-up. Nine patients progressed to total knee arthroplasty at a mean of 10.3-year post-osteotomy. The cumulative survival rate of the HTVO was 96% (95% CI

Fig. 13.10 Minimum
primary wedge resection

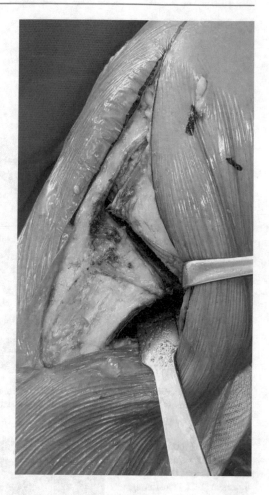

0.92–1.00) at 5 years, 87% (95% CI 0.80–0.94) at 10 years, and 60% (95% CI 0.47–0.74) at 15 years.

In regard to the 18 remaining knees, the Knee Society objective score improved from 53.4 (range, 14–80) to 72.1 (range, 43–95) ($p = 0.001$). The Knee Society function score improved from 78.8 (range, 30–100) to 91.7 (range, 70–100) ($p = 0.02$). The pain score (0–50 points) improved from 12.2 (range, 0–30) to 32.8 (range 10–45) ($p < 0.001$). UCLA score analyzing patients' activity levels improved from 6 (range, 4–9) to 8 (range, 4–9) ($p < 0.001$).

No major complications such as infection, thromboembolism, intra-articular fractures, neurovascular complications, hinge fracture, delayed, or nonunion were observed in this study. Painful hardware was removed in six patients. Two patients underwent partial lateral and medial meniscectomies after the osteotomy.

Five patients had preoperative femora valga (mLDFA <85°). Among these patients, two presented with early failure of the HTVO and underwent TKA after

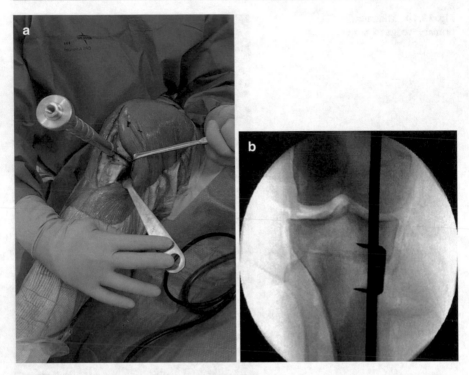

Fig. 13.11 (**a**) Osteotomy temporarily fixation with a surgical staple. (**b**) Fluoroscopy control showing osteotomy temporarily fixation with a surgical staple

Fig. 13.12 Fluoroscopy control with varus stress showing lateral collateral ligament (LCL) tensioning and pseudo-overcorrection

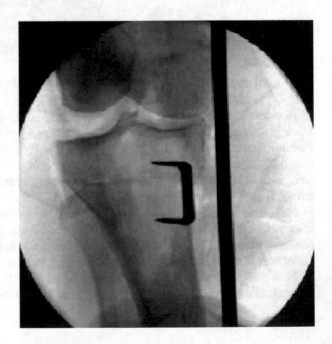

Fig. 13.13 Osteotomy
fixation with a four-hole
locking L-plate (NewClip
Technics, Nantes, France)

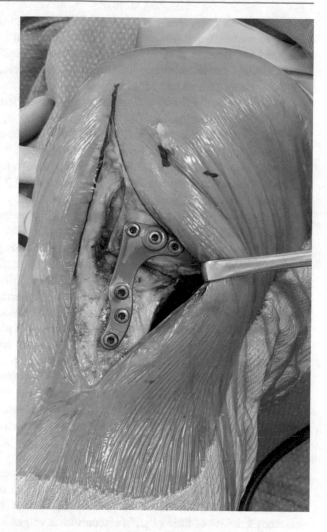

4.4 and 7 years of follow-up, respectively, and two patients had poor clinical outcomes at last follow-up.

In two patients, a postoperative joint line obliquity of more than 10° was recorded.
One patient reported recurrent pain with tibiofemoral instability 1 year after the
index procedure and underwent TKA at 4.4-year post-HTVO.

13.7 Literature

There is a paucity of studies in the literature focused on varus tibial osteotomies for
valgus arthritic knees. Only five studies reported on the results of varus closing-
wedge proximal tibial osteotomies [4–7, 12]. Some limitations of these studies were
small sample sizes, retrospective study designs, and no control groups. Additionally,

these series were heterogeneous in terms of surgical indication, surgical technique, clinical assessment, and follow-up. All of them reported a significant improvement in clinical and functional scores and lower rates of complication than open-wedge proximal tibial osteotomies and distal femoral osteotomies such as nonunion and common peroneal nerve palsy [13].

An early series, published by Jackson et al., was carried out in 11 patients with a mean of 31-month follow-up. The authors reported a significant improvement in pain without any specific complications [5]. Shoji and Insall reported on a series of 49 knees with a mean of 31.5-month follow-up (range, 13–69 months). The authors described 53% of patient reporting successful pain relief and 57% satisfactory results, but the mean preoperative valgus deformity was 21.5° (range, 13–30°), and all patients had a preoperative medial thrust [6]. Coventry reported on a series of 49 varus closing-wedge proximal osteotomies with a mean of 9.4-year follow-up (range, 2–7 years). Major pain relief was achieved in 77% of cases, and the authors did not find any evidence of neurovascular complications [4].

Varus tibial closing-wedge osteotomy was initially performed even in the setting of large valgus deformities, and overcorrection led to joint line obliquity and shear stresses generated by the femur on the tibia [4–7]. Coventry [4] also reported that a joint line horizontal obliquity of less than 10° was associated with good results. Shoji and Insall [6] recommended precise preoperative planning to facilitate accurate siting of the osteotomy. Chambat et al. [7] reported on a series of 47 patients at a mean of 7-year follow-up with 72% of patients experiencing good and very good functional outcomes. The authors stated that tibial osteotomies have an inherent advantage of efficacy in both flexion and extension.

Mirouse et al. [12] described only a 57% survival rate at 5-year follow-up. The authors reported a rate of 58. 2% of under- or overcorrection, and joint line obliquity greater than 10° was found in 26.3%. 71.4% of patients who underwent a TKA had had a miscorrection and 26.3% had had a joint line obliquity of more than 10°.

The site of the osteotomy (tibial or femoral) depends on the site of valgus deformity [14]. According to Hofmann et al., genu valgum originates from the distal femur in 22%, from the tibia in 45%, and from both in 33% [15]. Alghamdi et al. also recorded 53% of tibia valga in osteoarthritic valgus knees [16]. Normal values for tibial and femoral mechanical angles are between 85° and 90°. According to Shoji and Insall [6] and Coventry [4], high tibial varus osteotomies should not be performed when the valgus deformity exceeds 6° or if the planned postoperative joint line obliquity will exceed 10°. For greater accuracy, the femoral contribution in valgus deformity should be considered when the mechanical femoral angle is less than 85°.

13.8 Conclusion

Closing-wedge varus tibial osteotomies for lateral osteoarthritis provide good long-term functional and clinical results, with a low complication and revision rate. However, one must adhere to certain criteria for patient selection to increase the likelihood of achieving a good result. These are a preoperative femoral valgus deformity of less than 6°, a normal postoperative axis, and a postoperative joint line obliquity of less than 10°. In cases of femora valga with less than 85° of a femoral mechanical angle, femoral or combined osteotomies should be considered.

References

1. Jamali AA, Scott RD. Lateral unicompartmental knee arthroplasty. Tech Knee Surg. 2005;4(2):79.
2. Glyn-Jones S, Palmer AJR, Agricola R, Price AJ, Vincent TL, Weinans H, et al. Osteoarthritis. Lancet. 2015;386(9991):376–87.
3. Santaguida PL, Hawker GA, Hudak PL, Glazier R, Mahomed NN, Kreder HJ, et al. Patient characteristics affecting the prognosis of total hip and knee joint arthroplasty: a systematic review. Can J Surg. 2008;51(6):428–36.
4. Coventry MB. Proximal tibial varus osteotomy for osteoarthritis of the lateral compartment of the knee. J Bone Joint Surg Am. 1987;69(1):32–8.
5. Jackson JP, Waugh W. Tibial osteotomy for osteoarthritis of the knee. J Bone Joint Surg Br. 1961;43-B:746–51.
6. Shoji H, Insall J. High tibial osteotomy for osteoarthritis of the knee with valgus deformity. J Bone Joint Surg Am. 1973;55(5):963–73.
7. Chambat P, Selmi T, Dejour D, Denoyers J. Varus tibial osteotomy. Oper Tech Sports Med. 2000;8(1):44–7.
8. Ahlbäck S. Osteoarthrosis of the knee. A radiographic investigation. Acta Radiol Diagn (Stockh). 1968;(Suppl 277):7–72.
9. Miniaci A, Ballmer FT, Ballmer PM, Jakob RP. Proximal tibial osteotomy. A new fixation device. Clin Orthop Relat Res. 1989;246:250–9.
10. Puddu G, Cipolla M, Cerullo G, Franco V, Giannì E. Which osteotomy for a valgus knee? Int Orthop. 2010;34(2):239–47.
11. Collins B, Getgood A, Alomar AZ, Giffin JR, Willits K, Fowler PJ, et al. A case series of lateral opening wedge high tibial osteotomy for valgus malalignment. Knee Surg Sports Traumatol Arthrosc. 2013;21(1):152–60.
12. Mirouse G, Dubory A, Roubineau F, Poignard A, Hernigou P, Allain J, et al. Failure of high tibial varus osteotomy for lateral tibio-femoral osteoarthritis with <10° of valgus: outcomes in 19 patients. Orthop Traumatol Surg Res. 2017;103(6):953–8.
13. Haviv B, Bronak S, Thein R, Thein R. The results of corrective osteotomy for valgus arthritic knees. Knee Surg Sports Traumatol Arthrosc. 2013;21(1):49–56.
14. Marti RK, Verhagen RA, Kerkhoffs GM, Moojen TM. Proximal tibial varus osteotomy. Indications, technique, and five to twenty-one-year results. J Bone Joint Surg Am. 2001;83-A(2):164–70.
15. Hofmann S, Paszicneyk T, Mohajer M. A new concept for transposition osteotomies around the knee. Iatros Iatros. 2004;1(1):40–8.
16. Alghamdi A, Rahmé M, Lavigne M, Massé V, Vendittoli P-A. Tibia valga morphology in osteoarthritic knees: importance of preoperative full limb radiographs in total knee arthroplasty. J Arthroplasty. 2014;29(8):1671–6.

Surgical Technique: Sagittal Plane Correction

14

Guillaume Demey and David Dejour

14.1 Introduction

Stability of the knee is controlled by both soft tissue and bony elements, which are responsible for the overall balance of the joint on both coronal and sagittal plane. The main actors in the control of sagittal stability of the knee are anterior cruciate ligament (ACL), posterior cruciate ligament (PCL), posteromedial and posterolateral structures, the menisci, and the posterior tibial slope (PTS). Correction of the tibial slope may be performed in two different situations: anterior closing-wedge osteotomy to correct excessive PTS or anterior opening-wedge osteotomy to increase PTS and to correct a pathologic genu recurvatum. The aim of this chapter is to describe these two procedures. Tibial slope management during frontal high tibial osteotomy (HTO) will not be discussed in this chapter.

14.2 Anterior Tibial Closing-Wedge Osteotomy for Tibial Slope Correction

Several authors confirmed that an excessive PTS increases tensions within the ACL and exacerbates the risk of injury or failure after reconstruction [1–5]. The normal PTS is within the range of 5°–7°, depending on the measurement technique, and is considered pathologic if it exceeds 12° [1, 4, 5]. Correction of excessive slope is rarely indicated; however, it must be considered in patients with a failed ACL reconstruction combined with a tibial slope greater than 12° [4]. Anterior tibial closing-wedge osteotomy (also called deflexion osteotomy) is performed to reduce anterior

G. Demey (✉) · D. Dejour
Lyon Ortho Clinic, Clinique de la Sauvegarde, Lyon, France
e-mail: dr.demey@lyon-ortho-clinic.com; dr.dejour@lyon-ortho-clinic.com

© Springer Nature Switzerland AG 2020
S. Oussedik, S. Lustig (eds.), *Osteotomy About the Knee*,
https://doi.org/10.1007/978-3-030-49055-3_14

tibial translation induced by excessive PTS. This technique does not alter the position of the anterior tibial tuberosity. Preservation of the anterior tibial cortex in this region helps to limit postoperative hyperextension.

14.2.1 Surgical Technique

The patient is in supine position on a radiolucent table. A tourniquet is placed high on the thigh. A lateral post at the level of the tourniquet maintained leg position in the frontal plane, and a distal support held the knee at 90° of flexion, allowing full range of motion when desired.

The surgical approach is identical to the valgus medial-opening HTO (Fig. 14.1). The incision is anterior and approximately 1–2 cm medial to the tibial tuberosity. In many revision cases, previous incisions should be used for the approach.

The patellar tendon is exposed, and then the deep medial collateral ligament (MCL) and the fascia lata on Gerdy's tubercle are detached up to the posterior part of the tibia (Fig. 14.2). The level of the osteotomy always starts from the superior margin of the patellar tendon insertion, approximatively 4 cm below the joint line.

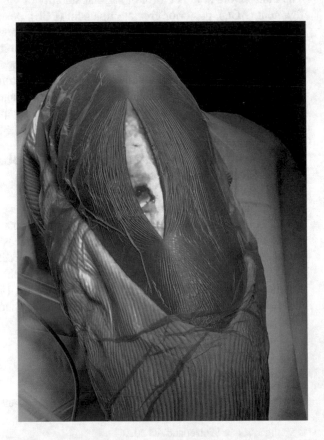

Fig. 14.1 Surgical approach: The incision is anterior and approximately 1–2 cm medial to the tibial tuberosity

Fig. 14.2 Exposure of the patellar tendon and partial detachment of the MCL and the fascia lata on Gerdy's tubercle

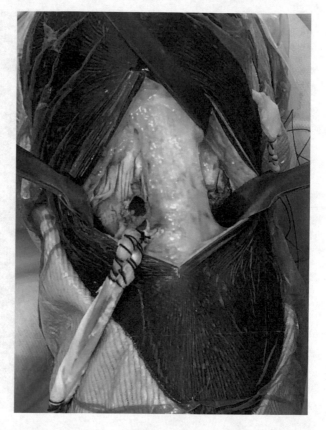

Two parallel K-wires are inserted under fluoroscopic control on both sides of the patellar tendon. The K-wires are placed with an upward direction and should meet the posterior tibial cortex near its junction with the PCL facet (Figs. 14.3, 14.4, and 14.5).

The anterior closing-wedge osteotomy is performed under the K-wires on both sides of the patellar tendon using the oscillating saw preserving a posterior hinge. The hinge should be centered at the junction of the PCL facet of the tibia with the posterior tibial cortex, just distal to the PCL insertion. An intact posterior cortex limits the risk of nonunion and protects the popliteal vascular structures.

A second osteotomy (the upper cut) is completed. It should begin between a few millimeters (depending on the planning) proximal to the first cut and converges posteriorly (Figs. 14.6, 14.7, and 14.8). An anterior wedge is resected to obtain a desired PTS between 0° and 5°. We considered that 1mm resection is equal to 1° correction, but the oscillating saw thickness should be taken into account (at least 2 mm as two cuts are performed). The bone wedge is resected, and the anterior closing-wedge osteotomy is compressed simply by extending the knee, thereby exerting pressure by the femoral condyles onto the anterior tibial plateau. In case of difficulty to compress the osteotomy, the posterior cortex could be weakened by drilling using a 3.2 mm drill.

Fig. 14.3 K-wires placement with an upward direction from the superior part of the tibial tubercle to the posterior tibial cortex (PCL facet)

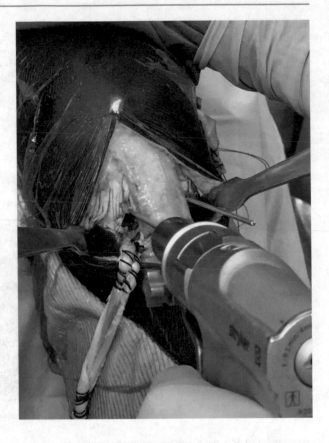

When the resected surfaces united, a new fluoroscopy control is obtained to assess the new PTS. If correction is appropriate, the osteotomy is fixed by two large staples, one on either side of the patellar tendon (Figs. 14.9 and 14.10). We emphasize that a more rigid fixation (e.g., fixation by plate) is not necessary as this osteotomy is naturally stable.

When planning the degree of correction, the calculation must take into consideration the measured bone abnormality but also the clinical abnormality. A patient with significant recurvatum will not tolerate a larger correction.

14.2.2 Postoperative Rehabilitation

Progressive nonaggressive rehabilitation is followed immediately after surgery, with passive and active motion exercises as tolerated by the patient. Range-of-motion exercises aimed at obtaining full extension but avoiding hyperextension, and there was no limitation in flexion. For the first 3 weeks, weight-bearing is not allowed. Immobilization in an extension brace for transfers is used. In case of

Figs. 14.4 and 14.5 Fluoroscopic
control is mandatory

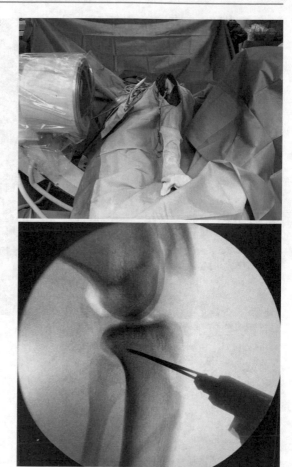

excessive postoperative hyperextension, the knee can be maintained in a brace with a slight flexion during 3–4 weeks. Reduction in knee swelling, quadriceps control, and recovery of range of motion are the main objectives. Over the 3 following weeks, weight-bearing is gradually allowed until day 45.

14.2.3 Reefing of Posteromedial Soft Tissues

In case of excessive hyperextension associated with anterior closing-wedge osteotomy, reefing of the posteromedial soft tissues is usually sufficient. Rarely, posterolateral reefing is also required.

Reefing is a combined procedure and performed by placing a retention suture in the superficial medial collateral ligament and oblique popliteal ligament and

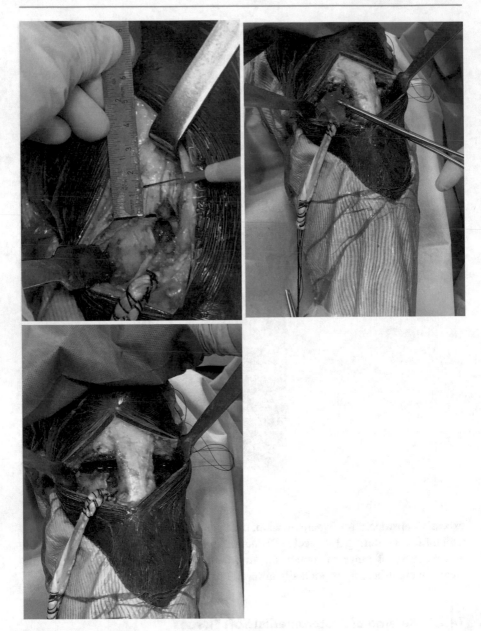

Figs. 14.6–14.8 The osteotomy is completed and the anterior wedge is resected

Fig. 14.9 A very stable
fixation of the osteotomy is
obtained by only
two staples

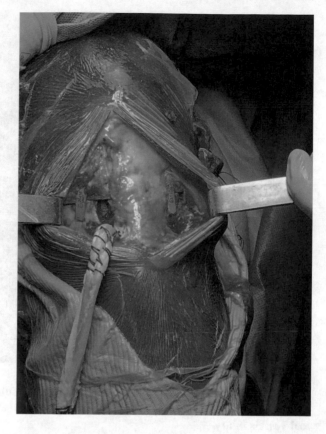

advancing the semimembranosus. This procedure is useful for control of anterior
tibial translation in single leg stance and control of recurvatum. Rehabilitation will
include bracing to block full extension for 45 days.

14.2.4 Tibial Tubercle Detachment

Detachment of the anterior tibial tubercle is not mandatory in our experience. First
of all, the distance from the superior margin of the patellar tendon insertion and
anterior aspect of the joint line is greater in patients with an excessive PTS. Thus, it
is easier to perform this procedure without tibial tubercle osteotomy in these
patients. There are also several advantages to avoid tibial tubercle detachment.
Preservation of the anterior tibial cortex in this region helps to limit postoperative
hyperextension. The bone contact area is greater in case of preservation of tibial
tubercle attachment increasing stability and fusion process. Iatrogenic complications related to the tibial tubercle osteotomy can be avoided (risk of wound problems, nonunion, range of motion, infection, etc.). At last, tibial tubercle is a great

Fig. 14.10 Fluoroscopic control after closing and fixation of the osteotomy. The posterior tibial slope is checked

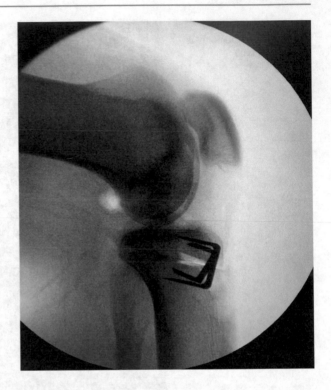

landmark for level of the osteotomy. The direction should start from the superior margin of the patellar tendon to the PCL insertion site, which protects from popliteal vessels injury.

14.2.5 Indications and Contraindications

The main indication for this procedure is increased sagittal plane posterior slope ≥12° in a patient with a failed ACLR (Figs. 14.11 and 14.12). Other relative indications include severe anterior instability as evidenced by a high-grade Lachman and pivot shift (3+) on physical examination in patients with single or multiple failed ACLRs. Measurements may be conducted on the lateral view of plain radiographs, ensuring there is sufficient visualization of the distal tibia (20 cm). Long-standing radiographs should also be obtained to rule out any significant genu varum or valgus malalignment. Contraindications for a decreasing slope anterior closing-wedge osteotomy include primary ACLR patients (excepted for very selective cases), genu recurvatum with significant knee hyperextension (e.g.,>10° where tightening of posterior capsular elements should be combined), posterior cruciate ligament (PCL) deficiency, significant genu varum malalignment, and end-stage tibiofemoral osteoarthritis.

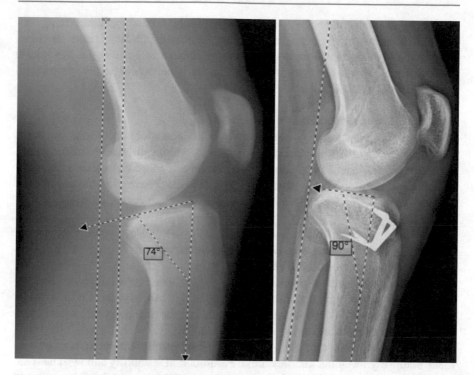

Figs. 14.11 and 14.12   Preoperative X-rays showing an important postoperative tibial slope of 16° associated with an important anterior tibial drawer. The postoperative x-rays show a very nice correction of the posterior tibial slope, a nice fusion of the osteotomy, and the disappearance of the anterior tibial drawer in full weight-bearing

14.3   Anterior Tibial Opening-Wedge Osteotomy for Genu Recurvatum

Osteotomy for correction of genu recurvatum is rarely indicated. Genu recurvatum is defined by knee hyperextension over 180° on femorotibial sagittal alignment. Genu recurvatum may be constitutional, congenital, or acquired [6–8]. Constitutional genu recurvatum is symmetrical, usually less than 15° and often asymptomatic. Pathologic genu recurvatum is acquired, symptomatic, and asymmetrical.

14.3.1   Etiology

There are three types of pathologic genu recurvatum [6]:

14.3.1.1   Bony Genu Recurvatum
The origin of bony recurvatum is usually the tibial superior metaphysis with inversion of the PTS in the sagittal plane. Deformity can be articular or extra-articular. The most frequent etiology is damage to the growth plate of the tibial tubercle. The most common mechanisms are direct trauma, fracture of the proximal tibia,

avulsion of the tibial tuberosity, osteomyelitis, patellar tendon graft harvesting, tibial tubercle transfer before physeal closure, Osgood-Schlatter disease sequelae, long period of immobilization, or tibial traction. Another rare etiology is hypoplasia of the lateral femoral condyle, which can cause hyperextension associated with excessive tibial external rotation.

14.3.1.2 Ligamentous Genu Recurvatum

Such recurvatum is caused by insufficiency of the posterior capsule and popliteus muscle, PCL rupture, or bicruciate injury (e.g., posterior dislocation of the knee). The origin of the ligamentous etiology may be an acute trauma or a chronic injury leading to posterior soft tissue insufficiency. Soft tissue deficiencies may involve the posterolateral and/or the posteromedial corner. In these cases, there is no PTS inversion.

14.3.1.3 Ligamentous and Bony Genu Recurvatum (Combined Recurvatum)

Bony deformation leads to insufficiency of the posterior capsuloligamentous tissues, but soft tissue injury can also lead to tibial slope inversion as in poliomyelitis sequelae. Patients with such sequelae experience quadriceps palsy and need hyperextension to lock the knee during walking.

Main symptoms are knee pain, femorotibial and patellofemoral instability, cosmetic deformity, swelling, and weakness. Femorotibial instability and weakness are caused by hyperextension, which decreases the patellofemoral joint lever arm and leads to atrophy of the quadriceps muscle. Hyperextension can also lead to patellofemoral instability because of a pseudopatella alta. In addition, patients are not able to walk on irregular ground and to practice sports. Lower limb length discrepancy can also be present. Indeed, a genu valgum is often present and can be associated with a pseudo-lengthening of the lower limb. On the other hand, a shortening can be caused by an early closure of the tibial superior growth plate.

14.3.2 Surgical Technique

Different tibial osteotomies have been described in the literature. Posterior closing-wedge osteotomy below the anterior tibial tubercle, with osteotomy of the fibula, was described by Irwin in 1942 [9]. Posterior closing-wedge osteotomy above the anterior tibial tubercle was described by Bowen et al. [10]. The distances between the osteotomy and the deformity and between the osteotomy and the articular surface are greater in the osteotomy below the tuberosity. This leads to a larger opening wedge and probably increases the risk of nonunion. Furthermore, this kind of procedure requires fibular osteotomy. Owing to those problems, this technique is not used anymore. Lexer [11] described anterior opening-wedge osteotomies above the anterior tibial tubercle. Those procedures present less nonunion risk than the osteotomy below tibial tuberosity, but the limited thickness of the epiphyseal fragment leads to a higher risk of epiphyseal osseous necrosis. Furthermore, stability of the epiphyseal fragment may be insufficient because of the thin posterior hinge. Patellar height is also an issue because of lowering equal to the anterior graft thickness. Dome-shaped HTO has been proposed, using the principles of frontal tibial osteotomies. This procedure is technically demanding, less reproducible, and therefore rarely used.

Henri Dejour [12] modified the technique described by Lexer to prevent previous problems. It is an anterior opening-wedge procedure associated with a tibial tubercle detachment with proximal transfer to prevent patella infera. If required, a tightening of capsuloligamentous posterior elements can be performed in association with it.

The patient is in supine position on a radiolucent table. A tourniquet is placed high on the thigh. A lateral post at the level of the tourniquet maintained leg position in the frontal plane, and a distal support held the knee at 90° of flexion, allowing full range of motion when desired. Fluoroscopy will be used during the procedure.

The incision is vertical, from the lower part of the patella to the tibial tubercle, at the medial border of the patellar tendon (Fig. 14.13). Through this incision, the anterior tibial tubercle and the patellar tendon are exposed. The tibial tubercle is detached; the goal is to detach a fragment of 6 cm in length including anterior tibial tuberosity (Fig. 14.14). The first osteotomy line is lateral and horizontal and must reach the cancellous bone. The medial line is almost vertical and medial. The distal

Fig. 14.13 Vertical incision from the lower part of the patella to the tibial tubercle, at the medial border of the patellar tendon

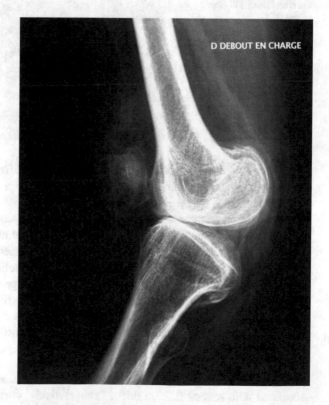

D DEBOUT EN CHARGE

Fig. 14.14 Detachment of the tibial tubercle with a 6cm length

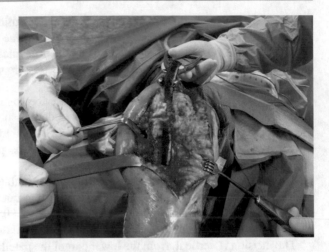

Fig. 14.15 Direction of the osteotomy marked with two pins up to the anterior tibial tuberosity side by side with the patellar tendon and oriented toward the tibial insertion fibers of the PCL

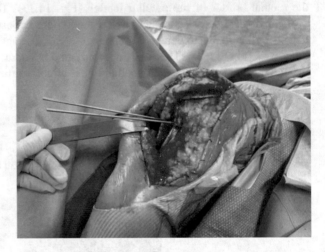

transverse osseous cut is performed softly to avoid tibial fracture. Then, this osseous fragment is detached using osteotomes. All the peripheral capsuloligamentous structures attached to the epiphysis are left intact.

The direction of the osteotomy is marked with two pins up to the anterior tibial tuberosity side by side with the patellar tendon and oriented toward the tibial insertion fibers of the PCL (Fig. 14.15). Those pins are inserted approximately 4 cm below the tibial articular surface. Ideally, those pins should meet the inferior part of the PCL fibers, under the tibial articular surface and proximal to the tibiofibular joint to avoid fibula osteotomy. Pins must exit above the tibial capsule to conserve a posterior hinge. It is recommended to check the position of the pin using fluoroscopy. The osteotomy is proximal to the proximal tibiofibular joint so there is no need for a fibular osteotomy.

The osteotomy is performed with an oscillating saw placed under the pins to avoid joint damage. The posterior cortex must be preserved and is progressively weakened with several 3.2mm drills. Preoperatively, correction must be carefully

Fig. 14.16 Gentle
opening of the osteotomy
using several osteotomes

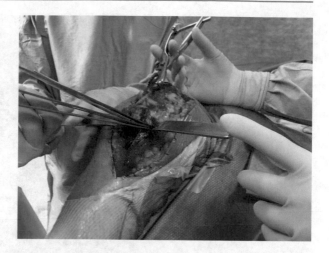

checked. The anterior opening-wedge osteotomy is done using osteotomes. Subsequently a Lambotte osteotome (thickness 2 mm, corresponding with approximately 2° of angular correction) is introduced into the osteotomy. A second osteotome is then introduced below the first. To gently open up the osteotomy, several more osteotomes are introduced between the two firsts (Fig. 14.16). Preoperatively, tibial varization is the natural tendency. To avoid such varization, osteotomes should be located on the medial side of the osteotomy. Posterior capsuloligamentous elements allow a good stability to this osteotomy. Nevertheless, we always use two staples on the sides of the patellar tendon. The anterior gap is filled using a secure bone allograft (Osteopure®) (Figs. 14.17 and 14.18). The opening wedge is very stable because of the posterior capsuloligamentous hinge. The tibial tubercle is reinserted and fixed with two cortical 4.5 mm screws, one above and one below the osteotomy. If the upper screw is closed to the osteotomy, it is possible to place both screws under the osteotomy. For preserving patellar height, the tibial tubercle is moved proximally of a height equal to the thickness of the osteotomy.

Another fluoroscopy control is necessary to check the PTS correction and the patellar height (Fig. 14.19). In the case of a bony or a soft tissue recurvatum deformity, the PTS will be corrected until normal alignment is achieved (no hyperextension clinically) (Figs. 14.20 and 14.21); sometimes, slight overcorrection (into a flexion deformity) will be required, since there is always a risk of secondary posterior soft tissue stretching. The recurvatum deformity following poliomyelitis needs special consideration: in such knees, slight undercorrection is required, since, with the quadriceps palsy, the knee can be locked only in hyperextension.

14.3.3 Tightening of Posterior Capsular Elements

Tightening posterior capsuloligamentous soft tissue elements is indicated when posterior ligaments and capsule are stretched. Three main procedures exist. The first one consists of detaching the posterior femoral capsular insertion and then reattaching it more proximally with anchors or using a transfemoral tunnel. The second one

Figs. 14.17 and 14.18 Two staples are fixed on the sides of the patellar tendon. The anterior gap is filled using a secure bone allograft

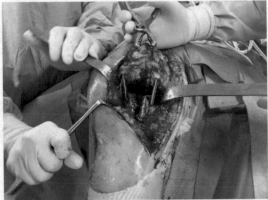

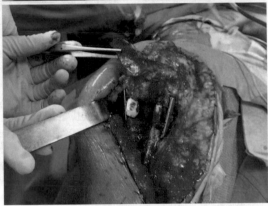

Fig. 14.19 Fluoroscopy control checking the PTS correction and the patellar height

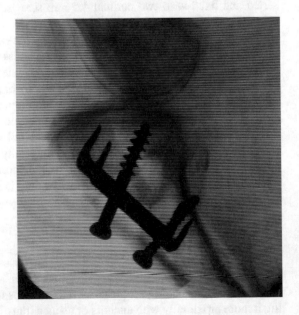

Figs. 14.20 and 14.21 In the case of a bony or a soft tissue recurvatum deformity, the PTS will be corrected until normal alignment is achieved (no hyperextension clinically). Figure 14.20 shows a very significative hyperextension. Figure 14.21 shows a very nice correction obtained with the bony procedure (without reefing)

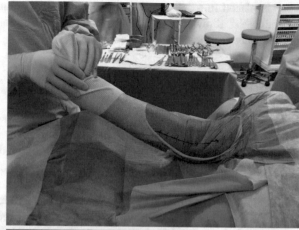

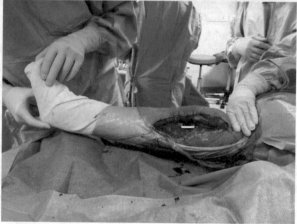

consists of sectioning the posterior knee capsule and performing a suture with a shift. The third one was described by Judet and Judet [13]. Two parallelepipedic bone blocks with their capsular femoral insertions are detached using a medial and lateral approach. These bone blocks have a square section from 9 to 14 mm, which depends on the amount of recurvatum to correct. Then both bone blocks are rotated 90° and reinserted in their initial place. This procedure allows a capsular tightening with bone fixation.

14.3.4 Postoperative Management

The day after surgery, rehabilitation may be started. Passive motion is allowed between 5° and 95° using continuous passive motion. We avoid full extension and flexion greater than 95° for 4 weeks, to protect the osteotomy during the time of osseous consolidation. Weight-bearing is allowed after 45 days. For 45 days, the knee is placed in a splint at 10°. This surgical technique is relatively simple and reproducible, allows very accurate correction, and is safe concerning the common peroneal nerve. Rapid healing is the rule.

14.3.5 Indications

Surgical indication depends on the degree of hyperextension, the clinical examination, and the etiology of the recurvatum. Surgical indication is discussed in cases of a painful or unstable knee with hyperextension of 15° and only when the growth plate is closed. Nevertheless, not all patients with knee recurvatum with hyperextension of 15° need to be treated with an operation. Surgical correction must be planned on an x-ray of the contralateral knee or with an x-ray of the pathologic knee before trauma. Peroperatively, the surgeon must verify that extension is complete. The surgeon must never accept any preoperative fixed flexion. Isolated opening-wedge osteotomy is indicated for isolated osseous recurvatum with reversed tibial slope. Osseous recurvatum with more than 20° of hyperextension and following constitutional hyperlaxity may require surgery. Conservative treatment such as physiotherapy, kinesitherapy, and wearing high-heel shoes must be tried first. In cases of posterior capsular stretching, the role of the osteotomy is to protect ligamentous tightening. Indeed, Vicenzi et al. reported poor results for isolated osteotomy in patients with ligamentous recurvatum. Furthermore, it is possible to add some valgus in the osteotomy plan when varus thrust, posteromedial joint narrowing, and posterolateral knee instability are associated with knee recurvatum. Correction of the entire recurvatum has to be done in every case except for patients with poliomyelitis who need only a partial correction because they use hyperextension for locking their knee to walk.

14.4   Conclusion

Sagittal plane correction osteotomies are rarely indicated, but knee surgeons should know how and when to use them. Correction of excessive posterior tibial slope must be discussed at the time of the second revision ACL reconstruction. It should be considered as of the first revision ACL reconstruction as this can reduce risks of recurrent failure in patients with predisposing risk factors. Surgical indications for genu recurvatum obey strict rules. Before surgery, knee recurvatum must be analyzed to identify a ligamentous part. If needed, a complementary posterior soft tissue tightening is performed. These procedures of closing- and opening-wedge osteotomy are reliable and safe and correct the osseous deformity.

References

1. Giffin JR, Vogrin TM, Zantop T, Woo SL, Harner CD. Effects of increasing tibial slope on the biomechanics of the knee. Am J Sports Med. 2004;32:376–82.
2. Hohmann E, Bryant A, Reaburn P, Tetsworth K. Is there a correlation between posterior tibial slope and non-contact anterior cruciate ligament injuries? Knee Surg Sports Traumatol Arthrosc. 2011;19:S109–14.
3. Fening SD, Kovacic J, Kambic H, McLean S, Scott J, Miniaci A. The effects of modified posterior tibial slope on anterior cruciate ligament strain and knee kinematics: a human cadaveric study. J Knee Surg. 2008;21:205–11.
4. Dejour D, Saffarini M, Demey G, Baverel L. Tibial slope correction combined with second revision ACL produces good knee stability and prevents graft rupture. Knee Surg Sports Traumatol Arthrosc. 2015;23:2846–52.
5. Sonnery-Cottet B, Mogos S, Thaunat M, et al. Proximal tibial anterior closing wedge osteotomy in repeat revision of anterior cruciate ligament reconstruction. Am J Sports Med. 2014;42:1873–80.
6. Demey G, Lustig S, Servien E, Neyret P. Genu recurvatum osseux. EMC—Appareil locomoteur. 2013;8(4):1–9.
7. Lecuire F, Lerat JL, Bousquet G, et al. Le genu recurvatum et son traitement par ostéotomie tibiale. Rev Chir Orthop Repartrice Appar Mot. 1980;66:95–103.
8. Balestro JC, Lustig S, Servien E, Carmody D, Neyret P. Opening wedge tibial osteotomy in genu recurvatum. Tech Knee Surg. 2009;8(2):126–35.
9. Irwin CE. Genu recurvatum following poliomyelitis: controlled method of operative correction. JAMA. 1942;120:277–9.
10. Bowen JR, Morley DC, McInerny V, et al. Treatment of genu recurvatum by proximal tibial closing-wedge/anterior displacement osteotomy. Clin Orthop Relat Res. 1983;179:194–9.
11. Lexer E. Die gesamte wiederherstellungs chirurgie. Leipzig Bart JA. 1931:551–3.
12. Dejour D, Khun A, Dejour H. Ostéotomie tibiale de déflexion et laxité chronique antérieure à propos de 22 cas. Rev Chir Orthop. 1998;84:28.
13. Judet J, Judet H. Genu recurvatum par lésion du cartilage de conjugaison supérieur du tibia. Communication à la 49e réunion annuelle de la SOFCOT. Rev Chir Orthop. 1975;61:296–300.

Patient-Specific Instrumentation (PSI) for High Tibial Osteotomy (HTO)

15

Thomas Tampere, Mathias Donnez, Christophe Jacquet, Philippe Berton, Matthieu Ollivier, and Sébastien Parratte

15.1 Introduction

High tibial osteotomy (HTO) is nowadays a well-accepted joint-preserving procedure for the treatment of early-stage unicompartmental knee osteoarthritis (OA) or overload of the medial compartment related to proximal tibial varus malalignment. The goal of this treatment is to unload the medial compartment of the knee by shifting the load axis of the lower extremity from the medial compartment toward the center of the knee [1–4].

T. Tampere
Department of Orthopaedic Surgery, Ghent University Hospital, Ghent, Belgium
e-mail: thomas.tampere@uzgent.be

M. Donnez
Newclip Technics, Haute-Goulaine, France

Department of Orthopaedics and Traumatology, APHM, CNRS, ISM, Sainte-Marguerite Hospital, Institute for Locomotion, Aix Marseille University, Marseille, France
e-mail: mdonnez@newcliptechnics.com

C. Jacquet
Department of Orthopaedics and Traumatology, APHM, CNRS, ISM, Sainte-Marguerite Hospital, Institute for Locomotion, Aix Marseille University, Marseille, France

P. Berton
Newclip Technics, Haute-Goulaine, France
e-mail: pberton@newcliptechnics.com

M. Ollivier
Department of Orthopaedics and Traumatology, APHM, SNRS, ISM, Sainte-Marguerite Hospital, Institute for Locomotion, Aix Marseille University, Marseille, France

S. Parratte (✉)
Department of Orthopaedics and Traumatology, APHM, CNRS, ISM, Sainte-Marguerite Hospital, Institute for Locomotion, Aix Marseille University, Marseille, France

Department of Orthopaedic Surgery, International Knee and Joint Centre, Abu Dhabi, UAE
e-mail: sebastien@parratte.fr

© Springer Nature Switzerland AG 2020
S. Oussedik, S. Lustig (eds.), *Osteotomy About the Knee*,
https://doi.org/10.1007/978-3-030-49055-3_15

There are however several pitfalls in today's popularized osteotomy techniques. Conventional procedures for osteotomy rely on 2D preoperative planning and the intraoperative use of 2D fluoroscopy; this can potentially cause measuring errors due to rotation of the knee or a flexion deformity. Furthermore, the conventional rule of thumb of one degree of correction for each millimeter of osteotomy opening is an oversimplification as one should take the length of the lower limb, the width of the tibial plateau, and the depth of the osteotomy into account [5–8]. According to Gebhard et al. [9], the ideal axis correction is difficult to obtain, and postoperative under- and overcorrection regularly occur. Traditional perioperative measurement techniques, such as the mathematical, rod, or cable method, have shown both low reproducibility and intra-observer variability and incorrect radiologic measurement. Small deviations in weight-bearing axis generally result in large changes in load distribution over the knee joint, which can lead to further cartilage degeneration, lateral compartment overload, and unsatisfactory results following HTO [10, 11].

The angular correction must be optimal in all three spatial planes for the osteotomy to be effective, and numerous studies have shown that accuracy of correction relative to preoperative planning is the most important factor determining a successful HTO outcome [5]. In conventional techniques, it is hard to precisely control the degree of correction, and there is a potential risk to inadvertently increase tibial sagittal slope. It is shown that for varus knees with medial compartment osteoarthritis, best results are achieved when the anatomic lower limb axis is corrected to 8–10° of valgus, according to a weight-bearing line passing through the lateral plateau at 62–66% of its width [6–8]. Van den Bempt et al. showed in a recent review on accuracy of coronal limb alignment correction after HTO that conventional techniques fall short, with a tendency toward undercorrection. Accordingly, only in 23–50% of conventional cohorts, the accepted range of accuracy was reached [5].

Appropriate predictive surgical planning is essential to achieve the ideal correction angle. Thus, with the advance of new technologies in orthopedic surgery aiming for improving surgical accuracy and improving the comfort of the surgeon, different techniques have been proposed to optimize surgical steps such as computer-assisted or patient-specific ancillaries as an alternative to conventional techniques. Computer navigation seemed to tackle the problems of inaccuracy, but results are contradictory [11, 12]. Some reports showed improved results in correction of mechanical axis alignment with significantly better control over the tibial slope when compared to conventional methods, but these improvements have not yet been reflected in clinical outcome. Navigation allows real-time visualization in 3D, but it remains expensive, and digital registration of the lower limb prolongs the operation [13, 14]. Moreover, we have seen computer-assisted surgery being used intraoperatively to control the overall frontal alignment of the lower limb axis; however, it has not been able to demonstrate an ability to control the degrees of correction required within the osteotomy itself. In the aforementioned review of computer navigation in HTO, it appeared that at least 75% of corrections fell into the accepted range of accuracy [5].

There is emerging evidence that the introduction of a patient-specific instrumentation based on preoperative 3D CT scan templating now offers the possibility to use patient-specific cutting guides allowing accurate control of the correction during the procedure for both the frontal and the sagittal planes. The principle is simple: a 3D model of the bone is created, and the osteotomy and the ideal position of the screw and the plate are simulated (Figs. 15.1, 15.2, and 15.3). From this simulation, a patient-specific jig is designed and printed to perform the cut, to guide the drilling of the screw holes, and to place two protective K-wires. The surgeon receives a planning, the patient-specific jig, and information about length of the screws (Fig. 15.4). Accuracy of these systems has been demonstrated in

Fig. 15.1 Simulation of the mechanical axis of the lower limb before and after the osteotomy. This simulation is based on a CT scan of the lower limb, visualizing the hip, the knee, and the ankle

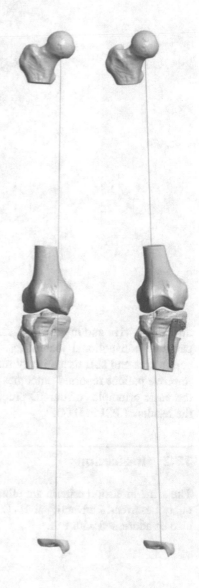

Fig. 15.2 Simulation of the osteotomy in the coronal plane. The best-fit position of the plate on the proximal tibia is determined

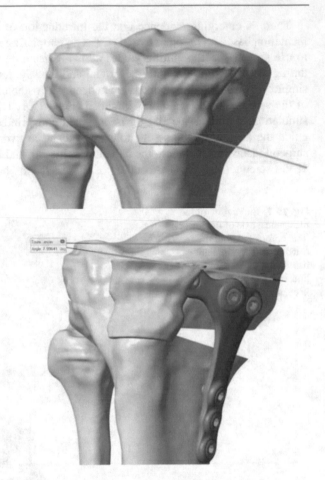

different in vivo and in vitro studies, with superior correction accuracy when compared to conventional techniques. In a final step, integration of dynamic gait parameters and soft tissue laxity may further reduce problems of inaccuracy and improve patient-reported outcomes [15]. The goals of this chapter are to present the basic principles of the 3D preoperative planning, the surgical technique, and the results of PSI in HTO.

15.2 Indications

The same inclusion criteria are eligible for opening-wedge PSI HTO as for previously described conventional HTO. More complex multi-planar deformities can also be addressed with PSI.

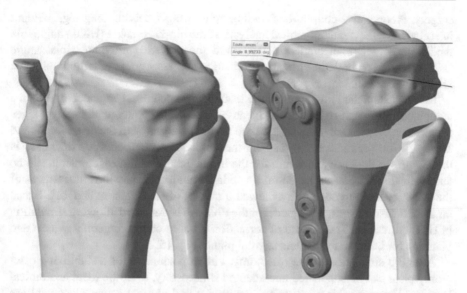

Fig. 15.3 Simulation of the osteotomy in the sagittal plane. Preoperative planning and PSI allow perfect control of the pre- and postoperative slope of the proximal tibia

Fig. 15.4 Simulation of the osteotomy allows preoperative determination of the ideal plate position and the screw length

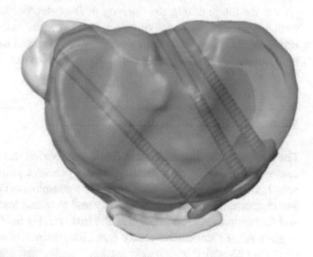

15.3   Preoperative Planning

Preoperative planning for PSI HTO is essential and is based on a thorough physical examination and imaging studies. Significant aspects of the patient's history should include previous injury and all prior treatment and/or surgical procedures to the extremity. Physical examination features inclusion of patient's gait and stance, patellar tracking, range of motion, and ligamentous stability. Limb length discrepancy, ankle deformity, and instability should be determined and considered before surgery. Preoperative conventional radiographs (weight-bearing long leg, A/P and lateral views) allow radiographical analysis of the hip-knee-ankle (HKA) angle, the medial proximal tibial angle (MPTA), and the posterior proximal tibial angle (PPTA). Based on both the clinical examination and assessment of radiographs, the surgeon defines the targeted correction.

In a next step, the virtual templating is made by a dedicated engineer, based on a computed tomography (CT) scan by means of a dedicated protocol including images centered on the femoral head, on the knee (with visualization of the distal femur and 15 cm of the proximal tibia), and on the ankle. The required slice thickness is 0.625 mm for the knee and 2 mm for the hip and ankle. All measurements can be automatically reproduced based on a validated algorithm; previous assessment of the accuracy and reproducibility showed a margin of error <2 mm and <1°. Based on these measurements, a 3D model of the tibia can be rendered allowing simulation of HTO correction. The amount of correction is based on the surgeon's request and planning for both the frontal and sagittal plane (Fig. 15.1).

After 3D simulation of the osteotomy, virtual positioning of a stabilizing osteotomy plate can be conducted and adapted if necessary, to fit the ideal anatomical location. Based on this positioning, screw size and optimal screw placement are defined. Additionally, two K-wires can be virtually positioned: the first one to protect the lateral tibial hinge while performing the saw cut and the second one to protect the hinge during the opening of the osteotomy. After approval of the final virtual construct by the surgeon, a patient-specific cutting jig (Newclip Technics, Haute-Goulaine, France) is designed and 3D-printed to guide the cut, to drill the final screw holes, and to position the two K-wires used to protect the hinge (Figs. 15.1–15.4).

15.4   Surgical Technique

The patient is installed under anesthetic supervision in supine position on a radiolucent operating table with padding of the pressure points. After spinal or general anesthesia is administered, a bilateral knee examination is performed to evaluate for any concurrent ligamentous instability and to assess knee range of motion. A thigh and foot support is used to position the involved leg in 90° of flexion. No tourniquet is used. After preoperative safety checklist, disinfection, and sterile draping, landmarks are identified with a skin marker. Patella, patellar tendon, joint line, and the tuberosity are marked; and both the anterior and posterior edges of the tibia are identified. When indicated, arthroscopic surgery is performed to address associated intra-articular lesions.

A standard surgical approach for HTO can be used with a 7 cm incision in between the anterior tibial crest and the posteromedial tibial margin from 1 cm proximal to the joint line ending just distal to the tibial tuberosity. The incision is carried through the skin, and dissection proceeds through the subcutaneous tissue until the anterior aspect of the proximal tibial and sartorial fascia is exposed. A sharp dissection to the bone is performed; the common hamstring insertion (pes anserine) and superficial medial collateral ligament (MCL) are subperiosteally peeled off the bone and retracted posteriorly. One should aim to elevate this tissue in a thick sleeve to allow repair over the osteotomy site. The larger the angular correction must be, the more the hamstrings and MCL should be released distally. Note that an adequate release allows opening of the osteotomy and facilitates insertion of the bone graft if used. If the release is too limited, there is a risk of tearing the lateral cortical hinge which may jeopardize complete bone healing. The tissue of the posteromedial tibia is elevated, and a blunt (radiolucent) retractor is placed around the posteromedial proximal tibia along the posterior cortex to protect the posterior neurovascular structures. In a last step, the tibial tubercle and its bursa are identified with anterior and lateral retraction of the patellar tendon.

The patient-specific cutting guide (Newclip Technics, Haute-Goulaine, France) is then positioned along the medial tibial flare on the preoperative determined ideal anatomical location. In our implants, an anterior bracket is provided to place posterior to the patellar tendon, and two distal posterior brackets fit the tibial posterior surface to ensure stability and best fit (Figs. 15.5 and 15.6). Final position of the

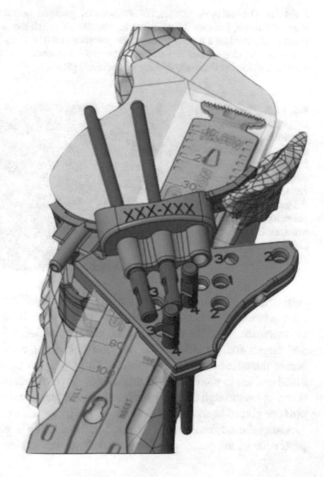

Fig. 15.5 Two posterior brackets fit around the posterior border of the tibia to provide stability and a perfect fit on the proximal tibia. A 2.2 mm K-wire is placed in the posterior proximal bracket to secure the jig to the bone. It also determines the orientation and the position of the cut as it is placed 1 mm below the actual cut and targets the fibula. A hinge pin can be inserted into the posterior distal bracket to protect the hinge. An anterior bracket is provided to place posterior to the patellar tendon as protection during sawing

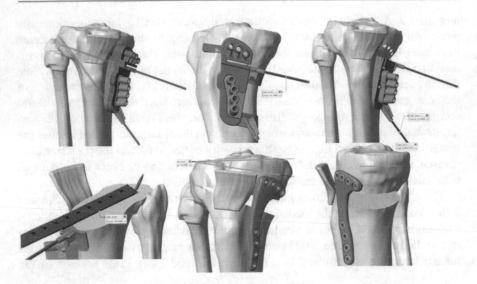

Fig. 15.6 Optimal positioning and fit of the cutting guide on the proximal tibia (Newclip Technics, Haute-Goulaine, France). A stabilizing K-wire goes through the posterior proximal bracket; the hinge is protected by a K-wire placed in the posterior distal bracket. The distal K-wire prevents the saw to cut the hinge. After application of the plate, a perfect correction in the frontal and sagittal plane is obtained as determined in the preoperative plan

Fig. 15.7 The PSI guide fits perfectly on the proximal tibia through a standard anteromedial incision for HTO. The screw holes are pre-drilled, and temporary pins hold the guide into place. The posterior K-wire provides extra stability. The hinge pin is already removed in this picture

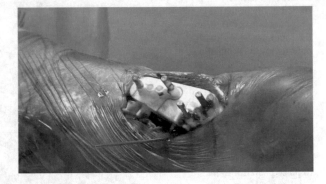

cutting guide should be confirmed with fluoroscopy. First, a 2.2 mm pin is placed in the posterior proximal bracket; this pin secures the jig to the bone and determines the orientation and the position of the cut as it is placed 1 mm below the actual cut and targets the fibula head. Its position is computed in a patient-specific way to obtain the accurate hinge position. A hinge pin can be inserted into the posterior distal bracket to protect the hinge. Finalization of fixation is done by pre-drilling the screw holes through the jig; two monocortical (proximal) and two bicortical (distal) pins are placed to secure the position of the jig on the tibia (Fig. 15.7).

Using the dedicated slot of the jig, the saw blade is guided during the cut, with protection of the posterior neurovascular structures. Note that the slot is closed on the anterior side to avoid cutting the anterior and lateral side of the tibia (Fig. 15.5). The upper part of the patient-specific cutting guide can be removed to finalize the cut, and an anterior/vertical slot of the jig should be used to guide the biplanar below the tibial tuberosity. The osteotomy is finalized when the saw blade is in contact with the hinge pin (Fig. 15.6). Gradual opening of the cut is supported by a laminar spreader until the holes of the plate are aligned with the pre-drilled holes on the tibia, confirming an adequate correction in both the frontal and sagittal plane. The screws are then inserted through the plate to secure the construct. As the screw length is measured on the virtual preoperative planning, intraoperative screw sizing is no longer required.

15.5 Postoperative Rehabilitation

Postoperatively, standard X-ray examination should be conducted to verify the osteotomy, plate, and screw position. A standard rehabilitation protocol is implemented with allowance of free range of motion and weight-bearing as tolerated with the use of crutches. Patients are allowed to return to their recreational activities at 6 months.

Pearls	Pitfalls
• Easy to use	• Need for additional imaging (CT)
• Improves accuracy (3D planning)	• Requires the involvement of the surgeon to analyze and confirm the planning by an engineer
• Cost-efficient (with disposable set)	• Time required to design and produce the PSI
• Reduction of intraoperative fluoroscopy	
• Reproducible	

15.6 Results

There is a plethora of publications commenting on a variety of topics around HTO, with only little homogeneity on solid outcome data of different techniques. Results of HTO vary across the literature, but in general there is good evidence to show that HTO provides good relief of pain and restoration of function for medial arthritis of the knee. Long-term results of HTO, however, depend on the accuracy of the correction [15]. A recent systematic review which reported on whether postoperative correction was within an "acceptable range" concluded that today's used HTO techniques seem to bear a surprisingly low accuracy with respect to the targeted angle [5].

Long-term outcome results on patient-specific cutting guides for HTO are lacking, due to the innovative and emerging character of this technology in orthopedics. Available publications on this subject are showing promising results as the learning curve only takes ten cases for a decrease in operating time, eight cases for an improvement in surgeon comfort levels, and nine cases for a reduction in the number of fluoroscopic images needed during HTO. Furthermore, it was shown that there is no learning curve to achieve an accurate correction when compared to preoperative planning [16]. The largest series was recently published by Chaouche et al. in 2019 reporting on 100 patients who underwent PSI HTO with a mean follow-up of 2 years. They withheld perfect correlation of corrected angles matched to the preoperative planning, with significant improvement of KOOS scores when compared to the preoperative situation ($p < 0.0001$) [17].

Victor et al. were one of the first proving that PSI in osteotomies around the knee adds accuracy to the technique with mean deviation between the planned wedge angle and the executed angle of $0°$ (SD 0.72) in the coronal plane and $0.3°$ (SD 1.14) in the sagittal plane. A postoperative difference of $0.3°$ was seen in hip-knee-ankle angle when compared to the preoperative planning [18]. Several recent papers confirm that PSI in HTO improves accuracy drastically which might benefit long-term clinical outcome [15–20]. In 2014, Munier et al. showed in a pilot study that in 95% of patients an accurate correction (<2% difference) was achieved according to the preoperative planning [19]. Yang et al. confirmed improvement of correction accuracy in their series of PSI HTO [20]. Donnez et al. reached in a recent in vitro study high accuracy with a minimal pre- and postoperative difference of $0.2°$ (SD 0.3) in the frontal plane and -0.1 (SD 0.5) in the sagittal plane [21].

15.7 Conclusions

In appropriately indicated patients, medial opening-wedge HTO is a proven safe and effective treatment for younger, active patients with symptomatic medial compartment OA associated with varus alignment. Today's conventional HTO techniques embrace low accuracy with respect to the targeted angle. 2D preoperative planning might introduce technical and corrective errors; a shift toward 3D rendering and imaging might increase surgical accuracy. It is notable that, even with perfect preoperative planning, the practical difficulty remains in extrapolation of the plan to the actual surgical procedure. In a first phase, computed navigation techniques were introduced to tackle the problem of inaccuracy. Because of time-consuming related issues and the need for registration and application of trackers, PSI might be the solution to address these issues. With incorporation of 2D and 3D preoperative planning to create PSI jigs, it is now possible to yield outcomes close to the planning. Compared to computed navigation, PSI guides are reliable, accurate, and cost-saving and don't necessitate continuous tracking and registration. PSI might be timesaving, radiation-reducing, and easy to use. Future directions may be incorporation of gait pattern data, musculoskeletal dynamics modelling, joint kinematics, and joint contact mechanics in preoperative planning and in the search for the precise patient-specific corrective angle for the realignment procedure.

References

1. Day M, Wolf B. Medial opening wedge high tibial osteotomy for medial compartment arthrosis/overload. Clin Sports Med. 2019;38:331–49.
2. Hoorntje A, Witjes S, Kuijer P, Koenraadt K, van Geenen R, Daams J, Getgood A, Kerkhoffs G. High rates of return to sports activities and work after osteotomies around the knee: a systematic review and meta-analysis. Sports Med. 2017;47:2219–44.
3. Webb M, Dewan V, Elson D. Functional results following high tibial osteotomy: a review of the literature. Eur J Orthop Surg Traumatol. 2018;28:555–63.
4. Yan J, Mushal V, Kay J, Khan M, Simunovic N, Ayeni O. Outcome reporting following navigated high tibial osteotomy of the knee: a systematic review. Knee Surg Sports Traumatol Arthrosc. 2016;24:3529–55.
5. Van den Bempt M, Van Genechten W, Claes T, Claes S. How accurately does high tibial osteotomy correct the mechanical axis of an arthritis varus knee? A systematic review. Knee. 2016;23:925–35.
6. Miniaci A, Ballmer F, Ballmer P, Jakob R. Proximal tibial osteotomy. A new fixation device. Clin Orthop. 1989;(246):250–9.
7. Dugdale T, Noyes F, Styer D. Preoperative planning for high tibial osteotomy. The effect of lateral tibiofemoral separation and tibiofemoral length. Clin Orthop Relat Res. 1992;(274):248–64.
8. Fujisawa Y, Masuhara K, Shiomi S. The effect of high tibial osteotomy on osteoarthritis of the knee. An arthroscopic study of 54 knee joints. Orthop Clin North Am. 1979;10:585–608.
9. Gebhard F, Krettek C, Hüfner T, Grützner P, Stöckle U, Imhoff A, et al. Reliability of computer-assisted surgery as an intraoperative ruler in navigated high tibial osteotomy. Arch Orthop Trauma Surg. 2011;131:297–302.
10. Hankemeier S, Mommsen P, Krettek C, Jagodzinski M, Brand J, Meyer C, et al. Accuracy of high tibial osteotomy: comparison between open- and closed wedge technique. Knee Surg Sports Traumatol Arthrosc. 2010;18:1328–33.
11. Stanley J, Robinson K, Devitt B, Richmond A, Webster K, Whitehead T, et al. Computer assisted alignment of opening wedge high tibial osteotomy provides limited improvement of radiographic outcomes compared to fluoroscopic alignment. Knee. 2016;23:289–94.
12. Bae D, Song S, Yoon K. Closed-wedge high tibial osteotomy using computer-assisted surgery compared to the conventional technique. J Bone Joint Surg Br. 2009;91:1164–71.
13. Picardo N, Khan W, Johnstone D. Computer-assisted navigation in high tibial osteotomy: a systematic review of the literature. Open Orthop J. 2012;6:305–12.
14. Lee D, Han S, Oh K, Lee J, Kwon J, Kim J, et al. The weight-bearing scanogram technique provides better coronal limb alignment than the navigation technique in open high tibial osteotomy. Knee. 2014;21:451–5.
15. Jones G, Jaere M, Clarke S, Cobb J. 3D printing and high tibial osteotomy. Effort Open Rev. 2018;3:254–9.
16. Jacquet C, Sharma A, Fabre M, Ehlinger M, Argenson J, Parratte S, Ollivier M. Patient-specific high-tibial osteotomy's 'cutting-guides' decrease operating time and the number of fluoroscopic images taken after a brief learning curve. Knee Surg Sports Traumatol Arthrosc. 2019; https://doi.org/10.1007/s00167-019-05637-6.
17. Chaouche S, Jacquet C, Fabre-Aubrespy M, Sharma A, Argenson J, Parratte S, Ollivier M. Patient-specific cutting guides for open wedge high tibial osteotomy: safety and accuracy analysis of a hundred patients continuous cohort. Int Orthop. 2019; https://doi.org/10.1007/s00264-019-04372-4.
18. Victor J, Premananthan A. Virtual 3D planning and patient specific surgical guides for osteotomies around the knee: a feasibility and proof-of-concept study. Bone Joint J. 2013;95:153–8.
19. Munier M, Donnez M, Ollivier M, Flecher X, Chabrand P, Argenson J, Parratte S. Can three-dimensional patient-specific cutting guides be used to achieve optimal correction for high tibial osteotomy? Pilot study. Orthop Traumatol Surg Res. 2017;103:245–50.

20. Yang J, Chen C, Luo C, Chang M, Lee O, Huang Y, Lin S. Clinical experience using a 3D-printed patient-specific instrument for medial opening wedge high tibial osteotomy. Biomed Res Int. 2018; https://doi.org/10.1155/2018/9246529.
21. Donnez M, Ollivier M, Munier M, Berton P, Podgorski J, Chabrand P, Parratte S. Are three-dimensional patient-specific cutting guides for open wedge high tibial osteotomy accurate? An in vitro study. J Orthop Surg Res. 2018;13:171–4.

Navigation for HTO

16

Sven Putnis, Thomas Neri, and Myles Coolican

16.1 Introduction

Success of an osteotomy around the knee relies on the ability to accurately translate a preoperative plan into a postoperative result to give the desired correction of alignment in both the coronal and sagittal planes. In this context of improving precision and adapting the correction to each patient, the use of computer navigation guidance is attractive. Navigation has been successfully implemented in knee arthroplasty with the benefits of giving accurate real-time corrections allowing greater intraoperative control and better management of multiple surgical variables [1]. In reality, if there is a surgical procedure best suited to computer navigation, it is opening wedge high tibial osteotomy. The rationale for its use in HTO is based on understanding the advantages, technical principles, potential pitfalls and limitations. These areas and the current clinical outcomes of this surgical technique for HTO and other knee osteotomies are described in this chapter.

S. Putnis
Avon Orthopaedic Centre, Bristol, UK

Sydney Orthopaedic Research Institute, Sydney, NSW, Australia

T. Neri
University Hospital of Saint-Etienne, University of Lyon, Lyon, France

Sydney Orthopaedic Research Institute, Sydney, NSW, Australia

M. Coolican (✉)
Sydney Orthopaedic Research Institute, Sydney, NSW, Australia
e-mail: myles@mylescoolican.com.au

© Springer Nature Switzerland AG 2020
S. Oussedik, S. Lustig (eds.), *Osteotomy About the Knee*,
https://doi.org/10.1007/978-3-030-49055-3_16

16.2   Advantages

16.2.1 Improved Accuracy

HTO is a technically demanding procedure, and accuracy of correction is a key factor for achieving successful limb realignment and appropriate unloading of the
medial compartment. Surgical imprecision of only a few degrees may result in the
failure of the osteotomy with poor clinical results [2]. In addition, there is not necessarily a set target point for correction in all patients with evidence for an individualised approach [3]. Achieving this patient-specific accuracy therefore implies three
conditions: a reliable surgical technique with a stable fixation [4]; accurate preoperative planning of correction [5]; and a precise control of the intraoperative alignment correction. The first condition has been better controlled since the development
of reliable osteotomy techniques [6] and strong fixation assured by a locking plate
[4]. Improved accuracy of preoperative planning of limb alignment and subsequent
calculation of the correction to perform during the osteotomy has been seen with the
development of digital measurement systems and most recently three-dimensional
assessment systems allowing the measurement of the coronal, sagittal and rotational
component of a deformity [7, 8].

   Reaching the same level of accuracy during the procedure remains challenging.
Historically, many techniques have been used to determine intraoperative alignment
correction, such as long alignment rods, cables, grids or fluoroscopic confirmation.
However, there are many potential limitations, such as a bent alignment cable, mis-
placed guide position, suboptimal or low-quality fluoroscopy image, limb rotation,
obstruction with the tourniquet in obese patients and no sagittal assessment [5, 9,
10]. Intraoperative errors in calculating the mechanical axis can lead to a number of
potential complications. Inaccurate correction in the coronal plane risks creating a
proximal tibial deformity, which could affect a future revision to total knee arthroplasty (TKA); [11] under-correction risks OA progression [12], with patient dissatisfaction [13]; and over-correction can lead to rapid degeneration of the lateral
compartment [14] and risks patellar baja or subluxation [15]. An inadvertent change
in the sagittal plane can manifest as alteration to the posterior tibial plateau slope
with potential clinical repercussions, especially in an ACL deficient knee [16–19].
To avoid these issues, other techniques have been proposed: gap measurement [20],
patient-specific instrumentation [21], and computer navigation.

   Computer navigation systems have been developed to improve both the accuracy
and precision of orthopaedic procedures. With these aims, this system was firstly
developed for the spine and then for joint replacement procedures [22]. It has been
shown to be effective for accurate restoration of neutral alignment in patients undergoing TKA [23], suggesting that computer-assisted systems may be used for knee
osteotomy to help surgeons to determine the intraoperative adequacy of alignment
correction [24]. By providing a more precise analysis of limb alignment and a
capacity to make multiplane measurements in real time, navigation systems have
been increasingly used in HTO [25–30] and in distal femoral osteotomy [11, 31].

Computer navigation improves accuracy (the degree of closeness to the target angle value) and precision (the reliability of consistently obtaining the planned correction and to the capacity to reduce outliers) [32], both required to obtain the ideal correction [33]. The lower incidence of instrumental errors and the ability to calculate full anatomical and mechanical axis from the hip to the ankle have been proven in a number of studies and can compensate for the shortcomings of preoperative radiographic planning [25–30, 34].

Unlike conventional techniques, a navigation system allows an intraoperative assessment of limb alignment throughout the entire range of motion and not just with the knee in full extension [35]. The navigated osteotomy can be individually tailored to the exact pattern of osteoarthritis or malalignment of the knee in different functional positions [3]. The ability to give real-time measurements provides many advantages [35]. Fine adjustments can be made and quantified during creation and fixation of the osteotomy. Soft tissue laxity can be measured and accounted for in the correction, providing dynamic information on the ligament balancing (information on medial or lateral soft tissue) throughout range of motion or simulated load-bearing. Fixation strength and integrity of the cortical hinge can be tested. Song et al. demonstrated that accurate control of the position of the cortical hinge and the dynamic assessment of the plastic deformation of the opposite cortex when using navigation guidance can help to avoid hinge fractures in osteotomy [36]. Given the possibility to easily check the intraoperative alignment, navigation systems also allow a reduction in the use of fluoroscopy and therefore decreased radiation exposure.

Navigation allows accurate assessment of sagittal alignment, avoiding inadvertent alteration of the tibial posterior slope angle [17–19] and aiding more complex osteotomies, such as double-level (tibia and femur) or multiplanar osteotomies for severe deformation or knee instability [11]. Lustig et al. demonstrated there was a significant increase in bony tibial slope in both compartments following medial opening wedge HTO and that the tibial change was larger in the medial compartment compared with the lateral compartment [17]. Noyes et al. reported that even a small gap error of 1 mm could result in a change of the posterior slope of approximately 2° [18].

These benefits of navigation have also developed into a teaching tool, allowing clear explanation of the procedure and to shorten the learning curve, and a research instrument to accurately record intraoperative correction angles or kinematics [36].

16.2.2 Clinical Outcome

Whilst the theoretical advantages related to the enhanced precision and accuracy have been demonstrated for HTO, it still remains debatable whether these improvements lead to enhanced clinical outcomes [37–39]. Many case series of navigated HTO have shown good outcomes in terms of postoperative coronal alignment and clinical outcomes [25–30]. Results concerning tibial slope control have been conflicting, but many studies used the first software versions which did not allow good assessment of sagittal alignment [36].

There are few comparative investigations of the outcome of navigated osteotomy versus conventional techniques, and closer scrutiny of the literature reveals methodological deficiencies. Amongst them, the main limitation is due to a change in surgical technique over time with the introduction of navigation at a time where there were concurrent changes in surgical techniques and fixation methods. Ribeiro et al. in a controlled clinical study concluded that the navigation system allowed a significantly better control of tibial slope and a better Lysholm outcome score compared to a conventional HTO technique, but the conventional group was based on an older series with different internal fixation plates [25]. Recently, a retrospective study also proposed a comparison between both techniques [40]. The group comparison was based on surgeon preference (some of them used navigation; others used conventional instrumentation). The authors concluded that navigation allowed greater success in achieving the desired correction value in coronal plane and reduced outliers. Akamatsu et al. in a comparative study of HTO with and without a combined CT-based and image-free navigation system reported that navigation restored normal coronal and sagittal plane knee joint alignment more frequently when compared with a conventional technique [41].

In summary, as concluded by recent meta-analyses [37, 39, 42] and literature reviews [36, 38, 43], navigation systems increase the accuracy and the reliability of the correction, but there is currently no clear evidence that this leads to improved clinical outcomes or longer survivorship.

16.3 Surgical Technique

16.3.1 Technical Principles

Navigation systems can broadly be divided into two types: image-based systems depending on either preoperative CT scans or intraoperative fluoroscopy and, more commonly, imageless systems using intraoperative data acquisition to build an anatomic model [35]. Imageless systems have become more popular because of less irradiation, reduced cost and the ability to provide real-time measurements and adjustments [35].

The setup of navigation system requires two steps: instrument calibration and femoral and tibial bony fixation of pins with markers (either active or passive). After registration of anatomical landmarks and determination of hip/knee/ankle joint centre, a 3D model of the lower limb is created including the coronal and the sagittal axes. Obtaining these data at the beginning, during and at the end of surgery allows the surgeon to assess the effect of a procedure on the axis, knee laxity and range of motion [35].

As with every procedure, navigated osteotomy requires technical knowledge and a learning curve. In the following part, a detailed surgical technique of a navigated HTO, based on 10 years of experience, will be presented [17].

16.3.2 Preoperative Assessment

Preoperative planning is undertaken with a long leg weight-bearing alignment film. The width of the plateau is calculated and the current mechanical axis assessed. Fujisawa's point (defined as 62% of the entire width measured from the medial side) is used to plan the mechanical axis [44]. With digital imaging, the thickness of the required wedge is calculated. These measurements will then be correlated with the navigation measurements obtained intraoperatively. Preoperative MRI is routinely undertaken to evaluate the lateral and patellofemoral articular cartilage.

16.3.3 Navigation Setup

A large operating room is required to set up all the equipment, including arthroscopic tower, navigation camera, navigation and osteotomy instruments and fluoroscopy image intensifier C-arm and screen. The patient is placed supine with a thigh tourniquet and side support setup to support the knee at 90°. Footrests are to be used with caution as they can push the knee into recurvatum as the fixation plate is applied.

16.3.4 Diagnostic and Therapeutic Arthroscopy with Landmark Registration

A knee arthroscopy is firstly performed, for systematic examination (cartilage, menisci, cruciate ligament, synovium) of the knee and confirmation that the lateral and patellofemoral compartments are relatively well preserved. This also permits treatment of any intra-articular pathology, such as meniscal tears or chondral defects.

16.3.5 Navigation Registration with Arthroscopic Assistance

After instrument calibration, percutaneous partially threaded 3.0mm pins are placed into the tibial shaft and distal femur femoral allowing the attachment of the trackers with care to position the tibial pins distal to the intended position of the plate.

The centre of the hip is registered by circumduction movements (Fig. 16.1a). Knee arthroscopy is then performed to register intra-articular landmarks necessary to calculate the limb axis. With a pointing device introduced through the anteromedial portal, the centre of the distal femur (intramedullary entry point) and the centre of the proximal tibia (ACL footprint) are registered (Fig. 16.1b). Other landmarks of the knee are then also digitised to allow creation of the sagittal and coronal planes. The centre of the ankle is calculated from the registration of the medial and lateral malleoli (Fig. 16.1c).

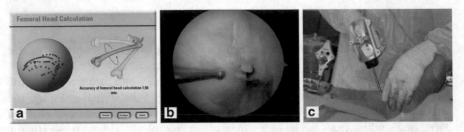

Fig. 16.1 Determining limb alignment using the (**a**) hip centre by circumduction, (**b**) knee centre with a pointing device registering arthroscopically and (**c**) ankle centre using surface malleoli landmarks

This completes the registration process, and the software calculates the mechanical femoral and tibial axes and displays the mechanical alignment through the full range of motion (Fig. 16.2), and this is then correlated to preoperative imaging. Ligament balancing and the ROM are also recorded in order to refer back to when the post-osteotomy values are obtained. Full extension is measured by lifting the patient's leg by the heel gradually off the table, and alteration of this value is an accurate surrogate for alteration of the tibial slope.

16.3.6 Medial Opening Wedge HTO

A 10 cm incision is made midway between the tibial tubercle and the posteromedial tibial border, beginning 1 cm inferior to the joint line and extending distally. The sartorius fascia is sharply divided in line with the skin incision followed by posterior reflection of sartorius, gracilis, semitendinosis and the superficial medial collateral ligament with its underlying periosteal attachment. The patellar tendon and retropatellar bursa are exposed anteriorly and protected. This achieves a subperiosteal exposure of the proposed site for the osteotomy. Under fluoroscopy, a 2-mm guide pin is advanced under from the medial side slightly oblique to the axial plane above the tibial tuberosity and towards the tip of the fibula, sitting 15 mm distal to the lateral tibial plateau to prevent the osteotomy from disrupting the joint. The osteotomy is made immediately distal to the guide pin to centre the hinge of the osteotomy at the proximal tibiofibular joint. The osteotomy is performed under fluoroscopy using an oscillating saw for the outer medial and anterior cortices and completed with osteotomes, carried to within 5–8 mm of the lateral cortex.

16.3.7 Navigated Opening and Osteotomy Fixation

A laminar spreader is placed posteriorly, and the osteotomy opens until the desired alignment of mechanical valgus in full extension is achieved. The posterior opening is measured and checked to be in line with preoperative calculations, after which

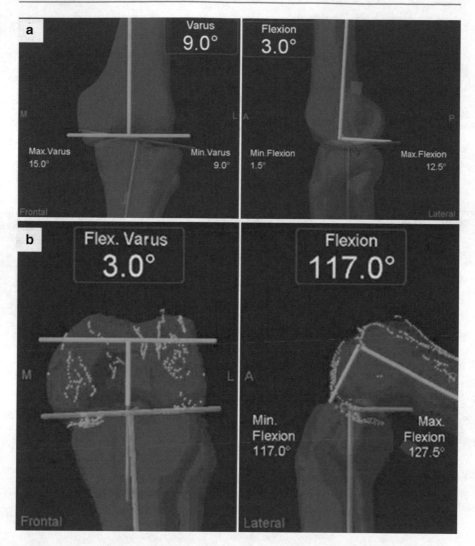

Fig. 16.2 Intraoperative assessment of the malalignment in coronal and sagittal planes (**a**) in extension and (**b**) throughout the entire range of motion

allograft is inserted, and a locking plate is secured in place with three to four screws proximally and three to four distally taking care to hold the knee aligned in both planes confirmed with navigation. Maintenance of tibial slope is confirmed by ensuring the greatest extension measured prior to the osteotomy remains when using the same pre-correction technique.

The gap filling and fixation position are checked by fluoroscopy, and final coronal and sagittal alignment is checked and recorded (Fig. 16.3).

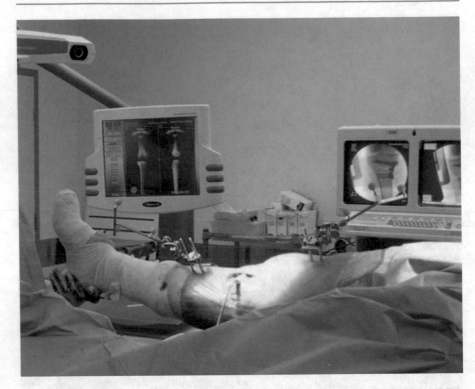

Fig. 16.3 Intraoperative view of the final alignment check after a navigated medial opening wedge HTO

16.3.8 Postoperative Plan Regimen

The postoperative rehabilitation programme includes mobilisation touch weight-bearing on the day of surgery with a knee brace set from 0–90° of flexion, followed by 4 weeks of gradual progression to full weight-bearing and brace removal at 4–6 weeks.

16.3.9 Potential Navigation Pitfalls

Surgeons have to be aware of potential pitfalls such as registration failures, line of sight issues and mechanical or software malfunctions [36]. Surgeons have to therefore be comfortable with conventional techniques, in case such issues with the navigation system occur intraoperatively.

The mechanical axis and angle values are calculated from registered landmarks and require careful registration. The computer cannot compensate for inaccuracies [27, 45]. This limitation should be considered, because the navigation system cannot identify features without surgeon definition. A careful check that the intraoperative navigation data (coronal and sagittal alignment, maximum flexion and extension values) correlate with those values collected preoperatively. A marked discrepancy should result in repeat registration of all landmarks.

Navigation trackers are supported with transosseous pins which must be securely fixed. If there is movement of the trackers, all measurements may be inaccurate. To avoid this issue, bicortical fixation in the diaphyseal areas is recommended [46].

For navigation systems using passive reflective markers, surgeons need to avoid contamination with blood that can block reflection and transmission.

Despite best efforts some measurements errors due to computer, camera or trackers can occur [36, 45]; however with newer navigation systems, these errors are calculated as less than 1 mm [36, 45]. We recommend that every displayed value is checked. Navigation is an accurate and helpful tool, but cannot be considered to be a foolproof technology. A regular comparison with the initial intraoperative data (coronal and sagittal angles, maximal flexion and extension values) and the preoperative data is necessary.

There is a potential discrepancy between the non-weight-bearing navigated value of pre-osteotomy alignment and standing loaded radiographic preoperative value [47]. Yaffe et al. reported a difference of 8° between navigated and radiographic measurement values [48]. To avoid this magnitude of error, we recommend dynamic range of coronal alignment under applied varus and valgus force and simulated weight-bearing by applying a varus external force during the registration step until the navigated value of the preoperative alignment is close to matching the radiographic value. This position and force is then mimicked post-osteotomy. For the amount of correction expected, a further check with the preoperative templated plan is also recommended [47].

For the sagittal alignment, the post-osteotomy maximal degree of extension should match the pre-osteotomy value [17]. If it is increased, the tibial slope has most likely been increased, and the correction should be re-evaluated. Whilst this may be appropriate and intended for patients with a PCL deficiency, an increase in tibial slope can exacerbate pain and instability in patients with an ACL deficient knee.

16.4 Limitations

Navigated surgery can be time-consuming especially during a surgeons learning curve, with an additional cost of theatre time, so justification should be sought before recommending the use of this technology [32, 49]. Often considered by surgeons as the main limitation, use of navigation requires setup (calibration, bony fixation) and registration, leading to additional theatre time from 10 to 30 min [49]. This longer time has the potential to be associated with an increased incidence of surgical site infection [50].

High-cost technologies increase economic burden. Goradia et al. indicated that only high-volume centres can support this additional cost [51]. Paradoxically, navigated surgery is more beneficial for low-volume surgeons, who may have only a limited access to this technology [27, 51].

In addition to complications related to the osteotomy procedure (cortical hinge or intra-articular fracture, delayed union, loss of correction) [52], navigation systems have to be considered as a procedure by itself with its own complications [49]. Specific complications of navigation are however uncommon and mainly related to the use of reference array pins, including additional incisions for insertion of pins increasing the risk of wound complications including infection [49], iatrogenic fracture around the pins [46], neurovascular injury during insertion of pins and heterotopic ossification [53]. Gebhard et al. highlighted that the complication rate is related to surgeon experience and that navigation requires a learning curve [27]. The majority of mistakes are related to registration failures and navigation system malfunctions/misuse [33].

16.5 Discussion and Conclusions

Despite encouraging results for the use of navigation in knee osteotomies, some questions remain unresolved.

The ideal alignment in the coronal, sagittal and axial planes necessary to give optimal symptom relief after high tibial osteotomy remains controversial. Navigation is a tool allowing a more accurate and precise osteotomy, but does not provide all the information required to restore physiological alignment and kinematics. With more data and longer follow-up of navigated osteotomies, we will likely know more in the future about the ideal final alignment. Biomechanical studies and in particular gait analysis will help to define ideal alignments in each plane to provide individualised optimal conditions for articular cartilage health and symptom relief.

Navigation is an intraoperative guide which allows only simulated weight-bearing assessment of limb alignment. Further studies analysing the relationship between supine alignment, simulated weight-bearing with navigation and dynamic full weight-bearing are needed.

Computer-assisted surgery remains an added cost and is mainly available in high-volume centres although it may be more beneficial for low-volume surgeons. Reduced price and increased availability are therefore necessary.

In order to decrease the learning curve and prevent the potential pitfalls, new software which is easier and simpler to use will be developed.

Navigation represents an accurate and reliable tool for the surgeon performing knee osteotomy for OA and ligament instability. This technique provides intraoperative real-time guidance of the degree of correction for coronal and sagittal alignment throughout the entire range of motion. The accuracy and the precision of the final correction angle in realignment osteotomies provided by computer-assisted surgery are now well recognised in the literature. The clinical benefits however remain unclear, requiring further clinical follow-up, including an ongoing discussion related to the ideal alignment and more dynamic assessment.

References

1. van der List JP, Chawla H, Joskowicz L, Pearle AD. Current state of computer navigation and robotics in unicompartmental and total knee arthroplasty: a systematic review with meta-analysis. Knee Surg Sports Traumatol Arthrosc. 2016;24(11):3482–95.
2. Sharma L, Song J, Felson DT, Cahue S, Shamiyeh E, Dunlop DD. The role of knee alignment in disease progression and functional decline in knee osteoarthritis. JAMA. 2001;286(2):188–95.
3. Feucht MJ, Minzlaff P, Saier T, Cotic M, Südkamp NP, Niemeyer P, et al. Degree of axis correction in valgus high tibial osteotomy: proposal of an individualised approach. Int Orthop. 2014;38(11):2273–80.
4. Staubli AE, De Simoni C, Babst R, Lobenhoffer P. TomoFix: a new LCP-concept for open wedge osteotomy of the medial proximal tibia—early results in 92 cases. Injury. 2003;34(Suppl 2):B55–62.
5. Dugdale TW, Noyes FR, Styer D. Preoperative planning for high tibial osteotomy. The effect of lateral tibiofemoral separation and tibiofemoral length. Clin Orthop. 1992;274:248–64.
6. Lobenhoffer P, Agneskirchner JD. Improvements in surgical technique of valgus high tibial osteotomy. Knee Surg Sports Traumatol Arthrosc. 2003;11(3):132–8.
7. Schröter S, Ihle C, Mueller J, Lobenhoffer P, Stöckle U, van Heerwaarden R. Digital planning of high tibial osteotomy. Interrater reliability by using two different software. Knee Surg Sports Traumatol Arthrosc. 2013;21(1):189–96.
8. Sailhan F, Jacob L, Hamadouche M. Differences in limb alignment and femoral mechanical-anatomical angles using two dimension versus three dimension radiographic imaging. Int Orthop. 2017;41(10):2009–16.
9. Krettek C, Miclau T, Grün O, Schandelmaier P, Tscherne H. Intraoperative control of axes, rotation and length in femoral and tibial fractures. Technical note. Injury. 1998;29(Suppl 3):C29–39.
10. Saleh M, Harriman P, Edwards DJ. A radiological method for producing precise limb alignment. J Bone Joint Surg Br. 1991;73(3):515–6.
11. Saragaglia D, Chedal-Bornu B, Rouchy RC, Rubens-Duval B, Mader R, Pailhé R. Role of computer-assisted surgery in osteotomies around the knee. Knee Surg Sports Traumatol Arthrosc. 2016;24(11):3387–95.
12. Cerejo R, Dunlop DD, Cahue S, Channin D, Song J, Sharma L. The influence of alignment on risk of knee osteoarthritis progression according to baseline stage of disease. Arthritis Rheum. 2002;46(10):2632–6.
13. Ribeiro CH, Severino NR, Fucs PM de MB. Preoperative surgical planning versus navigation system in valgus tibial osteotomy: a cross-sectional study. Int Orthop. 2013;37(8):1483–6.
14. Sim JA, Kwak JH, Yang SH, Choi ES, Lee BK. Effect of weight-bearing on the alignment after open wedge high tibial osteotomy. Knee Surg Sports Traumatol Arthrosc. 2010;18(7):874–8.
15. Dowd GSE, Somayaji HS, Uthukuri M. High tibial osteotomy for medial compartment osteoarthritis. Knee. 2006;13(2):87–92.
16. Nerhus TK, Ekeland A, Solberg G, Sivertsen EA, Madsen JE, Heir S. Radiological outcomes in a randomized trial comparing opening wedge and closing wedge techniques of high tibial osteotomy. Knee Surg Sports Traumatol Arthrosc. 2017;25(3):910–7.
17. Lustig S, Scholes CJ, Costa AJ, Coolican MJ, Parker DA. Different changes in slope between the medial and lateral tibial plateau after open-wedge high tibial osteotomy. Knee Surg Sports Traumatol Arthrosc. 2013;21(1):32–8.
18. Noyes FR, Goebel SX, West J. Opening wedge tibial osteotomy: the 3-triangle method to correct axial alignment and tibial slope. Am J Sports Med. 2005;33(3):378–87.
19. Bae DK, Ko YW, Kim SJ, Baek JH, Song SJ. Computer-assisted navigation decreases the change in the tibial posterior slope angle after closed-wedge high tibial osteotomy. Knee Surg Sports Traumatol Arthrosc. 2016;24(11):3433–40.

20. Schröter S, Ihle C, Elson DW, Döbele S, Stöckle U, Ateschrang A. Surgical accuracy in high tibial osteotomy: coronal equivalence of computer navigation and gap measurement. Knee Surg Sports Traumatol Arthrosc. 2016;24(11):3410–7.
21. Donnez M, Ollivier M, Munier M, Berton P, Podgorski J-P, Chabrand P, et al. Are three-dimensional patient-specific cutting guides for open wedge high tibial osteotomy accurate? An in vitro study. J Orthop Surg. 2018;13(1):171.
22. Delp SL, Stulberg SD, Davies B, Picard F, Leitner F. Computer assisted knee replacement. Clin Orthop. 1998;354:49–56.
23. Petursson G, Fenstad AM, Gøthesen Ø, Dyrhovden GS, Hallan G, Röhrl SM, et al. Computer-assisted compared with conventional total knee replacement: a multicenter parallel-group randomized controlled trial. J Bone Joint Surg Am. 2018;100(15):1265–74.
24. Lee D-H, Nha K-W, Park S-J, Han S-B. Preoperative and postoperative comparisons of navigation and radiologic limb alignment measurements after high tibial osteotomy. Arthroscopy. 2012;28(12):1842–50.
25. Ribeiro CH, Severino NR, Moraes de Barros Fucs PM. Opening wedge high tibial osteotomy: navigation system compared to the conventional technique in a controlled clinical study. Int Orthop. 2014;38(8):1627–31.
26. Akamatsu Y, Mitsugi N, Mochida Y, Taki N, Kobayashi H, Takeuchi R, et al. Navigated opening wedge high tibial osteotomy improves intraoperative correction angle compared with conventional method. Knee Surg Sports Traumatol Arthrosc. 2012;20(3):586–93.
27. Gebhard F, Krettek C, Hüfner T, Grützner PA, Stöckle U, Imhoff AB, et al. Reliability of computer-assisted surgery as an intraoperative ruler in navigated high tibial osteotomy. Arch Orthop Trauma Surg. 2011;131(3):297–302.
28. Heijens E, Kornherr P, Meister C. The role of navigation in high tibial osteotomy: a study of 50 patients. Orthopedics. 2009;32(10 Suppl):40–3.
29. Iorio R, Vadalà A, Giannetti S, Pagnottelli M, Di Sette P, Conteduca F, et al. Computer-assisted high tibial osteotomy: preliminary results. Orthopedics. 2010;33(10 Suppl):82–6.
30. Reising K, Strohm PC, Hauschild O, Schmal H, Khattab M, Südkamp NP, et al. Computer-assisted navigation for the intraoperative assessment of lower limb alignment in high tibial osteotomy can avoid outliers compared with the conventional technique. Knee Surg Sports Traumatol Arthrosc. 2013;21(1):181–8.
31. Saragaglia D, Mercier N, Colle P-E. Computer-assisted osteotomies for genu varum deformity: which osteotomy for which varus? Int Orthop. 2010;34(2):185–90.
32. Young SW, Safran MR, Clatworthy M. Applications of computer navigation in sports medicine knee surgery: an evidence-based review. Curr Rev Musculoskelet Med. 2013;6(2):150–7.
33. Picardo NE, Khan W, Johnstone D. Computer-assisted navigation in high tibial osteotomy: a systematic review of the literature. Open Orthop J. 2012;6:305–12.
34. Lo WN, Cheung KW, Yung SH, Chiu KH. Arthroscopy-assisted computer navigation in high tibial osteotomy for varus knee deformity. J Orthop Surg Hong Kong. 2009;17(1):51–5.
35. Matsumoto T, Nakano N, Lawrence JE, Khanduja V. Current concepts and future perspectives in computer-assisted navigated total knee replacement. Int Orthop. 2019;43(6):1337–43.
36. Song SJ, Bae DK. Computer-assisted navigation in high tibial osteotomy. Clin Orthop Surg. 2016;8(4):349–57.
37. Wu Z-P, Zhang P, Bai J-Z, Liang Y, Chen P-T, He J-S, et al. Comparison of navigated and conventional high tibial osteotomy for the treatment of osteoarthritic knees with varus deformity: a meta-analysis. Int J Surg Lond Engl. 2018;55:211–9.
38. Yan J, Musahl V, Kay J, Khan M, Simunovic N, Ayeni OR. Outcome reporting following navigated high tibial osteotomy of the knee: a systematic review. Knee Surg Sports Traumatol Arthrosc. 2016;24(11):3529–55.
39. Kim HJ, Yoon J-R, Choi GW, Yang J-H. Imageless navigation versus conventional open wedge high tibial osteotomy: a meta-analysis of comparative studies. Knee Surg Relat Res. 2016;28(1):16–26.

40. Chang J, Scallon G, Beckert M, Zavala J, Bollier M, Wolf B, et al. Comparing the accuracy of high tibial osteotomies between computer navigation and conventional methods. Comput Assist Surg. 2017;22(1):1–8.
41. Akamatsu Y, Kobayashi H, Kusayama Y, Kumagai K, Saito T. Comparative study of opening-wedge high tibial osteotomy with and without a combined computed tomography-based and image-free navigation system. Arthrosc J Arthrosc Relat Surg. 2016;32(10):2072–81.
42. Han S-B, Kim HJ, Lee D-H. Effect of computer navigation on accuracy and reliability of limb alignment correction following open-wedge high tibial osteotomy: a meta-analysis. Biomed Res Int. 2017;2017:3803457.
43. Hasan K, Rahman QA, Zalzal P. Navigation versus conventional high tibial osteotomy: systematic review. Springerplus. 2015;4(1):271.
44. Fujisawa Y, Masuhara K, Shiomi S. The effect of high tibial osteotomy on osteoarthritis of the knee. An arthroscopic study of 54 knee joints. Orthop Clin North Am. 1979;10(3):585–608.
45. Khadem R, Yeh CC, Sadeghi-Tehrani M, Bax MR, Johnson JA, Welch JN, et al. Comparative tracking error analysis of five different optical tracking systems. Comput Aided Surg. 2000;5(2):98–107.
46. Bonutti P, Dethmers D, Stiehl JB. Case report. Clin Orthop. 2008;466(6):1499–502.
47. Kyung BS, Kim JG, Jang K-M, Chang M, Moon Y-W, Ahn JH, et al. Are navigation systems accurate enough to predict the correction angle during high tibial osteotomy? Comparison of navigation systems with 3-dimensional computed tomography and standing radiographs. Am J Sports Med. 2013;41(10):2368–74.
48. Yaffe MA, Koo SS, Stulberg SD. Radiographic and navigation measurements of TKA limb alignment do not correlate. Clin Orthop. 2008;466(11):2736–44.
49. Hankemeier S, Hufner T, Wang G, Kendoff D, Zeichen J, Zheng G, et al. Navigated open-wedge high tibial osteotomy: advantages and disadvantages compared to the conventional technique in a cadaver study. Knee Surg Sports Traumatol Arthrosc. 2006;14(10):917–21.
50. Iorio R, Pagnottelli M, Vadalà A, Giannetti S, Di Sette P, Papandrea P, et al. Open-wedge high tibial osteotomy: comparison between manual and computer-assisted techniques. Knee Surg Sports Traumatol Arthrosc. 2013;21(1):113–9.
51. Goradia VK. Computer-assisted and robotic surgery in orthopedics: where we are in 2014. Sports Med Arthrosc Rev. 2014;22(4):202–5.
52. Amendola A, Bonasia DE. Results of high tibial osteotomy: review of the literature. Int Orthop. 2010;34(2):155–60.
53. Citak M, Kendoff D, O'Loughlin PF, Pearle AD. Heterotopic ossification post navigated high tibial osteotomy. Knee Surg Sports Traumatol Arthrosc. 2009;17(4):352–5.

Part IV

Revision Surgery

Indications and Outcomes of Revision to Another HTO

17

Tomas Pineda, Mattia Basilico, Elliot Sappey-Marinier, and Sebastien Lustig

17.1 Introduction

High tibial osteotomy (HTO) is a common surgical option for osteoarthritic (OA) knees with varus or valgus deformity, especially in young and active patients [1, 2].

The goal of HTO is to transfer the weight-bearing load to the undamaged compartment.

However, the incidence of complications after HTO ranged from 1.9% to 55% [3–8], and clinical results deteriorate over time [9–16].

Intraoperative complications of HTO include neurovascular injury, under- or overcorrection of the lower limb alignment, fracture of the opposite cortical hinge, intra-articular fracture, and unintended change of the tibial posterior slope angle. Postoperative complications include non-union or delayed union of the osteotomy site, change of the patellar height, and infection.

Most complications are caused by surgical errors and can be avoided with a meticulous surgical technique. However, the avoidance of under- or overcorrection and change in the tibial posterior slope angle in every knee may not be easy.

The incidence of surgical failures in HTO has varied widely in previous studies, ranging from 9% to 62% for undercorrection and from 4% to 16% for overcorrection [17–24].

T. Pineda
Universidad de Chile, Santiago, RM, Chile

M. Basilico
Fondazione Policlinico Universitario A. Gemelli IRCCS, Università Cattolica del Sacro Cuore, Rome, Italy

E. Sappey-Marinier (✉) · S. Lustig
Department of Orthopaedic Surgery, Croix-Rousse Hospital, Lyon, France

© Springer Nature Switzerland AG 2020
S. Oussedik, S. Lustig (eds.), *Osteotomy About the Knee*,
https://doi.org/10.1007/978-3-030-49055-3_17

249

The complications after HTO might be divided in:

- Short-term complications, such as overcorrection
- Mid-term complications, such as undercorrection or non-union
- Long-term complications, such as the progression of osteoarthritis

Generally, unchanged pain is an unsatisfactory result. Nowadays TKA is considered the best alternative for painful knees after osteotomy.

Several studies focused on how high tibial osteotomy affects the outcome following TKA [25, 26].

Instead, less than 17% have a second osteotomy as treatment [27].

In this chapter, we focus on Indications and outcomes of revision to another HTO.

17.2   Overcorrection in Medial Opening-Wedge HTO

Valgization high tibial osteotomy (HTO) is considered as a successful procedure for varus osteoarthritis in young patient. This surgery allows to shift the weight-bearing axis into the nonaffected lateral knee compartment, decreasing the load on the medial compartment [28].

Two surgical techniques are available to correct the tibial varus deformity: the lateral closing-wedge HTO (LCW-HTO) and the medial opening-wedge HTO (MOW-HTO).

Initially the lateral closing-wedge high tibial osteotomy was more performed. In the last decades, medial opening-wedge HTO has become more popular, and the surgical technique was subject to continuous improvements over the years [29–31].

The reason of this increase is probably its more direct approach and the avoidance of exposing the lateral aspect of the knee and the peroneal nerve.

Generally, the tendency is to prefer the MOW-HTO in young patients with limited OA and the LCW-HTO in older patients with advanced OA [32].

Several studies have focused on the HTO long-term survival, showing that HTO provides symptomatic relief for approximately 10 years, but frequently it does not ensure a permanent pain relief [33, 34].

Many factors influence the outcome; first of all, a correct preoperative planning is essential. The radiologic work-up includes bipedal stance full leg films, bipedal stance at 45° of flexion view (schuss view), unipodal weight bearing, unipodal stance profile at 30° of flexion, and skyline view of the patella. All these radiographs are essential for obtaining information about the type of arthrosis, osteophytes, and deformities and for the measurement of the different angles and axes.

It is critical to have an accurate preoperative planning to obtain the desired degrees of correction. The best result of valgus osteotomy is obtained when a postoperative valgus axis ranging from 3° to 6° is reached, with a mechanical femorotibial angle included between 183° and 186° [35–37].

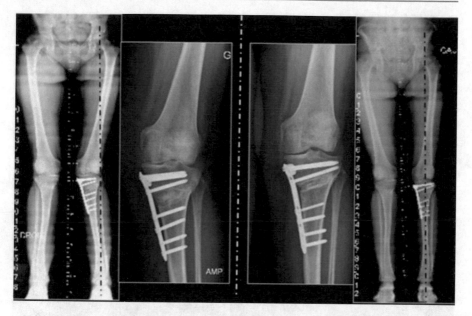

Fig. 17.1 Medial closing-wedge HTO after medial opening-wedge HTO overcorrection

When an osteotomy produces a correction greater than 6°, the weight-bearing axis of the leg is overcorrected, causing pain and discomfort to the patient. It can cause cosmetic issues and later development of lateral osteoarthritis.

The patient dissatisfaction may be such as to require a revision. Overcorrection is the first cause of short-term failure of osteotomies; it may be the result of incorrect planning or an inaccurate intraoperative execution.

After a medial opening-wedge HTO overcorrection, the correction is the less tricky: a medial closing-wedge high tibial osteotomy is suggested (Fig. 17.1). It allows to correct the leg alignment via the same approach of previous osteotomy.

First the previous plate is removed, and then using the osteotomy guide, the desired amount of bone is resected, according to the preoperative planning.

After compressing the osteotomy, the fixation is performed using a plate locked in screw.

17.3   Undercorrection in Medial Opening-Wedge HTO

A correction of the mechanical axis less than 2° of valgus can be considered as undercorrection [21, 38].

It can be the consequence of an incorrect planning or an inaccurate execution. But after an opening-wedge high tibial osteotomy, it is often due to loss of correction in the postoperative period. This is why undercorrection is the most important cause of medium-term failure after HTO: it causes recurrence of the varus

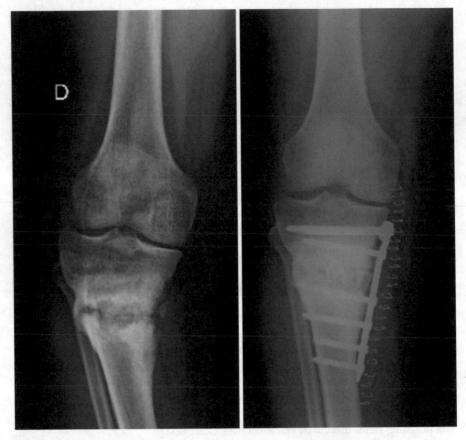

Fig. 17.2 Non-union after opening-wedge HTO treated with opening-wedge HTO revision placing a new plate

deformity with development of medial osteoarthritis over the time, until a revision surgery could be necessary [39].

In many cases this loss of correction can be related to a delayed union or a non-union (Fig. 17.2).

The non-union rates after HTO range between 0.5% and 1.1% [40].

When non-union is associated with undercorrection, an ongoing infection must be excluded: in this case a one-step revision can be performed.

The previous plate should be removed, the osteotomy is opened, and the fixation is performed using a locking plate. Before the osteosynthesis, the osteotomy should be filled up using autograft bone: it provides higher rates of clinical and radiographic union. The use of synthetic bone substitutes in OWHTO cannot be recommended [40].

Performing this revision, it is difficult to achieve the correct alignment due to previous surgical approach, the anatomical distortion of the proximal tibial metaphysis, and the related difficult to obtain a rigid and stable fixation.

17.4 Closing-Wedge Overcorrection

Closing-wedge HTO (CWHTO) remains an effective and successful treatment for unicompartment osteoarthrosis of the knee. Good results have been achieved in the literature over both the medium and long term, with a gradual deterioration in function and outcome over time [33, 41–47].

The reported advantages of this technique include better initial stability due to the compressive nature of the osteotomy leading to more immediate weight bearing and quicker bone healing.

However, the incidence of complications after CWHTO ranges widely between different series from 5.6% to 34% [33, 44–47].

Closing-wedge overcorrection could cause cosmetic problems and overloading of the lateral compartment [46].

Biomechanically, 70% of the load is borne by the medial compartment when the mechanical axis goes through the center of the knee. This load decreases to 50% for 4° of valgus with a further reduction to 40% for 6° of valgus [48].

Nevertheless, some authors achieved bad results with overcorrection [49, 50].

Given this data most authors recommend an alignment range between 2° and 6° of mechanical valgus [43, 49, 51–54].

At our institution the majority of closing-wedge overcorrected cases are treated by lateral opening-wedge high tibial osteotomy (LOWHTO) to obtain an alignment range between 2° and 6° of mechanical valgus; the technique has been described in detail in the chapter on LOWHTO. In cases of revision to another high tibial osteotomy, we prefer corticocancellous bone graft from the anterior iliac crest to provide higher rates of clinical and radiographic union, and we recommend a fixation with a locking plate to get a more rigid form of fixation.

Non-union after closing-wedge osteotomy is uncommon given the excellent healing potential due to the stability and metaphyseal bony apposition afforded by the technique [41, 44–46, 55, 56].

Nevertheless, it takes a relatively long time to achieve bone healing at the osteotomy site after CWHTO because of discrepancies between the area on the proximal and distal fragments. This creates difficulties in maintaining alignment until bone union is acquired.

In cases of non-union and overcorrection, in the absence of infection, we recommend a one-step revision. The procedure usually involves a more rigid form of fixation such as locking plates or a compressive type of external fixation, and the use of autologous bone graft is suggested.

17.5 Infection

Infection is rare after HTO. Anagnostakos et al. performed an interesting systematic literature review: analyzing a total of 2026 patients who underwent HTO, superficial infections were observed in 1–9 % and deep infections in 0.5–4.7 % of the cases.

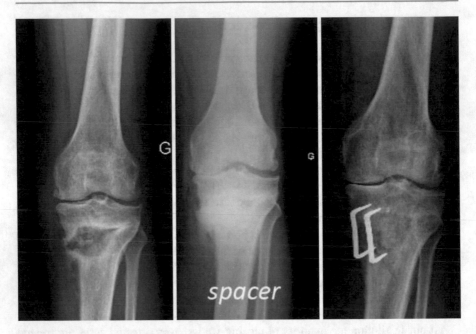

Fig. 17.3 A two-step surgical revision for infection after HTO

Several management options have been reported in the literature. Regarding superficial or deep infection, the treatment varied from oral or systemic antibiotics alone or combined with surgical revision, debridement, and hardware removal [57].

When the revision surgery indicated is a new osteotomy, a two-step revision is suggested. The first step consists in material removal and placing a spacer.

Only after infection eradication, the spacer can be removed, and a new osteotomy can be performed to achieve the correct leg alignment (Fig. 17.3).

17.6   Don't Forget the Sagittal Plane

The tibial posterior slope is extremely important for knee flexion, for the correct function of the cruciate ligaments and the normal knee kinematics in general. The physiologic range of slope of the tibial plateau is between 6° and 10° as stated by various authors [50, 58–60].

The effects of high tibial osteotomy on tibial slope have been widely debated. Agneskirchner et al., in a biomechanical study, demonstrated that after flexion osteotomy with an increase in the tibial slope, a statistically significant shift of the cartilage contact area and pressure load into the anterior half of the tibial plateau occurred. Accordingly, it was found that in the posterior part of the plateau, the tibiofemoral contact area and the contact pressure were significantly decreased as the tibial slope was gradually elevated [61].

Otherwise, modification of tibial slope is a source of instability and excessive anteroposterior tibial translation that may encourage the progression of osteoarthritis [49, 61, 62].

In clinical practice the most important factor that influence the posterior tibial inclination is the surgical technique.

According to most authors, medial opening-wedge high tibial osteotomy increases tibial slope by 3–4° [63–69], and lateral closing-wedge high tibial osteotomy decreases tibial slope by 3–5° [66, 70].

The tibial slope must be analyzed and studied in case of failed osteotomy as it may be the reason of the failure.

References

1. Habata T, Uematsu K, Hattori K, Kasanami R, Takakura Y, Fujisawa Y. High tibial osteotomy that does not cause recurrence of varus deformity for medial gonarthrosis. Knee Surg Sports Traumatol Arthrosc. 2006;14:962–7.
2. Lobenhoffer P. Importance of osteotomy around to the knee for medial gonarthritis: indications, technique and results. Orthopade. 2014;43:425–31.
3. Niemeyer P, Schmal H, Hauschild O, von Heyden J, Südkamp NP, Kostler W. Open-wedge osteotomy using an internal plate fixator in patients with medial-compartment gonarthritis and varus malalignment: 3-year results with regard to preoperative arthroscopic and radiographic findings. Arthroscopy. 2010;26:1607–16.
4. van den Bekerom MP, Patt TW, Kleinhout MY, van der Vis HM, Albers GH. Early complications after high tibial osteotomy: a comparison of two techniques. J Knee Surg. 2008;21:68–74.
5. Asik M, Sen C, Kilic B, Goksan SB, Ciftci F, Taser OF. High tibial osteotomy with Puddu plate for the treatment of varus gonarthrosis. Knee Surg Sports Traumatol Arthrosc. 2006;14:948–54.
6. Amendola A, Fowler PJ, Litchfield R, Kirkley S, Clatworthy M. Opening wedge high tibial osteotomy using a novel technique: early results and complications. J Knee Surg. 2004;17:164–9.
7. Kolb W, Guhlmann H, Windisch C, Kolb K, Koller H, Grützner P, Kolb K. Opening-wedge high tibial osteotomy with a locked low-profile plate. J Bone Joint Surg Am. 2009;91:2581–8.
8. Esenkaya I, Elmali N. Proximal tibia medial open-wedge osteotomy using plates with wedges: early results in 58 cases. Knee Surg Sports Traumatol Arthrosc. 2006;14:955–61.
9. Akizuki S, Shibakawa A, Takizawa T, Yamazaki I, Horiuchi H. The long-term outcome of high tibial osteotomy: a ten- to 20-year follow-up. J Bone Joint Surg Br. 2008;90:592–6.
10. Bonasia DE, Dettoni F, Sito G, Blonna D, Marmotti A, Bruzzone M, Castoldi F, Rossi R. Medial opening wedge high tibial osteotomy for medial compartment overload/arthritis in the varus knee: prognostic factors. Am J Sports Med. 2014;42:690–8.
11. DeMeo PJ, Johnson EM, Chiang PP, Flamm AM, Miller MC. Midterm follow-up of opening-wedge high tibial osteotomy. Am J Sports Med. 2010;38:2077–84.
12. Efe T, Ahmed G, Heyse TJ, Boudriot U, Timmesfeld N, Fuchs-Winkelmann S, Ishaque B, Lakemeier S, Schofer MD. Closing-wedge high tibial osteotomy: survival and risk factor analysis at long-term follow up. BMC Musculoskelet Disord. 2011;12:46.
13. Hui C, Salmon LJ, Kok A, Williams HA, Hockers N, van der Tempel WM, Chana R, Pinczewski LA. Long-term survival of high tibial osteotomy for medial compartment osteoarthritis of the knee. Am J Sport Med. 2011;39:64–70.
14. Koshino T, Yoshida T, Ara Y, Saito I, Saito T. Fifteen to twenty-eight years' follow-up results of high tibial valgus osteotomy for osteoarthritic knee. Knee. 2004;11:439–44.
15. Niinimaki TT, Eskelinen A, Mann BS, Junnila M, Ohtonen P, Leppilahti J. Survivorship of high tibial osteotomy in the treatment of osteoarthritis of the knee: Finnish registry- based study of 3195 knees. J Bone Joint Surg Br. 2012;94:1517–21.

16. van Raaij T, Reijman M, Brouwer RW, Jakma TS, Verhaar JN. Survival of closing-wedge high tibial osteotomy: good outcome in men with low-grade osteoarthritis after 10-16 years. Acta Orthop. 2008;79:230–4.

17. Hankemeier S, Mommsen P, Krettek C, Jagodzinski M, Brand J, Meyer C, Meller R. Accuracy of high tibial osteotomy: comparison between open and closed wedge technique. Knee Surg Sports Traumatol Arthrosc. 2010;18:1328–33.

18. Van den Bempt M, Van Genechten W, Claes T, Claes S. How accurately does high tibial osteotomy correct the mechanical axis of an arthritic varus knee? A systematic review. Knee. 2016;23:925–35.

19. Dexel J, Fritzsche H, Beyer F, Harman MK, Lutzner J. Openwedge high tibial osteotomy: incidence of lateral cortex fractures and influence of fixation device on osteotomy healing. Knee Surg Sports Traumatol Arthrosc. 2017;25:832–7.

20. Giffin JR, Vogrin TM, Zantop T, Woo SL, Harner CD. Effects of increasing tibial slope on the biomechanics of the knee. Am J Sports Med. 2004;32:376–82.

21. Iorio R, Pagnottelli M, Vadalà A, Giannetti S, Di Sette P, Papandrea P, Conteduca F, Ferretti A. Openwedge high tibial osteotomy: comparison between manual and computer assisted techniques. Knee Surg Sports Traumatol Arthrosc. 2013;21:113–9.

22. Brosset T, Pasquier G, Migaud H, Gougeon F. Opening wedge high tibial osteotomy performed without filling the defect but with locking plate fixation (TomoFixTM) and early weightbearing: prospective evaluation of bone union, precision and maintenance of correction in 51 cases. Orthop Traumatol Surg Res. 2011;97:705–11.

23. Lee DH, Han SB, Oh KJ, Lee JS, Kwon JH, Kim JI, Patnaik S, Shetty GM, Nha KW. The weightbearing scanogram technique provides better coronal limb alignment than the navigation technique in open high tibial osteotomy. Knee. 2014;21:451–5.

24. ElAzab HM, Morgenstern M, Ahrens P, Schuster T, Imhoff AB, Lorenz SG. Limb alignment after openwedge high tibial osteotomy and its effect on the clinical outcome. Orthopedics. 2011;34:622–8.

25. Virolainen P, Aro HT. High tibial osteotomy for the treatment of osteoarthritis of the knee: a review of the literature and a meta-analysis of follow-up studies. Arch Orthop Trauma Surg. 2004;124(4):258–61.

26. Preston S, Howard J, Naudie D, Somerville L, McAuley J. Total knee arthroplasty after high tibial osteotomy: no differences between medial and lateral osteotomy approaches. Clin Orthop Relat Res. 2014;472(1):105–10.

27. Odenbring S, Egund N, Knutson K, Lindstrand A, Taksvig L. Revision after osteotomy for gonarthrosis: a 10-19 year follow-up of 314 cases. Acto Orthop Scand. 1990;61(2):128–30.

28. Han JH, Yang JH, Bhandare NN, Suh DW, Lee JS, Chang YS, Yeom JW, Nha KW. Total knee arthroplasty after failed high tibial osteotomy: a systematic review of open versus closed wedge osteotomy. Knee Surg Sports Traumatol Arthrosc. 2016;24(8):2567–77.

29. Devgan A, Marya KM, Kundu ZS, Sangwan SS, Siwach RC. Medial opening wedge high tibial osteotomy for osteoarthritis of knee: long-term results in 50 knees. Med J Malaysia. 2003;58(1):62–8.

30. Hernigou P, Ma W. Open wedge tibial osteotomy with acrylic bone cement as bone substitute. Knee. 2001;8(2):103–10.

31. Koshino T, Murase T, Saito T. Medial opening-wedge high tibial osteotomy with use of porous hydroxyapatite to treat medial compartment osteoarthritis of the knee. J Bone Joint Surg Am. 2003;85-A(1):78–85.

32. Cerciello S, Lustig S, Servien E, Neyret P. Osteotomy for the arthritic knee: a European perspective. In: Scott WN, editor. Insall & Scott surgery of the knee. 6th ed. Philadelphia, PA: Elsevier; 2018. p. 1343–61.

33. Aglietti P, Buzzi R, Vena LM, Baldini A, Mondaini A. High tibial valgus osteotomy for medial gonarthrosis: a 10- to 21-year study. J Knee Surg. 2003;16(1):21–6.

34. Van Wulfften Palthe AFY, Clement ND, Temmerman OPP, Burger BJ. Survival and functional outcome of high tibial osteotomy for medial knee osteoarthritis: a 10-20-year cohort study. Eur J Orthop Surg Traumatol. 2018;28(7):1381–9.

35. Goutallier D, Hernigou P, Medevielle D, Debeyre J. Outcome at more than 10 years of 93 tibial osteotomies for internal arthritis in genu varum (or the predominant influence of the frontal angular correction). Rev Chir Orthop Reparatrice Appar Mot. 1986;72(2):101–13.
36. Goutallier D, Hernigou P, Medevielle D, Debeyre J. Long-term results of the treatment of medial femoro-tibial gonarthrosis by tibial valgisation osteotomy. Outcome of 93 osteotomies after more than 10 years. Mal Osteoartic. 1985;52(7–9):437–44.
37. Berman AT, Bosacco SJ, Kirshner S, Avolio A Jr. Factors influencing long-term results in high tibial osteotomy. Clin Orthop Relat Res. 1991;272:192–8.
38. Kim HJ, Yoon JR, Choi GW, Yang JH. Imageless navigation versus conventional open wedge high tibial osteotomy: a meta-analysis of comparative studies knee. Surg Relat Res. 2016;28(1):16–26.
39. Kamada S, Shiota E, Saeki K, Kiyama T, Maeyama A, Yamamoto T. Severe varus knees result in a high rate of undercorrection of lower limb alignment after opening wedge high tibial osteotomy. J Orthop Surg (Hong Kong). 2019;27(2):2.
40. Slevin O, Ayeni OR, Hinterwimmer S, Tischer T, Feucht MJ, Hirschmann MT. The role of bone void fillers in medial opening wedge high tibial osteotomy: a systematic review. Knee Surg Sports Traumatol Arthrosc. 2016;24(11):3584–98.
41. Insall JN, Joseph DM, Msika C. High tibial osteotomy for varus gonarthrosis. A long-term follow-up study. J Bone Joint Surg Am. 1984;66:1040–8.
42. Ivarsson I, Myrnerts R, Gillquist J. High tibial osteotomy for medial osteoarthritis of the knee. A 5 to 7 and 11 year follow- up. J Bone Joint Surg Br. 1990;72:238–44.
43. Coventry MB, Ilstrup DM, Wallrichs SL. Proximal tibial osteotomy. A critical long-term study of eighty-seven cases. J Bone Joint Surg Am. 1993;75:196–201.
44. Bettin D, Karbowski A, Schwering L, Matthiass HH. Time-dependent clinical and roentgeno-graphical results of Coventry high tibial valgisation osteotomy. Arch Orthop Trauma Surg. 1998;117:53–7.
45. Naudie D, Bourne RB, Rorabeck CH, Bourne TJ. The Install Award. Survivorship of the high tibial valgus osteotomy. A 10- to -22-year follow up study. Clin Orthop Relat Res. 1999;(367):18–27.
46. Sprenger TR, Doerzbacher JF. Tibial osteotomy for the treatment of varus gonarthrosis. Survival and failure analysis to twenty-two years. J Bone Joint Surg Am. 2003;85(3):469–74.
47. Wu LD, Hahne HJ, Hassenpflug T. A long-term follow-up study of high tibial osteotomy for medial compartment osteoarthrosis. Chin J Traumatol. 2004;7:348–53.
48. Kettelkamp DB, Wenger DR, Chao EY, Thompson C. Results of proximal tibial osteotomy. The effects of tibiofemoral angle, stance-phase flexion-extension, and medial-plateau force. J Bone Joint Surg Am. 1976;58:952–60.
49. Hernigou P, Medevielle D, Debeyre J, Goutallier D. Proximal tibial osteotomy for osteoarthritis with varus deformity. A ten to thirteen-year follow-up study. J Bone Joint Surg Am. 1987;69:332–54.
50. Shaw JA, Dungy DS, Arsht SS. Recurrent varus angulation after high tibial osteotomy: an anatomic analysis. Clin Orthop Relat Res. 2004;(420):205–12.
51. Fujisawa Y, Masuhara K, Shiomi S. The effect of high tibial osteotomy on osteoarthritis of the knee. An arthroscopic study of 54 knee joints. Orthop Clin North Am. 1979;10:585–608.
52. Jakob RP, Murphy SB. Tibial osteotomy for varus gonarthrosis: indication, planning, and operative technique. Instr Course Lect. 1992;41:87–93.
53. Koshino T, Tsuchiya K. The effect of high tibial osteotomy on osteoarthritis of the knee. Clinical and histological observations. Int Orthop. 1979;3:37–45.
54. Myrnerts R. Optimal correction in high tibial osteotomy for varus deformity. Acta Orthop Scand. 1980;51:689–94.
55. Cass JR, Bryan RS. High tibial osteotomy. Clin Orthop Relat Res. 1988;(230):196–9.
56. Vainionpaa S, Laike E, Kirves P, Tiusanen P. Tibial osteotomy for osteoarthritis of the knee. A five to ten-year follow- up study. J Bone Joint Surg Am. 1981;63:938–46.
57. Anagnostakos K, Mosser P, Kohn D. Infections after high tibial osteotomy. Knee Surg Sports Traumatol Arthrosc. 2013;21(1):161–9.

58. Chiu KY, Zhang SD, Zhang GH. Posterior slope of tibial plateau in Chinese. J Arthroplasty. 2000;15:224–7.
59. Insall JN. Total knee arthroplasty in rheumatoid arthritis. Ryumachi. 1993;33:472.
60. Lecuire L, Lerat JL, Bousquet G, et al. The treatment of genu recurvatum (author's translation). Rev Chir Orthop Reparatric Appar Mot. 1980;66:95–103.
61. Agneskirchner J, Hurschler C, Stukenborg-Colsman C, Imhoff A, Lobenhoffer P. Effect of high tibial flexion osteotomy on cartilage pressure and joint kinematics: a biomechanical study in human cadaveric knees. Arch Orthop Trauma Surg. 2004;124:575–84.
62. Liu W, Maitland ME. Influence of anthropometric and mechanical variations on functional instability in the ACL deficient knee. Ann Biomed Eng. 2003;31:1153–61.
63. El-Azab H, Halawa A, Anetzberger H, Imhoff AB, Hinterwimmer S. The effect of closed- and open-wedge high tibial osteotomy on tibial slope: a retrospective radiological review of 120 cases. J Bone Joint Surg Br. 2008;90:1193–7.
64. Marti C, Gautier E, Wachtl SW, Jakob R. Accuracy of frontal and sagittal plane correction in open-wedge high tibial osteotomy. Arthroscopy. 2004;20:366–72.
65. Noyes FR, Goebel SX, West J. Opening-wedge tibial osteotomy: the 3-Triangle method to correct axial alignment and tibial slope. Am J Sports Med. 2005;33:378–87.
66. El-Azab H, Glabgly P, Paul J, Imhoff AB, Hinterwimmer S. Patellar height and posterior tibial slope after open- and closed-wedge high tibial osteotomy: a radiological study on 100 patients. Am J Sports Med. 2010;38:323–9.
67. Bito H, Takeuchi R, Kumagai K, Aratake M, Saito I, Hayashi R, et al. Opening-wedge high tibial osteotomy affects both the lateral patellar tilt and patellar height. Knee Surg Sports Traumatol Arthrosc. 2010;18:955–60.
68. LaPrade RF, Oro FB, Ziegler CG, Wijdicks CA, Walsh MP. Patellar height. Sports Med. 2010;38:160–70.
69. Wang JH, Bae JH, Lim HC, Shon WY, Kim CW, Cho JW. Medial open-wedge high tibial osteotomy: the effect of the cortical hinge on posterior tibial slope. Am J Sports Med. 2009;37:2411–8.
70. Hohmann E, Bryant A, Imhoff AB. The effect of closed-wedge high tibial osteotomy on tibial slope: a radiographic study. Knee Surg Sports Traumatol Arthrosc. 2006;14:454–9.

Conversion of High Tibial Osteotomy to Total Knee Replacement

18

Branavan Rudran, Mazin Ibrahim, and Sam Oussedik

18.1 Introduction

High tibial osteotomy (HTO) is a globally recognised treatment for osteoarthritis (OA) of the knee with varus deformity, particularly in younger, active patients [1]. It was first conducted in 1958 to correct a varus deformity by lateral axis relocation [2]. Patients receiving HTO can benefit from natural joint preservation through realignment of the mechanical axis of the lower limb towards the healthy compartment, thereby decreasing the contact force through the affected compartment [3]. This ensures that the weight-bearing forces load the healthy knee compartment. HTO is now considered an important part of the treatment algorithm for the unstable knee.

Suitable limb alignment is pivotal to ensuring optimal surgical outcome from the procedure [4], emphasising the importance of long leg radiographs when planning the procedure. The clinical results of HTO have been shown to deteriorate over time, despite the initially promising results. Several studies with a mean age of 49.4 years to 62.9 years have reported a 5-year survival rate of HTO ranging from 75% to 98% and a 10-year survival from 51% to 98% [5–12]. Several knees may require conversion to total knee replacement (TKR) due to osteoarthritic changes or loss of the corrective angle. There is controversy in the literature as to the factors affecting the survival of HTO with intrinsic factors such as age, body mass index and OA grade being attributed as well as operative factors such as post-operative correction angle [8, 9].

B. Rudran
Chelsea and Westminster NHS Trust, London, UK
e-mail: B.rudran@imperial.ac.uk

M. Ibrahim
University College London Hospitals NHS Trust, London, UK

S. Oussedik (✉)
Orthopaedic Surgery Department, University College London Hospitals, London, UK

© Springer Nature Switzerland AG 2020
S. Oussedik, S. Lustig (eds.), *Osteotomy About the Knee*,
https://doi.org/10.1007/978-3-030-49055-3_18

The aim of this chapter is to provide an understanding of the indications and surgical approach to a TKR following a HTO. Another aim of this chapter is to review the results of revision TKR further to HTO.

18.2 Total Knee Replacement Following High Tibial Osteotomy

TKR has taken priority in recent years. The National Joint Registry in the United Kingdom showed an increase from 86,067 TKR 2010/2011 to 1,087,611 in 2015/2017 [13]. A TKR following an open-wedge or closed-wedge HTO can be complex, with possibility of excessive malunion from the initial procedure. This occurs with varus angulation of the knee over 10° and if the femoral mechanical axis is in varus [14]. Unsatisfactory surgical outcomes from HTO lead to a high probability in these young patients requiring a TKR. The main problem arises from valgus hypercorrection of the tibial epiphysis, resulting in valgus tibial mechanical axis and an oblique joint line [15].

It is important to know the rate of conversion of HTO to TKR and the reasons behind this to have an informed consent during patient's consultation for the surgical treatment with HTO. The indications for TKR remain the same; however there are specific indications for a TKR following HTO which can be progression of arthritis in the knee leading to loss of the correctable alignment or failure of the HTO due to variety of reasons.

18.3 Indications for TKR Following HTO

A revision of HTO to TKR can be considered when there is failure of the HTO. There are intraoperative causes of failure including neurovascular injury, under- or over-correction of the lower limb alignment, fracture of the opposite cortical hinge, intra-articular fracture and unintended change of the tibial posterior slope angle. There are also post-operative indications for considering a conversion to TKR following a failed HTO. These include progression of OA (of the medial compartment alone or with combination of the other compartments), delayed union or non-union of the osteotomy site and infection.

18.4 Intraoperative Indications for Failed HTO

18.4.1 Neurovascular Injury

A systematic review of the complications of high tibial osteotomy in unicompartmental OA of the knee reported EMG studies with 27% nerve damage of which reported symptomatic peroneal nerve injury was 3.3–11.9% [16]. It is widely accepted that the most common cause of nerve injury is iatrogenic damage of the deep peroneal nerve. Anatomical studies have confirmed that the extensor hallucis longus is the affected muscle, owing to its innervation by a singular branch of the deep peroneal nerve located 7–8 mm from the fibular styloid process [17, 18].

Georgoulis et al. [18] reported a 1.6% incidence of drop hallux further to closing-wedge high tibial osteotomy. Similarly in open-wedge high tibial osteotomy, a study of 55 patients who underwent post-operative CT scanning of the knee between 2009 and 2018 showed an increased risk of neurovascular injury due to the extended insertion trajectories of distal screws intersecting the interosseous membrane with the neurovascular bundle on its surface [19]. However, Song et al. in their review article mentioned about their unpublished data that their rate of nerve injury was 0% for 300 HTOs over 10-year period [20]. This illustrates the importance of understanding the potential risk of neurovascular injury and consequential failure of HTO, and this in turn can affect future conversion of HTO to TKR and the effect of that on functional outcomes.

18.4.2 Under or Overcorrection of Lower Limb Alignment

Satisfactory outcomes following HTO are dependent on appropriate alignment of the lower limb and correction of the deformity [7]. Despite meticulous preoperative planning producing adequate results [21], studies have shown considerable outliers in the clinical outcomes due to under- or overcorrection [22, 23]. A longitudinal study of 237 patients showed patients who had a varus alignment at baseline and had a fourfold increase in the odds of medial progression. Similarly, in valgus alignment, patients were found to have a fivefold increase in progression of OA. Undercorrection or overcorrection of the lower limb results in alignment of greater than 5° in either direction with a significantly higher deterioration in OA [24], and this speeds up the conversion of HTO to TKR.

18.4.3 Fracture of Opposite Cortical Hinge/ Intra-articular Fracture

An osteotomy is defined as a controlled fracture with a hinge of bone on the contralateral side maintaining stability. It is imperative during the procedure that there is no extension of the fracture of the opposite cortex or intra-articular region.

A retrospective radiological analysis of a randomised controlled trial of 87 patients to closing-wedge HTO and opening-wedge HTO showed that fracture of the opposite cortex was more common in the lateral closing-wedge technique than the medial opening-wedge technique. Interestingly, medial opening-wedge HTO was found to have less accurate correction at 1-year follow-up of statistical significance compared to a closing-wedge HTO with medial cortex fracture [25]. Miller et al. found that fracture to the lateral cortex causes increased micromotion at the osteotomy site and increased likelihood of non-union or malunion after medial HTO [26]. An option to optimise the valgus deformation prior to fracture would be to place a stress-relieving hole to reduce the risk of intra-articular fracture.

18.4.4 Unintended Change of the Posterior Tibial Slope Angle

HTO is used to correct coronal alignment of the proximal tibia and, however, can cause unintentional alteration in the posterior tibial slope. Studies suggest that after medial open-wedge HTO the posterior tibial angle increases [23, 27]. A radiographical study of 120 osteotomies (60 open-wedge, 60 closed-wedge) assessed for the posterior tibial slope before, after and before the removal of hardware. In the closed-wedge group, the mean slope was 5.7° before the operation, 2.4° after the operation and 2.7° at the time of removal of hardware. In the open-wedge group, the results were 5.0, 7.7 and 8.1, respectively. The reduction in the posterior tibial angle in closed-wedge HTO and the increased angle in open-wedge HTO was of statistical significance [28]. Similarly, Brouwer et al. [13] showed a statistical difference of 6.4° post-operatively in the posterior tibial slope. This showed that the geometry of the tibia is affected post-operatively in open-wedge HTO.

Unintentional increase in the posterior tibial slope has been shown to malalign the kinematics of the knee and results in instability in the sagittal plane. Cadaveric studies have shown increasing the slope causes an anterior shift in tibial resting position, which is exacerbated by loading the joint [29, 30].

18.5   Post-operative Complications

18.5.1 Non-union/Delayed Union of the Osteotomy Site

The risk of non-union and delayed union in HTO is varied depending on the surgical approach. Earlier studies have shown the risk of non-union in closed-wedge technique to be between 1.6% and 5.6% [10, 31–36] and delayed union up to 6.6% [31]. More recently, open-wedge HTO has become a viable alternative with the advantage of no fibular osteotomy, no muscle or nerve damage and improved reliability for leg length. Despite the perceived advantages in surgical approach, the risk of non-union has been reported to be similar with a non-union rate up to 5.4% [31, 34, 37].

There are multiple factors contributing to bone healing that lead to delayed union or non-union. These include non-variable and variable risk factors. Advanced age, female gender and poor bone quality have been found to be non-variable risk factors that increase the probability of non-union [38, 39]. Variable risk factors including smoking, drug, alcohol and obesity have been found to be significantly linked to non-union in fractures [40, 41]. A retrospective study of 186 medial open-wedge HTOs showed patients who developed non-union to have a statistically significant tobacco use and higher BMI [32]. Non-union can cause collapse of the osteotomy side and recurrence of deformity and further progression of arthritis and hence increase progression rate to TKR.

18.5.2 Progression of Arthritis

The demographics of patients who undergo high tibial osteotomy for medial compartment OA are younger [6]. Therefore, there is a propensity for the disease process to advance resulting in the requirement for a TKA. A population-based study of 2671 patients showed 32.3% of patients underwent a subsequent TKA after a median of 6 years. A prospective cohort study of 298 patients with a mean follow-up of 5.2 years showed that there was improved pain in the midterm following HTO; however there was a radiological progression of the disease state with increased joint space narrowing and a minimum increase of 1 Kellgren-Lawrence score classification in 48% of patients [42]. This corroborates with studies into radiological grading of OA having a significant correlation with the clinical outcome of HTO [43]. This shows that although HTO provides symptomatic relief in younger patients, there is continual progression in OA.

18.5.3 The Procedure and Challenges of TKR Following HTO

When planning for a TKR with a pre-existing HTO, certain factors need to be considered and planned for appropriately. These are skin and soft tissue scaring, fixation devices, deformity including patella, bone stock and finally ligament insufficiency especially MCL.

18.5.3.1 Skin

When considering the incision site, it is important to appreciate that a scar is present from the initial high tibial osteotomy, which can be vertical or horizontal. Conventionally, the previous scar is used when appropriate with a corresponding transverse scar at 90° [25]. It is important to note that a large skin bridge should be created of roughly 8 cm from the old and new scar [25] (Fig. 18.1). Vertical scars are challenging in the knee, and this should be considered and thought of carefully to protect especially the lateral flap due to the nature of the blood supply and the lymphatic drainage, which is medially based [20]. It is always advisable to include the most lateral vertical scar into the incision to obtain the desired arthrotomy exposure which is in the majority of the cases through the medial parapatellar; however, surgeons with experience in lateral parapatellar approach might opt to use this approach especially in valgus-aligned knees [20].

18.5.3.2 Hardware Removal

The introduction of new implants with locking plates and biomaterials has meant it is crucial to remove the fixation devices prior to a TKR. This is primarily done by removing the fixation device using the same incision as a single-stage procedure. For the removal of bulky plates using a separate incision and soft tissue dissection, a staged process should be considered to ensure a safe removal of fixation devices

Fig. 18.1 An example of
the incision for a total knee
replacement following
high tibial osteotomy [44]

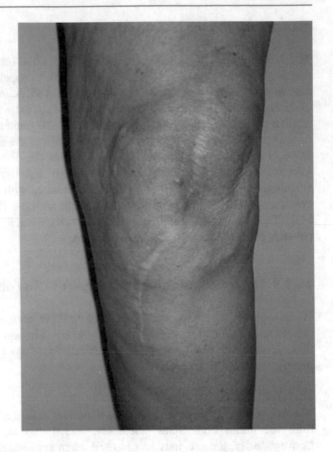

and suitable consequential TKR. It is possible that the hardware can be left if this doesn't interfere with the insertion of tibial baseplate nor causes tethering to the tissue that affects soft tissue release; however new designs of plates with their screws are more prominent, and in most of the cases, they need to be removed [20].

Performing a TKR after a HTO presents certain challenges, in particular the patella, ligamentous balancing and correction of potential deformity from the osteotomy.

18.5.4 Patella and Soft Tissue Scarring

The patella height as well as infrapatellar and periosteal site adhesions to the patella tendon can result in difficulty everting the patella. Everting the patella and patella baja is the main challenge during TKR following HTO [20]. Erak et al. 2011 found 27% of cases to have patella baja in a 33 patient series of TKR following medial opening-wedge tibial osteotomy [44]. Bastos Filho et al. [45] reported the incidence of additional procedures for the approach to TKR was up to 25% due to the difficulty in everting the patella during the procedure to TKR. Thus, careful step-wise release is important in preventing patella tendon injury. Patella baja problem can be worsened during TKR if a more lateral tibial cut is performed trying to achieve a 90° cut because in most HTO cases the medial side will be higher than the lateral side. This is especially in medial open-wedge osteotomy, where there is variance in the anatomy. Care should be taken to reduce the lateral cut and avoiding having thicker insert that will eventually worsen the patella baja problem [30]. Coming back to the issue of everting the patella, this can be overcome by a variety of ways including different extra surgical procedures including but not limited to quadriceps snip, VY plasty and tibial tubercle osteotomy in a similar fashion to those encountered during the surgical exposure of TKR revision cases [20]; however there are risks and complications from these procedures like quadriceps weakness that exacerbate the problem of patella baja, extensor lag and tibial tubercle non-union and/or migration [20]. In our experience, the senior author's surgical exposure doesn't include the necessity to evert the patella and instead prefers sub-luxing it following proper resurfacing, and this in our experience is adequate for the exposure in all our TKR cases.

18.5.5 Alignment and Preoperative Deformities

Coronal and sagittal plane deformities as well as tibial slope changes secondary to HTO are not uncommon. This can affect tissue balance in general and affect soft tissue in the knee rendering conversion to TKR a challenge [20]. Surgeons should be aware of these deformities and plan the procedure appropriately through adequate preoperative planning or intraoperative planning using navigation.

Most of the metaphyseal deformities can be corrected intraoperatively as the metaphysis is close to the surface and can be easily done [20].

Metaphyseal loss should be noted as well especially in closed-wedge osteotomy to avoid overcutting of the medial tibial plateau. Therefore it is better to start first with a smaller but adequate cut then cut more if required to avoid more loss of bone and the need for bigger poly insert thickness [20].

18.5.6 Ligaments Balance

Malalignment, over- or undercorrection and bone loss are factors contributing to ligament imbalance (laxity/tightness), which make conversion to TKR from HTO more challenging. Overall limb alignment post HTO and TKR can affect soft tissue balance especially ligament balance and specifically medial and lateral collateral and posterior cruciate ligaments. This can be different depending on the type of osteotomy conducted such as lateral collateral retraction in the case of lateral closed-wedge osteotomy and medial collateral insufficiency in case of open-wedge medial osteotomy which requires surgeon's attention to obtain the correct amount of required bone resection and achieving the required release and avoiding exacerbating the deformity [20]. Again the appropriate bone cuts for both tibia and femur are essential to obtain the correct rectangular flexion and extension gaps and avoid cutting both the tibia and femoral surfaces at 90° to the mechanical axis, which will yield a less parallel cut and exacerbate the ligament problems [20].

Another important consideration is the correction of tibial obliquity further to the HTO and ensuring appropriate ligamentous integrity in both terminal extension and flexion. At the time of conversion to TKR, there is a possibility of undercorrection and varus recurrence or overcorrection and valgus deformity.

Tibial mechanical axes greater than 100° with valgus deformity have an increased risk of ligamentous laxity. A study showed increased tibial mechanical axes have been found to lead to asymmetrical cut of 1.5 cm, creating ligamentous laxity [46]. To minimise this, an angulated cut of the tibial plateau should be taken with 10–12 mm of the medial plateau resected. This resection can defunction the medial collateral ligament, which increases laxity. Therefore, to balance the knee in extension, "pie crusting" is conducted where there is a release of the fascia lata. A systematic review of the literature found 77% of studies reported a higher rate of lateral release in TKR following HTO [47].

The distal femoral cut depends on the mechanical axis of the femur. A varus femur requires minimal femoral condylar resection to ensure correction of the medial laxity. This is achieved by the implant, which is thicker than the condyle, hence reducing laxity (Fig. 18.2). However, in a valgus femur, the medial femoral condyle should be resected to the same thickness as the implant. In cases of overcorrected valgus deformity, balance is particularly difficult. The realignment of the lower limb can affect the collateral ligaments and posterior cruciate ligament.

18.5.7 Implant Choice

Due to the aforementioned considerations, it has been advised that PCL-substituting implants are better to be used in converting HTO to TKR due to the effect of the new alignment and geometry on the function of PCL combined with poor-quality PCL secondary to OA; this has encouraged surgeons to use this technique and implant more than the cruciate-retaining counterparts with evidence to show early failure due to loosening in the PCL-retaining implants compared to the sacrificing one [48] and better functional outcome for the earlier more than the latter [49]. Resurfacing of the patella in this cohort of patients was found to be of better results compared to not resurfacing them in the setting of TKR following HTO. Finally in the presence of proximal tibial non-union, it was recommended to use the long-stem implants to allow for a stable and protected healing and union.

18.5.8 Navigation in TKR Following HTO

Computer navigation in knee surgery has gained popularity in the United Kingdom and North America. The intention is to provide more precise implantation by digitally mapping the anatomy and ensuring a precise excision of bone.

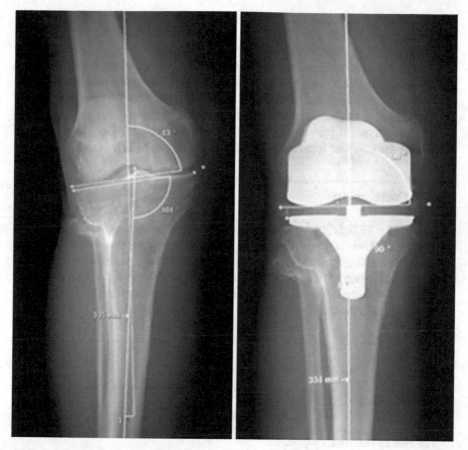

Fig. 18.2 The pre- and post-radiographs of an oblique joint line after closing-wedge HTO and a TKR with appropriate balancing

Several studies have suggested that there is an improvement in the kinematic alignment of the knee when navigation is used [50–52]. A multicentre randomised controlled trial of 190 patients comparing computer assisted with conventional total knee replacement showed that computer-assisted group had significantly better improvement in functional knee scores and improved pain relief [53].

In TKR following HTO, precision and planning are integral to ensuring an optimal outcome. A study of 58 patients comparing primary navigated TKR and navigated TKR following HTO showed comparable functional outcomes with similar Oxford Knee Score, Tegner and Lysholm and Knee Society Scores. Interestingly, significantly higher mediolateral ligamentous instability was seen in the navigated TKR following osteotomy compared to primary TKR [54]. The literature suggests that better trials are required to consider the influence of navigation; however, appreciation for the soft tissue and balancing of the joint are important for improved outcomes.

18.6   Future Directions

As we acknowledged that the failed HTO poses a challenge for surgeons in converting this to TKR, new directions have been implemented to improve overall outcomes following HTO. The birth of robotic surgery combined with its extensive preoperative planning might be the way forward in improving the outcomes further for this cohort of patients. A recent study from the Imperial College London discussed the use of 3D printing and 3D CT scanning preoperatively as a mean of optimising the outcome from revising HTO to arthroplasty [55].

18.7   Conclusion

In conclusion, TKR following HTO is a surgically demanding procedure in comparison to TKR without previous HTO. Surgeons must appreciate various factors including surgical approach, anatomical deformities and ligamentous imbalance. However, sound surgical steps and procedures and preoperative planning combined with the aid of computer navigation can improve the precision and reproducibility with appropriate outcomes for TKR after HTO in patients.

References

1. Jackson JP, Waugh W. Tibial osteotomy for osteoarthritis of the knee. Proc R Soc Med. 1960;53(10):888.
2. Santoso MB, Wu L. Unicompartmental knee arthroplasty, is it superior to high tibial osteotomy in treating unicompartmental osteoarthritis? A meta-analysis and systemic review. J Orthop Surg Res. 2017;12(1):50.
3. Herman BV, Giffin JR. High tibial osteotomy in the ACL-deficient knee with medial compartment osteoarthritis. J Orthop Traumatol. 2016;17(3):277–85.
4. Nha KW, Shin YS, Kwon HM, Sim JA, Na YG. Navigated versus conventional technique in high tibial osteotomy: a meta-analysis focusing on weight bearing effect. Knee Surg Relat Res. 2019;31(2):81–102.
5. Akizuki S, Shibakawa A, Takizawa T, Yamazaki I, Horiuchi H. The long-term outcome of high tibial osteotomy: a ten- to 20-year follow-up. J Bone Joint Surg. 2008;90(5):592–6.
6. Bonasia DE, Dettoni F, Sito G, Blonna D, Marmotti A, Bruzzone M, et al. Medial opening wedge high tibial osteotomy for medial compartment overload/arthritis in the varus knee: prognostic factors. Am J Sports Med. 2014;42(3):690–8.
7. DeMeo PJ, Johnson EM, Chiang PP, Flamm AM, Miller MC. Midterm follow-up of opening-wedge high tibial osteotomy. Am J Sports Med. 2010;38(10):2077–84.
8. Efe T, Ahmed G, Heyse TJ, Boudriot U, Timmesfeld N, Fuchs-Winkelmann S, et al. Closing-wedge high tibial osteotomy: survival and risk factor analysis at long-term follow up. BMC Musculoskelet Disord. 2011;12:46.
9. Hui C, Salmon LJ, Kok A, Williams HA, Hockers N, van der Tempel WM, et al. Long-term survival of high tibial osteotomy for medial compartment osteoarthritis of the knee. Am J Sports Med. 2011;39(1):64–70.
10. Naudie D, Bourne RB, Rorabeck CH, Bourne TJ. The Install Award. Survivorship of the high tibial valgus osteotomy. A 10- to -22-year follow-up study. Clin Orthop Relat Res. 1999;(367):18–27.

11. Billings A, Scott DF, Camargo MP, Hofmann AA. High tibial osteotomy with a calibrated osteotomy guide, rigid internal fixation, and early motion. Long-term follow-up. J Bone Joint Surg Am. 2000;82(1):70–9.
12. Niinimaki TT, Eskelinen A, Mann BS, Junnila M, Ohtonen P, Leppilahti J. Survivorship of high tibial osteotomy in the treatment of osteoarthritis of the knee: Finnish registry-based study of 3195 knees. J Bone Joint Surg. 2012;94(11):1517–21.
13. Brouwer RW, Bierma-Zeinstra SM, van Koeveringe AJ, Verhaar JA. Patellar height and the inclination of the tibial plateau after high tibial osteotomy. The open versus the closed-wedge technique. J Bone Joint Surg. 2005;87(9):1227–32.
14. Saragaglia D, Mercier N, Colle PE. Computer-assisted osteotomies for genu varum deformity: which osteotomy for which varus? Int Orthop. 2010;34(2):185–90.
15. Saragaglia D, Massfelder J, Refaie R, Rubens-Duval B, Mader R, Rouchy RC, et al. Computer-assisted total knee replacement after medial opening wedge high tibial osteotomy: medium-term results in a series of ninety cases. Int Orthop. 2016;40(1):35–40.
16. Atrey A, Morison Z, Tosounidis T, Tunggal J, Waddell JP. Complications of closing wedge high tibial osteotomies for unicompartmental osteoarthritis of the knee. Bone Joint Res. 2012;1(9):205–9.
17. Kirgis A, Albrecht S. Palsy of the deep peroneal nerve after proximal tibial osteotomy. An anatomical study. J Bone Joint Surg Am. 1992;74(8):1180–5.
18. Georgoulis AD, Makris CA, Papageorgiou CD, Moebius UG, Xenakis T, Soucacos PN. Nerve and vessel injuries during high tibial osteotomy combined with distal fibular osteotomy: a clinically relevant anatomic study. Knee Surg Sports Traumatol Arthrosc. 1999;7(1):15–9.
19. Itou J, Itoh M, Maruki C, Tajimi T, So T, Kuwashima U, et al. Deep peroneal nerve has a potential risk of injury during open-wedge high tibial osteotomy. Knee Surg Sports Traumatol Arthrosc. 2019;28(5):1372–9.
20. Song SJ, Bae DK, Kim KI, Lee CH. Conversion total knee arthroplasty after failed high tibial osteotomy. Knee Surg Relat Res. 2016;28(2):89–98.
21. Ribeiro CH, Severino NR, Cury Rde P, de Oliveira VM, Avakian R, Ayhara T, et al. A new fixation material for open-wedge tibial osteotomy for genu varum. Knee. 2009;16(5):366–70.
22. Sprenger TR, Doerzbacher JF. Tibial osteotomy for the treatment of varus gonarthrosis. Survival and failure analysis to twenty-two years. J Bone Joint Surg Am. 2003;85(3):469–74.
23. Marti CB, Gautier E, Wachtl SW, Jakob RP. Accuracy of frontal and sagittal plane correction in open-wedge high tibial osteotomy. Arthroscopy. 2004;20(4):366–72.
24. Sharma L, Song J, Felson DT, Cahue S, Shamiyeh E, Dunlop DD. The role of knee alignment in disease progression and functional decline in knee osteoarthritis. JAMA. 2001;286(2):188–95.
25. van Raaij TM, Brouwer RW, de Vlieger R, Reijman M, Verhaar JA. Opposite cortical fracture in high tibial osteotomy: lateral closing compared to the medial opening-wedge technique. Acta Orthop. 2008;79(4):508–14.
26. Miller BS, Dorsey WO, Bryant CR, Austin JC. The effect of lateral cortex disruption and repair on the stability of the medial opening wedge high tibial osteotomy. Am J Sports Med. 2005;33(10):1552–7.
27. Noyes FR, Barber-Westin SD, Hewett TE. High tibial osteotomy and ligament reconstruction for varus angulated anterior cruciate ligament-deficient knees. Am J Sports Med. 2000;28(3):282–96.
28. El-Azab H, Halawa A, Anetzberger H, Imhoff AB, Hinterwimmer S. The effect of closed- and open-wedge high tibial osteotomy on tibial slope: a retrospective radiological review of 120 cases. J Bone Joint Surg. 2008;90(9):1193–7.
29. Giffin JR, Vogrin TM, Zantop T, Woo SL, Harner CD. Effects of increasing tibial slope on the biomechanics of the knee. Am J Sports Med. 2004;32(2):376–82.
30. Rodner CM, Adams DJ, Diaz-Doran V, Tate JP, Santangelo SA, Mazzocca AD, et al. Medial opening wedge tibial osteotomy and the sagittal plane: the effect of increasing tibial slope on tibiofemoral contact pressure. Am J Sports Med. 2006;34(9):1431–41.

31. Warden SJ, Morris HG, Crossley KM, Brukner PD, Bennell KL. Delayed- and non-union following opening wedge high tibial osteotomy: surgeons' results from 182 completed cases. Knee Surg Sports Traumatol Arthrosc. 2005;13(1):34–7.

32. Meidinger G, Imhoff AB, Paul J, Kirchhoff C, Sauerschnig M, Hinterwimmer S. May smokers and overweight patients be treated with a medial open-wedge HTO? Risk factors for non-union. Knee Surg Sports Traumatol Arthrosc. 2011;19(3):333–9.

33. W-Dahl A, Robertsson O, Lohmander LS. High tibial osteotomy in Sweden, 1998–2007: a population-based study of the use and rate of revision to knee arthroplasty. Acta Orthop. 2012;83(3):244–8.

34. van den Bekerom MP, Patt TW, Kleinhout MY, van der Vis HM, Albers GH. Early complications after high tibial osteotomy: a comparison of two techniques. J Knee Surg. 2008;21(1):68–74.

35. Lobenhoffer P, Agneskirchner JD. Improvements in surgical technique of valgus high tibial osteotomy. Knee Surg Sports Traumatol Arthrosc. 2003;11(3):132–8.

36. Spahn G. Complications in high tibial (medial opening wedge) osteotomy. Arch Orthop Trauma Surg. 2004;124(10):649–53.

37. Valkering KP, van den Bekerom MP, Kappelhoff FM, Albers GH. Complications after tomofix medial opening wedge high tibial osteotomy. J Knee Surg. 2009;22(3):218–25.

38. Hak DJ, Fitzpatrick D, Bishop JA, Marsh JL, Tilp S, Schnettler R, et al. Delayed union and nonunions: epidemiology, clinical issues, and financial aspects. Injury. 2014;45(Suppl 2):S3–7.

39. Foulke BA, Kendal AR, Murray DW, Pandit H. Fracture healing in the elderly: a review. Maturitas. 2016;92:49–55.

40. Pearson RG, Clement RG, Edwards KL, Scammell BE. Do smokers have greater risk of delayed and non-union after fracture, osteotomy and arthrodesis? A systematic review with meta-analysis. BMJ Open. 2016;6(11):e010303.

41. Zura R, Xiong Z, Einhorn T, Watson JT, Ostrum RF, Prayson MJ, et al. Epidemiology of fracture nonunion in 18 human bones. JAMA Surg. 2016;151(11):e162775.

42. Huizinga MR, Gorter J, Demmer A, Bierma-Zeinstra SMA, Brouwer RW. Progression of medial compartmental osteoarthritis 2-8 years after lateral closing-wedge high tibial osteotomy. Knee Surg Sports Traumatol Arthrosc. 2017;25(12):3679–86.

43. Nha KW, Oh SM, Ha YW, Patel MK, Seo JH, Lee BH. Radiological grading of osteoarthritis on Rosenberg view has a significant correlation with clinical outcomes after medial open-wedge high-tibial osteotomy. Knee Surg Sports Traumatol Arthrosc. 2019;27(6):2021–9.

44. Erak S, Naudie D, MacDonald SJ, McCalden RW, Rorabeck CH, Bourne RB. Total knee arthroplasty following medial opening wedge tibial osteotomy: technical issues early clinical radiological results. Knee. 2011;18(6):499–504.

45. Bastos Filho R, Magnussen RA, Duthon V, Demey G, Servien E, Granjeiro JM, et al. Total knee arthroplasty after high tibial osteotomy: a comparison of opening and closing wedge osteotomy. Int Orthop. 2013;37(3):427–31.

46. Wolff AM, Hungerford DS, Pepe CL. The effect of extraarticular varus and valgus deformity on total knee arthroplasty. Clin Orthop Relat Res. 1991;271:35–51.

47. van Raaij TM, Reijman M, Furlan AD, Verhaar JA. Total knee arthroplasty after high tibial osteotomy. A systematic review. BMC Musculoskelet Disord. 2009;10:88.

48. Meding JB, Keating EM, Ritter MA, Faris PM. Total knee arthroplasty after high tibial osteotomy. A comparison study in patients who had bilateral total knee replacement. J Bone Joint Surg Am. 2000;82(9):1252–9.

49. Akasaki Y, Matsuda S, Miura H, Okazaki K, Moro-oka TA, Mizu-uchi H, et al. Total knee arthroplasty following failed high tibial osteotomy: mid-term comparison of posterior cruciate-retaining versus posterior stabilized prosthesis. Knee Surg Sports Traumatol Arthrosc. 2009;17(7):795–9.

50. Saragaglia D, Picard F, Chaussard C, Montbarbon E, Leitner F, Cinquin P. Computer-assisted knee arthroplasty: comparison with a conventional procedure. Results of 50 cases in a prospective randomized study. Rev Chir Orthop Reparatrice Appar Mot. 2001;87(1):18–28.

51. Bathis H, Perlick L, Tingart M, Luring C, Zurakowski D, Grifka J. Alignment in total knee arthroplasty. A comparison of computer-assisted surgery with the conventional technique. J Bone Joint Surg. 2004;86(5):682–7.
52. Jenny JY, Clemens U, Kohler S, Kiefer H, Konermann W, Miehlke RK. Consistency of implantation of a total knee arthroplasty with a non-image-based navigation system: a case-control study of 235 cases compared with 235 conventionally implanted prostheses. J Arthroplast. 2005;20(7):832–9.
53. Petursson G, Fenstad AM, Gothesen O, Dyrhovden GS, Hallan G, Rohrl SM, et al. Computer-assisted compared with conventional total knee replacement: a multicenter parallel-group randomized controlled trial. J Bone Joint Surg Am. 2018;100(15):1265–74.
54. Frohlich V, Johandl S, De Zwart P, Stockle U, Ochs BG. Navigated TKA after osteotomy versus primary navigated TKA: a matched-pair analysis. Orthopedics. 2016;39(3 Suppl):S77–82.
55. Jones GG, Clarke S, Jaere M, Cobb JP. Failed high tibial osteotomy: A joint preserving alternative to total knee arthroplasty. Orthop Traumatol Surg Res. 2019;105(1):85–8.

Outcomes of Total Knee Arthroplasty for Failed Osteotomy

19

Raj R. Thakrar, Mazin Ibrahim, and Fares S. Haddad

19.1 Introduction

Periarticular knee osteotomy surgery is a common surgical procedure for the management of isolated compartmental osteoarthritis of the knee joint in the young active individual. There are a number of studies reporting the successful outcome of osteotomy surgery with a 10-year survival rate following tibial osteotomy being reported as high as 98% in some studies [1] and dropping to a respectable 85% at 20 years in others [2].

Despite the initial successful outcome, however, deterioration in clinical results with time has become a challenging issue faced by the orthopaedic surgeon today. There are a number of factors that contribute to failure of osteotomy surgery to include patient age, preoperative osteoarthritis grade, BMI and range of motion [1, 2]. Whilst revision to arthroplasty surgery is a commonly performed procedure, a number of earlier studies have suggested suboptimal outcomes in terms of clinical function and survivorship when compared to primary arthroplasty surgery in the absence of previous osteotomy [3, 4]. This is thought to be, in part, related to the challenges around managing the soft tissue and bony anatomical distortion created by the previous surgery.

This chapter aims at reviewing the current literature on outcomes of total knee arthroplasty (TKA) surgery following failed osteotomy and furthermore discusses important surgical considerations that may influence these.

R. R. Thakrar (✉)
Lister Hospital, Stevenage, UK

M. Ibrahim · F. S. Haddad
University College London Hospital, London, UK

© Springer Nature Switzerland AG 2020
S. Oussedik, S. Lustig (eds.), *Osteotomy About the Knee*,
https://doi.org/10.1007/978-3-030-49055-3_19

19.2   Surgical Considerations and Surgical Outcomes

A number of key surgical factors influence the outcome of TKA post osteotomy. There is a general consensus in that TKA after previous osteotomy surgery is a technically demanding procedure, and this is evident through an increased reported surgical time when compared to cases of surgery without preceding osteotomy [5]. Part of the difficulty is achieving adequate surgical exposure. The surgical approach may often utilise previous scars, but it is important to appreciate that this may only be possible in 50% of cases [6]. Blood supply to the extensor surface of the knee is medially dominant, and, hence, in the case of multiple parallel scars, a more unconventional approach through the most lateral scar may have to be adopted.

Furthermore, due to scar tissue formation, subperiosteal exposure of the proximal tibia can be challenging. This combined with the development of scar tissue between the patella tendon and anterior tibia and thickened fat pad makes techniques such as patellar eversion after previous tibial osteotomy more difficult. As a result, a number of studies have reported an increased need for additional procedures such as tibial tubercle osteotomies in order to gain adequate exposure [6, 7]. Furthermore, malrotation of the proximal tibia with reference to the tibial shaft may occur following osteotomy surgery contributing to patellar instability, increasing the requirement for lateral release procedures [6].

Component fixation may also be compromised due to loss of metaphyseal bone stock following osteotomy surgery warranting the use of a more constrained stemmed prosthesis to provide greater mechanical stability of fixation. Previous analysis of the Swedish registry data demonstrated that high tibial osteotomy (HTO) to TKA conversions was 4.7 times more likely to use such a stemmed or revision implant. Interestingly, this figure was still significantly lower when compared to unicompartmental knee arthroplasty (UKA) to TKA conversions (23 times more likely). A possible explanation for this is a greater degree of metaphyseal bone loss observed in failed UKA when compared with proximal tibial osteotomy surgery [8].

19.3   Clinical Outcomes

19.3.1 Range of Movement

Traditionally it is considered that post-operative knee range of movement (ROM) is an important factor influencing patient satisfaction after TKA [9]. Preoperative flexion angle together with tibiofemoral alignment angle demonstrates a significant correlation with post-operative flexion achieved [10], with a reported recovery in knee range of motion following TKA plateauing at 12-month post-surgery [11]. A limited ROM to include a fixed flexion deformity may occur following osteotomy surgery. This may be attributed to a combination of soft tissue scarring and bony malalignment.

TKA for failed HTO improves overall mean ROM post-operatively [12]. When compared to control groups without prior osteotomy, however, there are reports in literature suggesting less flexion. Van Raaij et al. [12] in their series reported a median flexion angle of 110 achieved in the prior osteotomy group vs 120 degrees in their primary TKA group. No fixed flexion deformity was observed in either cohort. Similarly, observation of less flexion has also been reported by Haddad et al. [5]. Both sides emphasised that this difference did not reach clinical significance. In the more recent study, Efe et al. [13], however, did demonstrate a statistically significant difference in ROM between the two groups but interestingly failed to correlate this with any difference in overall functional outcome.

19.3.2 Functional Outcome Scores

Overall, functional outcome after TKA for failed prior osteotomy demonstrates a significant improvement when compared to preoperatively [14].

Historically, however, comparison studies between TKA with prior osteotomy and without prior osteotomy have reported poorer functional outcome scores. Mont et al. in 1994 described several risk factors for predicting poor outcomes in knee arthroplasty following failed tibial osteotomy to include occupation as a labourer, multiple prior knee procedure, reflex sympathetic dystrophy after osteotomy surgery and workers' compensation patients [10].

Interestingly, as with ROM, very few of these studies have shown a statistically significant difference when comparing the two groups. At midterm follow-up, Efe et al. reported no significant difference in the visual analogue scale (VAS), the Western Ontario and McMaster Universities Osteoarthritis Index (WOMAC), University College London Activity score (UCLA), Feller's Patellar Score and SF-36 score. These findings have been echoed by other similar patient-matched studies discussed thus far. Huang et al. [15] reported outcomes in 17 patients at a mean follow-up of 59.4 months. They concluded that previous HTO did not have a negative effect on the outcome of TKA and reported 94% of patients having excellent or good results with no difference in knee or function score. More recently, Jabalameli et al. [16] in their prospective series of 25 cases reinforced the results of the aforementioned studies again reporting no significant difference between the two groups' clinical scores.

Importantly, review of the literature suggests that where inferior results of TKA post-tibial osteotomy in comparison to without prior osteotomy are reported, these are often based on an unmatched cohort of patients [17–19].

19.4   Radiological Outcomes

19.4.1 Component Position

There is an increase in emphasis in literature on the significance of component alignment in TKA surgery and its impact on implant survivorship [20–23]. The radiographic assessment of the mechanically aligned TKA will often demonstrate the joint to be in 4–6° of valgus (tibiofemoral angle) with optimal range reported as 2–7° by Fang et al. [24]. The anatomical alignment of the femoral component usually lies in 5–9° of valgus relative to the long axis of the femur [25]. The tibial component is placed perpendicular to the long axis of the tibia. Ritter et al. reported in their series of 6070 TKAs with a minimum follow-up of 2 years that implant failure was most likely to occur if placed <90° relative to the tibial axis (i.e. valgus) and the femoral component >8° valgus [22].

Invariably, osteotomy surgery will contribute to some degree of bony malalignment and joint line distortion. In the coronal axis, a valgus knee secondary to osteoarthritis (OA) is likely to be associated with valgus malalignment of both tibia and femur (Fig. 19.1). In contrast to this, valgus alignment post osteotomy for medial compartmental OA will be associated with a valgus tibia but likely varus femur from the primary OA diagnosis. Furthermore, slope adjustment (more often unintentional) will contribute to sagittal malalignment, with an increase in slope being commonly associated with medial open-wedge tibial osteotomies [26] (Fig. 19.2).

Fig. 19.1 Proximal tibial valgus deformity created by a medial open-wedge HTO

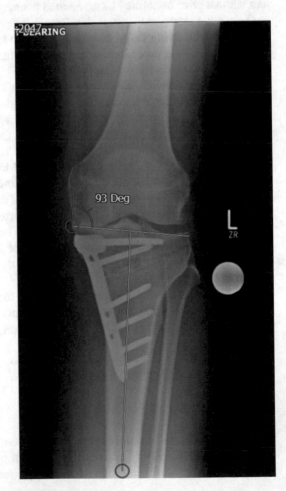

Fig. 19.2 Increased posterior slope following medial open-wedge HTO

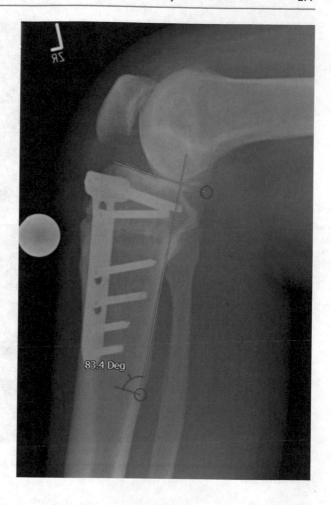

Despite this, however, there are a number of cohort studies comparing implant position of TKA post osteotomy vs without prior osteotomy, with little evidence of a statistically significant difference noted between the two groups [5, 13, 27]. It may therefore be proposed that a meticulous surgical technique leads to satisfactory radiological alignment of the TKA for a failed osteotomy (Fig. 19.3).

19.4.2 Patellar Height

Patella baja following high tibial osteotomy is a well-recognised phenomenon with reports in literature suggesting an incidence as high as 89% [28]. Particularly, after closing wedge osteotomy, there is secondary shortening of the patella tendon due to shortening of the distance between the tibial tubercle and tibial plateau. Other potential causes include contracture of the patella tendon secondary to post-op immobilisation and calcification within the tendon from a healing osteotomy.

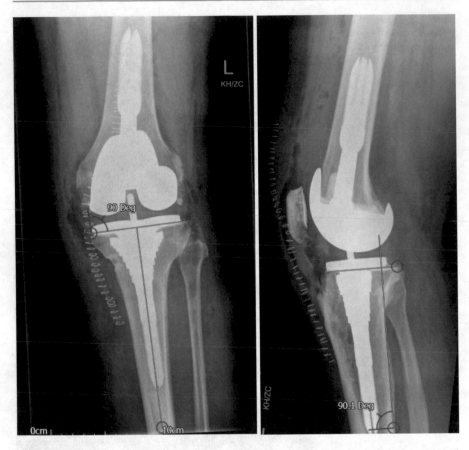

Fig. 19.3 Post-operative radiographs demonstrating restoration of posterior slope and mechanical axis of the tibia

Failure to address patella baja at the time of TKA surgery can lead to a decreased range of motion, a decrease extensor lever arm and subsequent increased energy expenditure, extensor lag and impingement of the patella against the tibial polyethylene or baseplate resulting in anterior knee pain [29]. A number of studies have identified the presence of patella baja in TKA for failed osteotomy. The exact clinical significance, however, remains unclear. Haddad et al. [5] in their series of 50 patients undergoing TKA for failed HTO identified a significantly higher proportion of patella baja when compared to their control (primary TKA) group (28 vs 6 cases $p < 0.02$). Despite this, however, they were unable to identify a discernible difference in outcomes from the point of view of patellofemoral symptoms, range of motion or knee scores between the two groups. More recently Amendola et al. reported a similar finding of a higher incidence of patella baja in the TKA post osteotomy group as compared to without prior osteotomy. In their series of 29 cases, the 3 patients with baja developed symptoms of anterior knee pain requiring further intervention in the form of secondary resurfacing of the patella [30].

Importantly, preoperative planning allows for identification of patella baja, and various different surgical techniques may be adopted to compensate for this. Proximal placement of the patellar button during resurfacing versus increasing tibial resection to distalise the joint line by 5 mm is one of the recognised approaches. Van Raaij et al. demonstrated this very well in their series of 14 TKAs following failed HTO. Preoperative comparison of patellar height to their control group of no prior osteotomy identified a significant degree of patella baja in the osteotomy cohort, which was adequately corrected at the time of surgery [12].

19.4.3 Radiolucency

Radiolucent lines are defined as radiolucent intervals found between the cement and bone interface. Preparation of bone surface prior to cementing together with the cementing technique used has an impact on the appearance of radiolucency. Within the tibial baseplate, peripheral radiolucent lines are a frequent appearance, with a tendency to resolve with time [10]. Progression of radiolucency, however, is associated with early failure. The presence of radiolucent lines may facilitate entry of joint fluid and wear debris contributing to progressive osteolysis.

Once again, the clinical relevance of these radiological findings remains questionable. There are reports in the literature of a higher prevalence of radiolucent lines in TKA following prior osteotomy when compared to without prior osteotomy. Parvizi et al. [17] reported a statistically significant increase in radiolucent lines in TKA following HTO as part of their subgroup analysis. Interestingly, this in isolation was not reported as correlating with an increased failure rate of the implant, and instead the authors attributed the higher failure rate to the patient demographic in the osteotomy group, being a younger more active and heavier population. Efe et al., in their matched-pair analysis, reported a similar higher incidence of nonprogressive radiolucent lines following prior HTO; however, they failed to demonstrate a statistically significant difference between the two groups.

Possible explanation for an increased radiolucency may be related to poor cementing technique with a lack of attention given to preparation of bone and pressurisation of the cement into the previously osteotomised sclerotic bone. Nonetheless, despite this increased prevalence of radiolucent line, the prosthetic survival rate after TKA in individuals who have had a previous osteotomy still remains high [17].

19.5 Implant Survivorship of TKA Following Prior Osteotomy Surgery

Due to factors such as difficult surgical exposure and ligament imbalance, there is potential risk of compromise to the precision and accuracy of the surgical technique, which in turn could influence implant survivorship in the long term [31]. In addition, previous osteotomy surgery may result in coronal and sagittal malalignment which in turn may influence patellar tracking resulting in rotatory instability and furthermore contribute to mechanical failure of the implant [32]. Despite this, however, in recent literature, there have been a number of large registry studies reporting positive results of long-term survivorship of TKA following tibial osteotomy in the order of 91–93% at 10 years [33, 34].

One such study by Badawy et al. [33] reported survival analysis of TKA in the Norwegian Arthroplasty Register. Their results identified a 10-year survival of 92.6% with a RR of 0.97. This was comparable to the survival analysis of their control group (no prior osteotomy) with no statistically significant difference noted between the two groups. Furthermore, Niinimäki et al. [34] in their analysis of the Finnish Arthroplasty Register reported a similar Kaplan-Meier survivorship of 92% at 10 years.

Though the overall survivorship results are promising, it is important to note that a number of studies have reported a higher overall revision rate in TKA following prior HTO. One study by Parvizi et al. [17] in 2004 reported their outcomes of TKA using a cemented unicondylar system for the management of failed proximal tibial osteotomies in 166 cases. They documented an 8% revision rate at a mean follow-up of 5.9 years. In their series, the common causes of revision included polyethylene wear (four cases) and component loosening (six cases). A similarly higher failure rate of TKA following HTO has also been reported by Haslam et al. [35]. They reported a failure rate of 20% in the TKAs following osteotomy vs 8% in their control group at a mean follow-up of 6 years after the index procedure. Again, in their series, the most common cause of failure was component loosening (four cases). Though on initial review these results may be somewhat worrying, when put into perspective, the risk of revision of TKA after prior unicompartmental knee replacement (UKA) still remains significantly higher when compared to that of prior HTO (2.3 vs 1.4) [8].

It is difficult to ascertain from current literature as to whether the type of osteotomy influences the survivorship of the subsequent TKA. This is mainly due to the heterogeneity in the methodology of many of the published reviews on the subject matter. With relation to proximal tibial osteotomies, Robertsson and W-Dahl [8] reported a significantly higher revision rate of TKA after prior closing wedge osteotomy when compared with open-wedge osteotomy. These results, however, have not been echoed in other studies carrying out similar subgroup analysis [36].

19.6 Future Directions

We are now in the era of using robotic-assisted surgery to achieve the optimal knee arthroplasty. This technology is promising in improving implant alignment and position with reported decreased pain, improved early functional recovery and reduced time to hospital discharge when compared with conventional jig-based TKA [37]. Robotic-assisted surgery may therefore be the solution to improve outcomes for TKA following failed osteotomy in a similar fashion to the navigated knee arthroplasty results as reported by Saragaglia et al. [38]. They, in a medium-term comparative study, reported results of TKA after medial opening-wedge osteotomy versus without prior osteotomy using a computer-assisted navigation system. Reassuringly, no statistically significant differences between these two groups with relation to the International Knee Society score (IKS), patient satisfaction, hip-knee-ankle angle and the tibial mechanical alignment were identified. As with much of the current literature on this subject matter, however, there lacks high-quality randomised control trials in order to draw concrete conclusions.

19.7   Conclusion

TKA for failed osteotomy is a technically challenging procedure. Previous surgery may influence the outcomes of subsequent knee replacement, but thus far there is little concrete evidence in the literature to suggest that prior osteotomy surgery has a significant detriment on the outcome of the future arthroplasty surgery. Osteotomy surgery, on the other hand, plays an important role in the management of compartmental osteoarthritis in a young active patient, in whom arthroplasty surgery is otherwise contraindicated. Many surgeons would therefore propose that the slight increased risk in failure and decrease in functional outcome of TKA following prior osteotomy reported in current literature are a balanced compromise in order to reap the benefits of joint preservation in the young individual.

References

1. Akizuki S, Shibakawa A, Takizawa T, Yamazaki I, Horiuchi H. The long-term outcome of high tibial osteotomy: a ten- to 20-year follow-up. J Bone Joint Surg Br. 2008;90(5):592–6. Available from: http://online.boneandjoint.org.uk/doi/10.1302/0301-620X.90B5.20386. Accessed 20 Oct 2018.
2. Flecher X, Parratte S, Aubaniac J-M, Argenson J-NA. A 12–28-year follow-up study of closing wedge high tibial osteotomy. Clin Orthop Relat Res. 2006;452:91–6. Available from: https://insights.ovid.com/crossref?an=00003086-200611000-00018. Accessed 20 Oct 2018.
3. Katz MM, Hungerford DS, Krackow KA, Lennox DW. Results of total knee arthroplasty after failed proximal tibial osteotomy for osteoarthritis. J Bone Joint Surg Am. 1987;69(2):225–33. Available from: http://www.ncbi.nlm.nih.gov/pubmed/3805083. Accessed 20 Oct 2018.
4. Windsor RE, Insall JN, Vince KG. Technical considerations of total knee arthroplasty after proximal tibial osteotomy. J Bone Joint Surg Am. 1988;70(4):547–55. Available from: http://www.ncbi.nlm.nih.gov/pubmed/3356722. Accessed 20 Oct 2018.
5. Haddad FS, Bentley G. Total knee arthroplasty after high tibial osteotomy a medium-term review. 2000. Available from: https://ac-els-cdn-com.libproxy.ucl.ac.uk/S0883540300787894/1-s2.0-S0883540300787894-main.pdf?_tid=a9ee4403-963d-49bc-a5df-2cc868cb79f3&acdnat=1540066505_28d40e9fa6dfe57df0b03ca9f39b57eb. Accessed 20 Oct 2018.
6. Nizard RS, Cardinne L, Bizot P, Witvoet J. Total knee replacement after failed tibial osteotomy: results of a matched-pair study. J Arthroplast. 1998;13(8):847–53. Available from: http://www.ncbi.nlm.nih.gov/pubmed/9880174. Accessed 20 Oct 2018.
7. Karabatsos B, Mahomed NN, Maistrelli GL. Functional outcome of total knee arthroplasty after high tibial osteotomy. Can J Surg. 2002;45(2):116–9. Available from: http://www.ncbi.nlm.nih.gov/pubmed/11939653. Accessed 20 Oct 2018.

8. Robertsson O, W-Dahl A. The risk of revision after TKA is affected by previous HTO or UKA. Clin Orthop Relat Res. 2015;473(1):90–3. Available from: http://www.ncbi.nlm.nih.gov/pubmed/24898530. Accessed 20 Oct 2018.
9. Mutsuzaki H, Takeuchi R, Mataki Y, Wadano Y. Target range of motion for rehabilitation after total knee arthroplasty. J Rural Med. 2017;12(1):33–7. Available from: http://www.ncbi.nlm.nih.gov/pubmed/28593015. Accessed 28 Oct 2018.
10. Mont MA, Alexander N, Krackow KA, Hungerford DS. Total knee arthroplasty after failed high tibial osteotomy. Orthop Clin North Am. 1994;25(3):515–25. Available from: http://www.ncbi.nlm.nih.gov/pubmed/8028892. Accessed 21 Oct 2018.
11. Zhou Z, Yew KSA, Arul E, Chin P-L, et al. Recovery in knee range of motion reaches a plateau by 12 months after total knee arthroplasty. Knee Surg Sports Traumatol Arthrosc. 2015;23(6):1729–33. Available from: http://www.ncbi.nlm.nih.gov/pubmed/25178534. Accessed 21 Oct 2018.
12. Van Raaij TM, Bakker W, Reijman M, Verhaar JAN. The effect of high tibial osteotomy on the results of total knee arthroplasty: a matched case control study. BMC Musculoskelet Disord. 2007;8:74.
13. Efe T, Heyse TJ, Boese C, Timmesfeld N, et al. TKA following high tibial osteotomy versus primary TKA—a matched pair analysis. BMC Musculoskelet Disord. 2010;11(1):207. Available from: http://bmcmusculoskeletdisord.biomedcentral.com/articles/10.1186/1471-2474-11-207. Accessed 17 Oct 2018.
14. Gupta H, Dahiya V, Vasdev A, Rajgopal A. Outcomes of total knee arthroplasty following high tibial osteotomy. Indian J Orthop. 2013;47(5):469–73. Available from: http://www.ncbi.nlm.nih.gov/pubmed/24133306. Accessed 21 Oct 2018.
15. Huang HT, Su JY, Su KN, Tien YC. Total knee arthroplasty after failed dome osteotomy. Kaohsiung J Med Sci. 2002;18(10):485–91. Available from: http://www.ncbi.nlm.nih.gov/pubmed/12517064. Accessed 21 Oct 2018.
16. Jabalameli M, Rahbar M, Moradi A, Hadi H. The mid-term outcome of total knee arthroplasty in patients with prior high tibial osteotomy: a prospective study. Shafa Orthop J. 2016. Available from: http://shafaorthoj.com/en/articles/4133.html. Accessed 21 Oct 2018.
17. Parvizi J, Hanssen AD, Spangehl MJ. Total knee arthroplasty following proximal tibial osteotomy: risk factors for failure. J Bone Joint Surg Am. 2004;86-A(3):474–9. Available from: http://www.ncbi.nlm.nih.gov/pubmed/14996871. Accessed 20 Oct 2018.
18. Noda T, Yasuda S, Nagano K, Takahara Y, et al. Clinico-radiological study of total knee arthroplasty after high tibial osteotomy. J Orthop Sci. 2000;5(1):25–36. Available from: http://www.ncbi.nlm.nih.gov/pubmed/10664436. Accessed 21 Oct 2018.
19. Erak S, Naudie D, MacDonald SJ, McCalden RW, et al. Total knee arthroplasty following medial opening wedge tibial osteotomy. Knee. 2011;18(6):499–504. Available from: http://www.ncbi.nlm.nih.gov/pubmed/21138790. Accessed 21 Oct 2018.
20. Longstaff LM, Sloan K, Stamp N, Scaddan M, Beaver R. Good alignment after total knee arthroplasty leads to faster rehabilitation and better function. J Arthroplast. 2009;24(4):570–8. Available from: http://www.ncbi.nlm.nih.gov/pubmed/18534396. Accessed 30 July 2018.
21. Choong PF, Dowsey MM, Stoney JD. Does accurate anatomical alignment result in better function and quality of life? Comparing conventional and computer-assisted total knee arthroplasty. J Arthroplast. 2009;24(4):560–9. Available from: http://www.ncbi.nlm.nih.gov/pubmed/18534397. Accessed 30 July 2018.
22. Ritter MA, Davis KE, Meding JB, Pierson JL, et al. The effect of alignment and BMI on failure of total knee replacement. J Bone Joint Surg Am. 2011;93(17):1588–96. Available from: http://www.ncbi.nlm.nih.gov/pubmed/21915573. Accessed 30 July 2018.
23. Benjamin J. Component alignment in total knee arthroplasty. Instr Course Lect. 2006;55:405–12. Available from: http://www.ncbi.nlm.nih.gov/pubmed/16958475. Accessed 31 July 2018.
24. Fang DM, Ritter MA, Davis KE. Coronal alignment in total knee arthroplasty. J Arthroplast. 2009;24(6):39–43. Available from: http://www.ncbi.nlm.nih.gov/pubmed/19553073. Accessed 11 Aug 2018.

25. Allen AM, Ward WG, Pope TL. Imaging of the total knee arthroplasty. Radiol Clin N Am. 1995;33(2):289–303. Available from: http://www.ncbi.nlm.nih.gov/pubmed/7871170. Accessed 12 Aug 2018.
26. Ducat A, Sariali E, Lebel B, Mertl P, et al. Posterior tibial slope changes after opening- and closing-wedge high tibial osteotomy: a comparative prospective multicenter study. Orthop Traumatol Surg Res. 2012;98(1):68–74. Available from: http://www.ncbi.nlm.nih.gov/pubmed/22244250. Accessed 28 Oct 2018.
27. Orban H, Mares E, Dragusanu M, Stan G. Maedica—a journal of clinical medicine total knee arthroplasty following high tibial osteotomy—a radiological evaluation. 2011. Available from: https://www.ncbi.nlm.nih.gov/pmc/articles/PMC3150017/pdf/maed-06-23.pdf. Accessed 20 Oct 2018.
28. Scuderi GR, Windsor RE, Insall JN. Observations on patellar height after proximal tibial osteotomy. J Bone Joint Surg Am. 1989;71(2):245–8. Available from: http://www.ncbi.nlm.nih.gov/pubmed/2918009. Accessed 21 Oct 2018.
29. Chonko DJ, Lombardi AV, Berend KR. Patella baja and total knee arthroplasty (TKA): etiology, diagnosis, and management. Surg Technol Int. 2004;12:231–8. Available from: http://www.ncbi.nlm.nih.gov/pubmed/15455331. Accessed 21 Oct 2018.
30. Amendola L, Fosco M, Cenni E, Tigani D. Knee joint arthroplasty after tibial osteotomy. Int Orthop. 2010;34(2):289–95. Available from: http://link.springer.com/10.1007/s00264-009-0894-y. Accessed 21 Oct 2018.
31. Mason JB, Fehring TK, Estok R, Banel D, Fahrbach K. Meta-analysis of alignment outcomes in computer-assisted total knee arthroplasty surgery. J Arthroplast. 2007;22(8):1097–106. Available from: http://linkinghub.elsevier.com/retrieve/pii/S0883540307004573. Accessed 20 Oct 2018.
32. Callaghan JJ, O'rourke MR, Saleh KJ. Why knees fail: lessons learned. J Arthroplast. 2004;19(4 Suppl 1):31–4. Available from: http://www.ncbi.nlm.nih.gov/pubmed/15190546. Accessed 20 Oct 2018.
33. Badawy M, Fenstad AM, Indrekvam K, Havelin LI, Furnes O. The risk of revision in total knee arthroplasty is not affected by previous high tibial osteotomy. Acta Orthop. 2015;86(6):734–9. Available from: http://www.ncbi.nlm.nih.gov/pubmed/26058747. Accessed 20 Oct 2018.
34. Niinimäki T, Eskelinen A, Ohtonen P, Puhto A-P, et al. Total knee arthroplasty after high tibial osteotomy: a registry-based case–control study of 1,036 knees. Arch Orthop Trauma Surg. 2014;134(1):73–7. Available from: http://www.ncbi.nlm.nih.gov/pubmed/24276363. Accessed 20 Oct 2018.
35. Haslam P, Armstrong M, Geutjens G, Wilton TJ. Total knee arthroplasty after failed high tibial osteotomy. J Arthroplast. 2007;22(2):245–50. Available from: http://www.ncbi.nlm.nih.gov/pubmed/17275642. Accessed 20 Oct 2018.
36. Preston S, Howard J, Naudie D, Somerville L, Mcauley J. Symposium: 2013 Knee Society proceedings total knee arthroplasty after high tibial osteotomy no differences between medial and lateral osteotomy approaches. n.d. Available from: https://europepmc.org/backend/ptpmcrender.fcgi?accid=PMC3889445&blobtype=pdf. Accessed 17 Oct 2018.
37. Kayani B, Konan S, Tahmassebi J, Pietrzak JRT, Haddad FS. Robotic-arm assisted total knee arthroplasty is associated with improved early functional recovery and reduced time to hospital discharge compared with conventional jig-based total knee arthroplasty. Bone Joint J. 2018;100-B(7):930–7. Available from: http://www.ncbi.nlm.nih.gov/pubmed/29954217. Accessed 28 Oct 2018.
38. Saragaglia D, Massfelder J, Refaie R, Rubens-Duval B, et al. Computer-assisted total knee replacement after medial opening wedge high tibial osteotomy: medium-term results in a series of ninety cases. Int Orthop. 2016;40(1):35–40. Available from: http://www.ncbi.nlm.nih.gov/pubmed/25947901. Accessed 30 Oct 2018.

Printed in the United States
by Baker & Taylor Publisher Services